HOSPITAL

Shoulder Surgery

Shoulder Surgery

Edited by

Stephen A Copeland FRCS

Consultant Orthopaedic Surgeon
Royal Berkshire & Battle Hospitals NHS Trust
Royal Berkshire Hospital
Reading

WB Saunders Company Limited
London   Philadelphia   Toronto   Sydney   Tokyo

W. B. Saunders Company Ltd 24–28 Oval Road
London NW1 7DX

The Curtis Center
Independence Square West
Philadelphia, PA 19106-3399, USA

Harcourt Brace & Company
55 Horner Avenue
Toronto, Ontario M8Z 4X6, Canada

Harcourt Brace & Company, Australia
30–52 Smidmore Street
Marrickville, NSW 2204, Australia

Harcourt Brace & Company, Japan
Ichibancho Central Building, 22-1 Ichibancho
Chiyoda-ku, Tokyo 102, Japan

A catalogue record for this book is available from the British Library

ISBN 0-7020-2063-X

Typeset by Paston Press Ltd, Loddon, Norfolk
Printed in Great Britain by The Bath Press, Bath

Contents

Contributors

Louis U Bigliani MD, Chief, The Shoulder Service, New York Orthopaedic Hospital, Columbian Presbyterian Medical Center, New York, USA and Professor of Orthopaedic Surgery, College of Physicians and Surgeons, Columbia University, New York, USA.

Rolfe Birch M Chir FRCS, Orthopaedic Surgeon, Royal National Orthopaedic Hospital, Brockley Hill, Stanmore, Middlesex, UK.

Juan A Bruguera MD PhD CST(ORTH), Orthopaedic Senior Registrar, Shoulder Fellow Shoulder Unit, Orthopaedic Department, Royal Berkshire Hospital, Reading, Berks, UK.

Paul T Calvert MA FRCS, Consultant Orthopaedic Surgeon, St George's Hospital, Blackshaw Road, London, UK and Royal National Orthopaedic Hospital, Brockley Hill, Stanmore, Middlesex, UK.

Andrew Carr MA ChM FRCS, Consultant Orthopaedic Surgeon, Nuffield Orthopaedic Centre, Headington, Oxford, UK.

Veronica Conboy BSc FRCS Shoulder Fellow, Nuffield Orthopaedic Centre, Headington, Oxford, UK.

Christopher R Constant LLM MCh FRCS, Consultant Orthopaedic Surgeon, Addenbrooke's Hospital, Cambridge, UK.

Patrick M Connor MD, Fellow in Shoulder Surgery, The Shoulder Service, New York Orthopaedic Hospital, Columbian Presbyterian Medical Center, New York, USA.

Stephen A Copeland FRCS, Consultant Orthopaedic Surgeon, Royal Berkshire & Battle Hospitals NHS Trust, Royal Berkshire Hospital, Reading, UK.

Geert Declercq Orthopaedic Surgeon, Hospital O.L.V. Middelares, Deurne Antwerp, Belgium.

Phillip Duke MB BS FRACS, Consultant Orthopaedic Surgeon, Brisbane Hand & Upper Limb Clinic, Holy Spirit Hospital, Brisbane, Queensland, Australia.

Roger Emery MS FRCS Ed, Consultant Orthopaedic Surgeon, St Mary's Hospital, London, UK.

Simon P Frostick MA DM FRCS, Professor of Orthopaedic and Accident Surgery, University of Liverpool, Royal Liverpool University Hospital, Liverpool, UK.

Roger Hackney FRCS(ORTH) Dip Sports Med, Consultant Orthopaedic Surgeon, Royal Hospital, Haslar, Gosport, UK.

Paula Hourston MCSP BSc, Senior Physiotherapist, Shoulder Unit, Orthopaedic Department, Royal Berkshire Hospital, Reading, Berks, UK.

Cormac Kelly FRCS Ed (Orth), Consultant Orthopaedic Surgeon, Hand and Upper Limb Unit, Robert Jones & Agnes Hunt Hospital, Oswestry, Shropshire, UK and Royal Shrewsbury Hospital, Shrewsbury, Shropshire, UK.

Charles S Neer II MD, Professor of Clinical Orthopaedic Surgery, Emeritus, and Special Lecturer, Columbia University, New York and Consultant Orthopaedic Surgeon, Emeritus, Columbia-Presbyterian Medical Center, New York, USA.

Lars Neumann Consultant Orthopaedic Surgeon, The Nottingham Shoulder & Elbow Unit, Nottingham City Hospital, Nottingham, UK.

Mike J Simmons FRCR, Consultant Radiologist, Royal Berkshire Hospital, Reading, Berkshire, UK.

Don Wallace MA FRCS, Senior Registrar in Orthopaedic Surgery, Nuffield Orthopaedic Centre, Oxford, UK.

W Angus Wallace MB ChB FRCS Ed FRCS Ed (Orth), Professor of Orthopaedic Surgery, Head Dept of Orthopaedic & Accident Surgery, University Hospital, Queen's Medical Centre, Nottingham, UK.

Foreword

Mr Stephen A. Copeland, by organizing the Reading Shoulder Courses, has made an important contribution to the education of orthopaedic surgeons in the theory and practice of modern shoulder surgery. These courses have been given at regular intervals since 1984 and are always over-subscribed. In this work, *Shoulder Surgery*, Mr Copeland presents the up-to-date concepts of the most recent course for the whole world to benefit. It is important to emphasize that, although most of the twenty-one contributors participate in the course, they have put much more than their lecture into this book. Many present background, personal opinion, new material, and original ideas in addition to established concepts. This is valuable not only for students who want to learn about this field, but also for the most experienced shoulder surgeons.

The first seven chapters are on evaluation and diagnosis. The discussions on examination, biomechanics, and roentgen imaging are truly outstanding. The most frequent clinical problems are then discussed in detail including frozen shoulder, genohumeral instability, subacromial impingement, rotator cuff tears, the throwing arm, glenohumeral arthroplasty, neurological aspects, fractures and rehabilitation. It is important that the indications and technique for both arthroscopic procedures and open reconstruction are considered carefully and well.

The reader is frequently impressed with the refreshing brevity, style, and precise use of the English language in dealing with complex and controversial issues that have been precipitated by some recent authors against methods of proven value. The content of this book is timely for all surgeons and residents who contemplate doing shoulder procedures. Undoubtedly, many sections will be widely quoted and of lasting value.

Charles S Neer, II, MD
Professor Emeritus and Special Lecturer
in Orthopaedic Surgery
Columbia University, New York, NY

Founding President, American Shoulder and Elbow Surgeons

Preface

I first started the Reading Shoulder Surgery Course in 1982. At that time I felt that the training in shoulder surgery available to a young surgeon was inadequate. There was a general feeling that if one had learned how to do a Putti Platt stabilization of a shoulder, then training was complete! It was also taught that all painful shoulders get better within two years and therefore, nothing could be offered or should be done. This was plainly not the case and I felt that the scope of possibilities of shoulder surgery deserved a wider audience and understanding. The results of shoulder surgery in the main are predictable and very gratifying and it has always been an amazement to me that it was so slow in gaining more popular appeal. It is rewarding now to see the enormously increased interest in shoulder surgery. It is obvious each time the course is held, how much more sophisticated and better informed the audience has become.

The course has grown over the years and often the lecturers gave pre-prepared handouts to the delegates. These were always very popular, but inevitably there came a time when it was suggested that there was a need for a non-specialist-level book to capture the essence of shoulder surgery. The aim of this book is to stay true to the original aim of the course, i.e. to offer an understanding of shoulder pathology and the surgical treatments available. Each contributor has been asked to offer a review of their subject, but with their own view based on their experience.

Such a book can never be truly comprehensive, nor is it intended to be, but it is aimed at generating enthusiasm, interest and curiosity in this important area of orthopaedic surgery.

Stephen Copeland
1996

Acknowledgements

I would like to whole-heartedly thank all the contributors, past and present to the Reading Shoulder Surgery Course and to this book for their unstinting support and enthusiasm. I would also like to thank the stalwarts of the course who do not appear as contributors, but who have helped enormously over the years with teaching contributions, notably Ian Bayley, Ian Kelly, Tim Bunker and Michael Watson. There is no doubt that the popularity of the course was due in no small part to the support of the late Professor Lipmann Kessel and Dr Charles Neer who has supported every course that has been run since 1982. Professor Kessel initially generated my interest in shoulder surgery. This interest was confirmed and enormously aided by the teachings of Dr Charles Neer to whom I will be forever grateful.

1

Clinical Examination of the Shoulder

PT Calvert

INTRODUCTION

Nowhere is clinical evaluation more important than in the diagnosis of disorders of the shoulder. It should be possible to achieve an accurate diagnosis of a shoulder problem after a good history, thorough clinical examination and a standard set of plain radiographs. Further expensive investigations may help in defining the problems slightly more accurately but are extremely unlikely to be useful if, at the end of the clinical assessment, the clinician has no idea about the possible diagnosis or nature of the problem.

Complaints related to the shoulder fall into four broad categories. These are **pain, stiffness, instability** *and* **weakness**. It may not be immediately obvious which is the patient's chief complaint because there is a significant degree of overlap. It is quite helpful to say to the patient something along the lines 'tell me about the problem'. After a few minutes, a good idea of what is the chief complaint can be obtained and the patient can be directed by asking specific questions. Nevertheless, the clinician should, throughout the assessment, be mentally reviewing what is the patient's predominant problem. It is also important to remember that pain apparently experienced in the shoulder may be referred from pathology in structures outside of the shoulder. The most common example of this is shoulder pain referred from disease in the cervical spine. Other more generalized neurological disorders can present as pain or weakness in the shoulder, and one has to be aware of these possibilities. Therefore, a full evaluation of the shoulder always includes an examination of the cervical spine and, where appropriate, a neurological examination of the upper limbs.

General medical conditions may influence either the diagnosis or management. For example, the association of adhesive capsulitis and diabetes is well known but it is not always so well recognized that the prognosis for full recovery is less good in a diabetic patient than it is in those without this disorder. The general medical condition may also affect choice of treatment, particularly with regard to surgical risk and what is involved in the subsequent rehabilitation. An extreme example of this is the paraplegic; if one is contemplating any operative treatment on such a patient it is important to remember that this patient 'walks on his hands'. The patient will become extremely dependent on outside assistance if it is not possible for the shoulder to be used actively. Hence, advising the paraplegic to 'rest the arm' has very different implications to giving the same advice to a 19-year-old student with his non-dominant arm being affected.

Whether the patient is right- or left-handed is useful information. It is essential to know about the lifestyle and expectations of the patient. Clearly the management of a rotator cuff disorder in a top-level throwing athlete is totally different from that of a retired 80-year-old bank manager. It is not just sufficient to know about a patient's occupation but one must also know precisely what this involves. It is very clear that a plasterer will be involved in significant manual overhead activity but the term 'engineer' covers occupations ranging from purely desk work in the office to heavy manual labour.

There are many ways of taking a history and examining the shoulder and each individual must develop his own particular method. What is important is to be consistent and have a system so that nothing is omitted. In this chapter I am going to detail how I do a clinical evaluation of the shoulder.

HISTORY

Initially some simple basic information should be obtained. This should include the patient's chief complaint, which shoulder is involved, hand dominance, occupation and age.

Age

The age of the patient in itself gives a significant pointer to the possible diagnosis (Table 1.1). Patients in the second and third decades of life are most likely to have instability problems, and those in their 40s and 50s will have mainly rotator cuff impingement, adhesive capsulitis or inflammatory joint disease. In patients in the 60s and 70s full-thickness rotator cuff tears and degenerative joint disease tend to predominate. These are not absolute rules but are very good pointers to possible diagnoses. If, for example, one is proposing to make a diagnosis of rotator cuff impingement in the 22-year-old, then one should think very carefully and make absolutely certain that this diagnosis is correct; it is not uncommon at this age to have instability presenting as pain apparently caused by impingement.

Table 1.1. Age as a guide to diagnosis

Age (years)	Diagnosis
10–30	Instability
40–60	Impingement
	Adhesive capsulitis
	Inflammatory joint disease
60–80	Full-thickness cuff tears
	Osteoarthritis
	Cuff arthropathy

Pain

The most common presenting chief complaint is pain. Evaluating the painful shoulder one wants to know whether the onset was spontaneous or caused by a specific injury. If the patient says that there was an injury it is important to go into this in some detail. Frequently patients will say that their shoulder pain originated from a particular event but when this is investigated further it turns out that the specific episode happened several weeks prior to the onset of shoulder pain and has just been ascribed as the cause in retrospect. In terms of a traumatic onset, one is looking for significant injury which would have been expected to damage the shoulder. If there has been a traumatic event then precisely what happened in the event, where the pain was felt, how long it took to settle and what was done to alleviate it are essential parts of the history. If the pain arose spontaneously the timing of the onset should be known. Did it occur suddenly, as, for example, with neuralgic amyotrophy, or was it a gradual slow onset with intermittent exacerbation?

Enquiry should be made about where the pain is felt. Pain which is well localized to the top of the shoulder with the patient pointing at the acromioclavicular joint (Figure 1.1) is likely to arise from that structure. Pain originating from pathology in the subacromial region tends to be more difficult to localize and is usually felt in the region of the deltoid often radiating to the upper arm as far as the elbow (Figure 1.2). Sometimes this pain is felt over the lateral aspect of the elbow. The pain felt at the front and back of the shoulder more usually arises from pathology within the glenohumeral joint. In general terms pain radiating to the neck is unlikely to arise from intrinsic pathology within the shoulder, although occasionally the acromioclavicular joint can cause pain going to the base of the neck. In addition, pain radiating into the distal forearm and hand, particularly if it is associated with paraesthesia, is unlikely to be caused by intrinsic shoulder pathology and is more probably neurogenic in origin from the cervical spine. One does sometimes get pain radiating to the radial aspect of the forearm and even to the thumb with shoulder pathology;

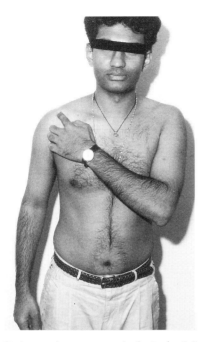

Fig. 1.1 Patient points to acromioclavicular joint as site of pain.

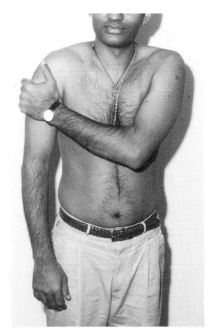

Fig. 1.2 Patient holds deltoid region indicating this as the site of pain when subacromial pathology is the source.

the precise mechanism of the this referral is not entirely clear.

When the pain occurs can be extremely useful information. Night pain is typical of full-thickness rotator cuff tears and severe impingement as well as of osteoarthritis or rheumatoid arthritis in the glenohumeral joint. Pain related to overhead activities is most likely caused by a milder degree of rotator cuff impingement or an instability problem.

Not only is it important to assess the site, periodicity and nature of the pain but it is also important to try and evaluate its severity. This is always difficult because pain is a subjective complaint. However, the presence or absence of night pain, degree of interference `with activities of either daily living or a sporting nature, the number of analgesics taken, the amount of time off work and methods used to alleviate the pain are all helpful in this regard. It can be useful to ask the patient to evaluate the pain on a visual analogue scale where zero is no pain and 10 is the worst pain imaginable. It is important when using such a scale to explain to the patient exactly

what is meant by zero or 10; patients who tell you immediately that 10 is their pain score should be regarded with a certain degree of suspicion. I usually explain to them that 10 is not possible since it equates to having one's leg removed with a blunt saw and no anaesthetic. Sudden onset of really agonizing pain should raise the suspicion of acute calcific tendinitis.

The response of the pain to any previous treatment may be useful information. For example, the pain associated with adhesive capsulitis seems to be frequently made worse by physiotherapy. With patients who have had injections it is important to know where the injection was placed and what was the immediate as well as the longer-term response.

Loss of movement

Patients do not usually complain specifically of stiffness and find it hard to distinguish between loss of active movement as opposed to passive restriction. What concerns the patient is the loss of function caused by the inability to place the hand where it is required. Sometimes the patient will say that they have observed that they cannot actively elevate the arm but if they lift it with the other hand they are able to elevate it fully. This immediately tells one that the patient either has a significant rotator cuff tear or some nerve lesion compromising the rotator cuff or deltoid. Again it is useful to know whether the onset of the loss of motion was sudden, for example following a fall, or whether the shoulder has got gradually stiffer. Clues about this can be obtained by asking the patient which activities have become impossible and when this occurred. Activities at waist level will be limited later than those at full stretch overhead; functions such as combing the hair will be prevented at an intermediate stage.

Instability

There is no easier diagnosis than the patient who presents to the casualty department with a clinically obvious and radiologically proven anterior dislocation of the shoulder following a significant fall or sporting injury. If this then goes on to recurrent anterior dislocation with further proven radiological episodes there is really no trouble in diagnosing the cause of the problem. Nevertheless it is important to know what sort of activities produce the episodes of instability. Movements associated with elevation extension and external rotation such as reaching up and behind or even reaching out in bed to, for example, turn off the alarm clock are indicative of anteroinferior instability. Even when the dislocation is proven it is worth finding out how easily the shoulder dislocates because this may well influence advice about treatment.

Frequently instability problems are not so easy to diagnose. In the first instance it is absolutely vital to establish whether there was a true traumatic episode. To classify the instability as being traumatic rather than atraumatic, the injury should have been sufficient to cause structural damage to a normal shoulder. Thus, going into a tackle on the rugby field with the arm outstretched and the opponent running through is a significant injury but swinging a tennis racquet overhead is not sufficient to cause

an initial episode of dislocation or subluxation in a normal shoulder. A history of fits or electrocution should immediately raise the suspicion of a posterior dislocation. For the acute posterior dislocation, the history, although important, is less important than is a careful physical examination.

Recurrent instability may be considerably more difficult to diagnose if there have not been proven episodes in which the shoulder has been shown to be frankly dislocated. These patients may well present with intermittent pain. They may describe a feeling of the shoulder 'coming out' or 'popping out'. It is then a question of establishing whether the true diagnosis is instability and, if that is the case, what is the direction. If one is backing probabilities, anterior instability is far more likely than is posterior. Nevertheless posterior instability is probably underdiagnosed and is quite easy to misdiagnose. With recurrent subluxation the exact history of the initial episode must be obtained. The cause of subsequent episodes and what happens after each one is essential information. Hence the patient who has intermittent episodes of the arm 'feeling dead' and dropping as he goes to serve overhead at tennis, with an inability to continue to serve followed by a day or so of pain in the shoulder, which gradually resolves, is absolutely typical of recurrent anterior subluxation. In contrast episodes of pain or 'popping out' associated with adduction across the chest, such as occurs with a backhand shot, are more likely to be posterior in direction. In the throwing athlete, who complains of pain when throwing, posterior instability should be considered as a possible diagnosis.

Weakness

Patients quite often complain that the shoulder is weak. This may not mean that there is actual weakness of specific muscles, but may just indicate they are unable to use it in the desired fashion. It is important to establish precisely what is meant by weakness. It is possible that it is pain which is limiting their ability to do normal activities or it may be genuine weakness. The analysis of weakness and precisely which muscles are weak is best achieved during the physical examination.

Previous treatment

If patients have had previous treatment, particularly if this is operative treatment, it is vital to go back and take a full history of the original complaint. This should be done as carefully as if the patient had never been treated because one of the causes of persistent symptoms following any intervention is that the original diagnosis was incorrect. One should then find out precisely what has been done and what was its effect on the symptoms. If there has been no change, then it is likely that either the diagnosis was wrong or the procedure was inappropriate for the condition or inadequately carried out. It is not uncommon to find that, although the patient is still complaining of, for example, pain, the nature of the pain has changed following the intervention. In that situation it may well be that the original problem was solved but a further one has either been caused or arisen.

Response to physiotherapy and exercise programmes should be detailed. It is possible that a treatment has been directed at the neck when the pathology is within the shoulder and vice versa: as far as the patient is concerned it is all physiotherapy which has failed to cure the problem. It is possible that there was an initial good response followed by a recurrence of symptoms; this is all useful information.

If the patient has received local steroid injections, the precise details of the site of injection and the effect should be elicited. It is remarkable how wide is the variation in the site of injection. If the diagnosis is one of acromioclavicular joint pain and the injection has been placed in the subacromial bursa or glenohumeral joint it will not be surprising to find that it had no effect. Patients will often say that an injection made no difference because long-term benefit has not been derived. When more detail is obtained it turns out that symptoms were relieved for a few weeks or months and then recurred; this type of information is highly relevant.

EXAMINATION

There is more than one way of conducting a clinical examination of the shoulder and each individual must develop their own particular system. Having done so one should use the same systematic routine. In that way vital clues will not be missed. There are a few general principles. Adequate exposure of the patient is essential. Men should be stripped to the waist. In women, all shoulder straps should be removed and one good way of retaining the patient's modesty is to cover the breasts with a triangular sling. During the course of the examination of the shoulder, it will be necessary to have the patient standing, sitting and lying. There should, therefore, be available a couch positioned in such a way that the clinician can access either side of it; many consulting rooms are set up in such a way that the examination couch is jammed into a corner of the room; this is totally unsatisfactory for examination of the shoulder. A chair or stool without arms should be available in the room because a number of the clinical tests are most easily done with the patient in a sitting position. The area used for examination should be such that the clinician can walk round the patient to examine both the shoulders both from in front and behind; one way of being able to examine the shoulder from the back and still observe what is going on in the front is to have a long mirror mounted on the wall; this is not essential but is useful.

Cervical spine

The clinical investigation should commence with an examination of the cervical spine (Figure 1.3). This ensures that it is not forgotten and allows one to analyse as far as possible whether any component of the pain arises from this source. The cervical spine is best examined from behind. It should be observed to ensure that the normal contour of the spine is present and that there is no scoliosis, abnormal kyphosis or lordosis. Then one should palpate along the spinous processes and the paraspinal muscles. Palpation should be carried out for tenderness in the belly of the trapezius

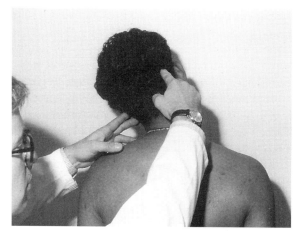

Fig. 1.3 Initial examination of the cervical spine.

muscle which, in the presence of neurogenic pain arising from the cervical spine, can be tender; this type of pain and tenderness is unlikely to arise from intrinsic pathology within the shoulder. Irritation of nerve roots may produce tenderness in the bellies of other muscles in the upper limb such as triceps, biceps or common extensor muscles. This tenderness is probably related to the motor end plates and can be an important clue to the source of apparent shoulder pain. The cervical spine is put through a full range of movement which includes flexion, extension, lateral flexion and rotation to both sides. It is important to ensure that the neck is taken to the extreme end of the available range of movement and note taken of whether this produces any of the patient's symptoms. In particular, if the pain arises from the structures in the cervical spine, lateral flexion combined with rotation may well reproduce the pain which frequently radiates to the scapula, especially the inferior angle, and one may be fortunate to reproduce the pain extending over the shoulder. If this occurs, the patient should be asked the question 'Do you recognize that as your type of pain?' As well as being useful diagnostically it also demonstrates to the patient that the source of the pain is the neck. Patients find it very hard to understand that pain experienced in the shoulder does not actually arise from some disease within that structure. If one can show that neck movement produces the pain it is easier for them to understand.

Observation

Having examined the cervical spine attention is turned to the shoulder. The first thing to do is to observe the general position and posture of the patient's upper body and shoulder (Figure 1.4). The clinician should observe whether the shoulders are lying at the same level, whether one is protracted forwards, whether there is any prominence or asymmetry of the scapula and whether the overall contour of the shoulder is normal and symmetrical; for example in a posterior dislocation, which is commonly missed, the humeral head will cause a small prominence posteriorly; careful clinical examination will ensure that this diagnosis is not missed.

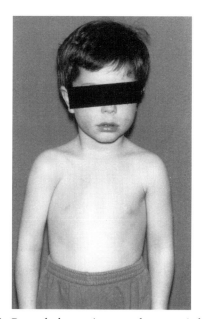

Fig. 1.4 General observation reveals congenital absence of the pectoralis major.

Muscle wasting

Muscle wasting can be an important clue to the diagnosis. Wasting of the deltoid as a result of disuse does occur but is less dramatic than the wasting caused by compromise of the circumflex nerve. In addition to local damage to this nerve it is important to consider such diagnoses as polio-myelitis; this is rarely seen in the UK today but worldwide is still a common disorder. Wasting of the spinati is one of the most important observational physical signs in the shoulder (Figure 1.5). It is easier to observe wasting of the infraspinatus than the supraspinatus. Significant wasting of the infraspinatus is likely to be caused by one of two types of diagnosis: the first, and most common, is a significant rotator cuff tear; the second is some compromise of the suprascapular nerve; there can be a nerve lesion more proximally but that is less likely to produce selective wasting of the infraspinatus. From a practical point of view, if there is marked wasting of the infraspinatus, the clinician should immediately be suspicious that there may be a rotator cuff tear.

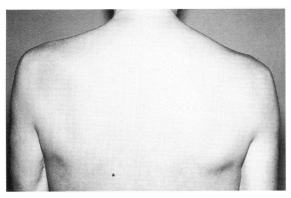

Fig. 1.5 Wasting of the left infraspinatus in a patient with a rotator cuff tear.

Scars

Scars from previous operations can give vital clues to both what was done at the time of the operation and to the residual problem. The site of the scar may lead to a suspicion of iatrogenic nerve damage. Sinuses are indicative of ongoing infection.

Palpation

Systematic palpation of the structures around the shoulder is the next step. The acromioclavicular joint is usually easy to identify. This should be palpated directly superiorly. It is also quite useful to stress the joint by grasping the clavicle between thumb and index finger and steadying the scapula with the other hand; then the clavicle can be gently moved in an anterior and posterior direction; if this reproduces the patient's type of pain it is significant. It is common to find tenderness just distal to the anterolateral acromion in patients who have problems with the rotator cuff. If there is a well-localized area of very acute tenderness, the possibility of a calcific tendonitis should be considered. Palpation is continued around just distal to the lateral part of the acromion until the posterior aspect of the shoulder joint is reached. Tenderness over the coracoid is rather non-specific and usually not helpful in achieving a diagnosis. Tenderness just lateral to the coracoid may be indicative of inflammation within the anterior capsule of the glenohumeral joint itself and is quite commonly found in patients with adhesive capsulitis. These patients may also have tenderness over the posterior joint line. Tenderness is a rather non-specific physical finding. It is just one indicator that there may be pathology in the region of the tenderness. The usefulness of muscle belly tenderness associated with neurogenic pain has already been discussed. If there is difficulty distinguishing between referred pain from extrinsic neurogenic sources as opposed to pain arising intrinsically within the shoulder, this can be a useful adjunctive clue. It is worth noting that it is not possible to specifically localize pathology to, for example, the long head of biceps as a result of tenderness in the region of the bicipital groove. It is hard enough to specifically localize the bicipital groove under direct X-ray control.

Palpation can also give clues as to abnormal contours or possible bony excrescences. The prominence of the humeral head posteriorly in association with either acute or chronic posterior dislocation has been mentioned. Exostoses may be palpable.

Movement

When it comes to movement some clinicians put the shoulder through the full available range of

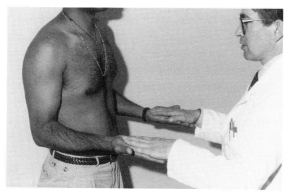

Fig. 1.6 Examiner stands in front of the patient observing contour of the biceps. Active flexion against resistance will emphasize a rupture of the long head of biceps.

active movement and then repeat the whole process for the passive range. It is more compact to do both at once but one should keep in mind precisely what one is testing at any particular moment. The examiner should stand in front of the patient and ask him to flex the elbows up to 90° so that the forearms are pointing directly anteriorly (Figure 1.6). The contour of the long head of biceps should be observed. The patient should be asked to actively flex the elbows against resistance. These two manoeuvres reveal whether the patient has a ruptured long head of biceps (Figure 1.7). If this is present it is usually an indication of underlying impingement and is an important clue. It may be an incidental finding. The patient should be asked to actively externally

rotate the arms keeping the elbows flexed at 90° (Figure 1.8). This gives a range of active external glenohumeral rotation. There is the opportunity to compare the two sides. When the patient has externally rotated as far as is possible, it should be observed whether it is possible to comfortably passively externally rotate any further; this gives the maximum range of passive external rotation. The examiner places his hands on the outside of the patient's wrist and asks the patient to resist keeping the arms in the position of external rotation. This gives a subjective indication of the strength of external rotation. Strength can be formally tested at the end with a spring balance or dynamometer if required. In this situation one is essentially comparing the two sides. There are a number of observations to make. Is the resisted external rotation weak, indicative of some dysfunction of the infraspinatus? When observing the resisted external rotation it is important to look at the humeral head and see whether it tends to ride up anterosuperiorly; if it does, it is an indication of rotator cuff dysfunction usually as result of a tear. Severe weakness can occasionally cause a similar appearance. The second thing to observe is whether resisted external rotation causes pain. If this occurs it suggests pathology in the rotator cuff and typically occurs with impingement but can also do so with calcific tendonitis and full-thickness rotator cuff tears. Of course, any glenohumeral pathology such as rheumatoid arthritis which creates an irritable joint will cause pain with this

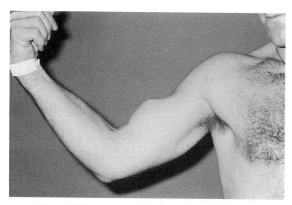

Fig. 1.7 Rupture of the long head of biceps.

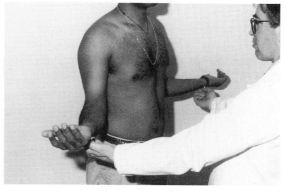

Fig. 1.8 Patient actively externally rotates shoulder with elbows flexed to 90°.

manoeuvre. During this procedure one can observe whether there is passive restriction of external rotation; this is indicative of pathology such as glenohumeral arthritis or true frozen shoulder.

Having investigated active and passive external rotation, the clinician should walk around behind the patient and ask him/her to place the hand up behind the back; how far the extended thumb will reach on the spinous processes can be assessed (Figure 1.9). This should first be carried out on the normal and then on the abnormal side. This is a composite movement of both internal rotation and extension. To formally assess pure internal rotation, the patient should be asked to straighten the arms beside the body; the medial and lateral epicondyles are then palpated and internally rotated keeping the fingers on the epicondyles; it is possible to see the degree of pure internal rotation; for most purposes the composite movement of putting the hand up behind the back is sufficient. Typically this is grossly restricted with diseases affecting the glenohumeral joint, such as arthritis or, in particular, adhesive capsulitis. However, lesser degrees of restriction are quite frequently seen with rotator cuff pathology and almost any condition causing pain in the shoulder. In high-class overhead athletes it is not uncommon to find a minor degree of restriction of internal rotation.

While standing behind the patient, it is useful to do the lift-off test (Figure 1.10). This was described by Gerber & Krushell.[1] It is a specific test for subscapularis function. The hand is placed at waist level behind the back and the patient asked to lift it away from the back towards the examiner who is standing behind him. This manoeuvre can then be resisted to assess the degree of power. If the patient is unable to actively lift off the hand from the back, then it should be passively held away to see whether the patient is able to maintain it in that position; if he cannot it will drop back on to the waist. If this happens with the lift-off test and particularly if there is a degree of increased passive external rotation, it is fairly certain that there is a tear of the subscapularis. Certainly by using this test it is possible to identify the subscapularis as being involved in rotator cuff disruption. This is important in planning the surgical approach and may lead to further investigation to identify the precise site of rotator cuff disruption.

External and internal rotation provide an idea of what is happening within the glenohumeral joint. If there is no passive rotation it can be anticipated that elevation will be mainly scapu-

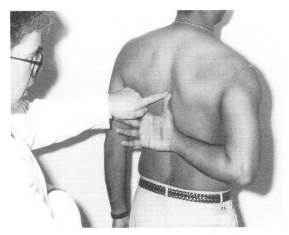

Fig. 1.9 Internal rotation behind the back. The spinous process which is reached by the thumb is used as a measure.

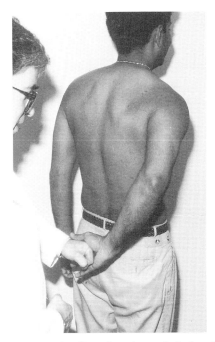

Fig. 1.10 Lift-off test for subscapularis function.

lothoracic. The conclusion will also have been reached that the pathology causing restriction of movement is affecting the glenohumeral joint.

The next step is to stay behind the patient and ask him/her to actively elevate the shoulder in a forward direction (Figure 1.11). The total range of forward elevation of the normal and abnormal side is compared. It is important not only to observe the range but also the rhythm of movement. Careful observation of what happens to the scapula both as the movement is initiated and as the arm goes upwards is required; does it move smoothly and evenly throughout the range or is there a sudden alteration of rhythm? Is there any suggestion of winging? If that is the case, then the serratus anterior should be formally tested by asking the patient to place the flat of both hands against the wall at shoulder level and gently press forwards keeping the elbows straight. While the patient is elevating the arm it is important to establish whether pain is produced and, if so, where in the range of movement does it occur. This manoeuvre is then repeated for pure abduction which is a functionally fairly useless movement, but is useful in terms of identifying painful arcs during the examination (Figure 1.12). If the patient experiences pain at some point during the range of elevation it is important to identify which part of the arc of movement causes pain. In broad general terms painful arcs which are maximal in the mid range of elevation are caused by subacromial pathology whereas a painful arc at the

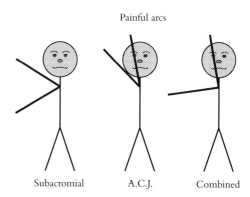

Painful arcs

Subacromial   A.C.J.   Combined

Fig. 1.12 Diagram illustrating painful arcs.

extreme top end of the range is more likely to be caused by acromioclavicular joint pathology. It is worth noting that a high painful arc can occur from subacromial pathology but tends to be referred down the deltoid rather than being localized to the acromioclavicular joint. There may well be combined pathology with pain arising from the acromioclavicular joint which is also causing subacromial impingement as a result of hypertrophic inferior osteophytes; in these circumstances a combined painful arc will be the result. The same movements should be observed from the front of the patient. It is possible that the patient will be unable to actively elevate the arm fully. If that occurs, a gentle attempt to passively raise the arm while holding the patient's wrist should be carried out. If there is full range of passive movement, then the most likely cause of the problem is a major rotator cuff disruption. Having passively raised the arm to the top of the range, it should be assessed whether the patient can hold the arm in that position. If it is impossible to raise the arm passively any more than the active range, an assessment should be made of whether the limitation is caused by pain or true restriction of movement; this can be difficult.

At this stage the basic examination consisting of look, feel and move has been completed and attention can be turned to specific tests. Not all of these will be done on every patient and the choice will depend on what the clinician thinks is the most likely diagnosis.

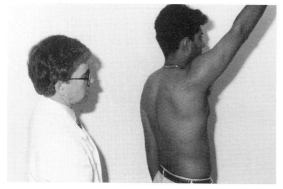

Fig. 1.11 Observation of forward elevation made from behind the patient.

Impingement sign and impingement test

This test is best done with the patient sitting. The examiner stands behind the patient with the left hand (if examining a right shoulder) on top of the acromion (Figure 1.13). The right hand is placed under the patient's elbow. A sharp downwards motion is applied to the left hand while a resisting axial force is applied to the right hand under the elbow. In this way the humeral head is compressed against the acromion. This is done with the arm in several positions of elevation and abduction. Neer & Walsh[2] originally described it with the arm in about 130° of forward elevation. It is significant if pain is produced similar to the patient's own pain. This is the impingement sign.

To do the impingement test local anaesthetic is infiltrated under the acromion into the subacromial bursa; usually about 5 ml is necessary. The test is then repeated. If the pain is abolished, that is a positive test. This sign and test were originally described as a diagnostic test for rotator cuff impingement. Of course anything which produces inflammation at any site between the acromion and the humeral head is likely to cause a positive impingement sign. If local anaesthetic into the bursa abolishes that, then it suggests that the problem is localized to the bursal side of the rotator cuff.

Laxity tests

These should be performed with the patient both sitting and lying. In the sitting position the following tests are carried out: sulcus sign, anterior drawer, posterior drawer.

Sulcus sign (Figure 1.14)

The examiner stands behind the patient and steadies the scapula between thumb and forefinger with the hand on top of the shoulder. Gentle downward traction in an axial direction is applied to the arm and the space between the lateral acromion and the humeral head is observed. If there is inferior laxity, this space will be seen to increase and a depression (sulcus) will appear between the acromion and the humeral head. It is difficult to quantify, but attempts have been

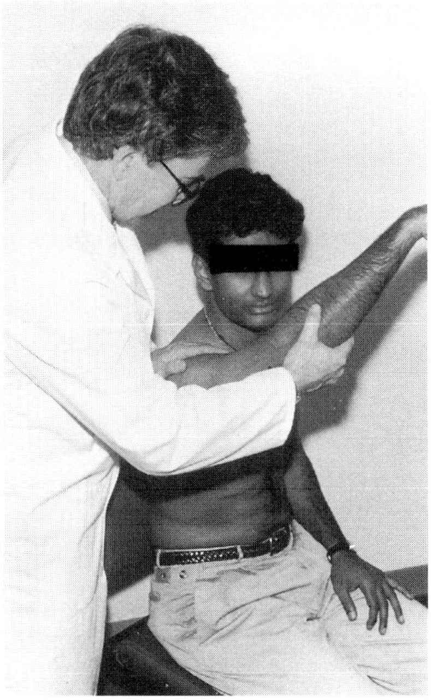

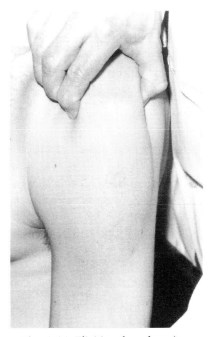

Fig. 1.13 Impingement test. Clinician applies sharp downward pressure on top of acromion while pushing upwards on the elbow with the other hand.

Fig. 1.14 Eliciting the sulcus sign.

made to do so by assessing whether the amount of downward movement is less than 1 cm, equal to, or greater than that amount.

Anterior and posterior drawer signs

The scapula is again steadied between thumb and forefinger with the hand on top of the shoulder. The right hand (if the right shoulder is being examined) grasps the humeral head between thumb, index and middle finger; the examiner attempts to translate the humeral head first in a forwards direction and then posteriorly. The amount of translation can be graded according to whether the humeral head remains centred, moves forwards towards but not on to the rim, up to the rim and finally over the rim. Some people attempt to quantify it in terms of the percentage translation but this is even more difficult. It is essential to compare the two sides.

Supine laxity tests (Figure 1.15)

The patient lies supine with the shoulder being tested just over the edge of the examination couch. The examiner gently grasps the patient's upper arm at about the level of the mid humerus; the patient's hand rests against the examiners body so that the elbow is flexed to 90°. The patient must be relaxed. The shoulder is then translated first in an anterior direction, i.e. up towards the ceiling and then posteriorly down towards the

floor. Once more an assessment is made of the degree of humeral translation in the glenoid.

Stability tests

These are also done both sitting and lying.

Anterior apprehension (sitting)

In the sitting position the patient relaxes and the examiner stands behind the shoulder to be examined. If a right shoulder is being examined, the left hand is placed with the palm on top of the shoulder and the fingers over the front in the region of the coracoid stabilize the scapula; the thumb rests on the back of the humeral head. The right hand gently grasps the patient's forearm and puts the shoulder into a position initially of 90° of abduction and external rotation (Figure 1.16). The shoulder is then extended and the thumb of the left hand gently pushes forward on the humeral head. A positive apprehension is when the patient resists with a reflex contraction of the pectoralis major; usually this is accompanied by a

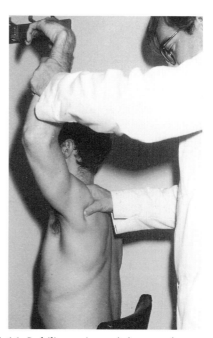

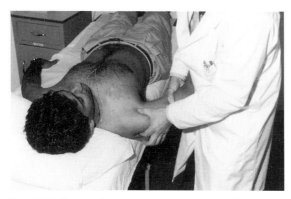

Fig. 1.15 Supine laxity tests – anterior and posterior translation.

Fig. 1.16 Stability testing – sitting anterior apprehension test.

statement that the manoeuvre has reproduced a feeling of the shoulder 'coming out'. This manoeuvre is repeated in 120° and 150° of elevation.

Posterior apprehension (sitting)

A posterior apprehension can also be performed in a sitting position. The left hand examining a right shoulder stabilizes the scapula. The right hand grasps the flexed elbow and places the shoulder in a position of approximately 90° of forward elevation and about 10° of adduction. In this position axial pressure is then applied along the humerus so that the humeral head is being pushed in a posterior direction; if the patient experiences pain or a feeling that the shoulder is 'coming out', this is a positive test. This is not a very reliable test and it is perfectly possible to have a negative posterior apprehension in the sitting position when there is indeed posterior instability.

Anterior apprehension (supine)

The patient is placed in a similar position for the lying down laxity tests. The examiner stands with the right side of his body against the patient's upper torso, facing the shoulder. The left hand gently grasps the forearm and places the shoulder into a position of abduction, external rotation and elevation. The right hand is placed around the humerus and, as the left hand abducts, externally rotates and extends the shoulder, the right hand gently pulls the humerus forwards. A positive apprehension is reflex resistance with contraction of the pectoralis major. In mild degrees of instability it is possible that the manoeuvre produces pain alone. This pain can be caused by impingement rather than instability and Jobe has described a relocation test to try to differentiate between these two diagnoses.

Jobe relocation test

The apprehension manoeuvre is repeated but with the examiner's right hand exerting posterior pressure on the upper humerus. This is designed to maintain the humeral head centred in the glenoid while placing the shoulder in a position

of abduction, extension and external rotation. If the pain is abolished by this relocation manoeuvre, then it suggests that instability is the cause, whereas if the pain remains unaltered, it is more likely to be some form of impingement.

Posterior apprehension (supine)

The posterior apprehension test is repeated in the same way as in the sitting position with the shoulder in 90° of forward flexion and slight adduction; axial pressure is directed along the humerus so that the humeral head is displaced posteriorly. Reproduction of the patient's symptoms is a positive.

The posterior drawer test in the lying position may also reproduce the patient's symptoms along with a subjective feeling that the shoulder is 'coming out'. If posterior instability is looked for carefully, then the rate of diagnosis rises.

Local anaesthetic tests

Although these may seem at first sight to be somewhat invasive, they are an integral and very important part of the clinical assessment of the shoulder. The principle of these tests is that local anaesthetic injected into the site where pathology is thought to arise should abolish the pain.

The two sites where this is most usefully applied are the acromioclavicular joint and the subacromial bursa. If the clinical features suggest pain arising from the acromioclavicular joint, then this hypothesis can be tested by injecting 1–2 ml of local anaesthetic into the acromioclavicular joint. This is best done from a direct superior approach. The clinician will feel the needle enter the joint and after a small amount has been injected it can be seen to return into the syringe when pressure is removed from the plunger; this tells the examiner that his injection is definitely in the correct position. After a few minutes the patient is re-examined. If the original high painful arc has been abolished, then it is fairly certain that the acromioclavicular joint is the source of the problem.

Similarly if it is thought that the pain arises from the subacromial region and there is a mid-range painful arc, local anaesthetic is injected into the subacromial bursa; abolition of the painful arc confirms the diagnosis. This is in many ways similar to the impingement test.

If there is doubt about whether the source of the pain is the glenohumeral joint, the test can be applied there but it is less often necessary in this site.

Biceps tendon tests

These are neither specific nor reliable. Yergasson's test is performed by placing the patient's forearm in full pronation with the elbow flexed to 90° and then asking him to try to supinate against resistance. A positive test is when the patient experiences pain in the biceps region.

Thoracic outlet tests

It is important to consider thoracic outlet compression as a possible diagnosis in the patient who has pain in an atypical distribution particularly if it radiates to the distal forearm and hand and is associated with vague neurological symptoms. The three standard tests are Adson's test, the hyperabduction test and the costoclavicular manoeuvre.

Adson's test is carried out by holding the patient's wrist whilst feeling the radial pulse. The shoulder is extended and the patient rotates the head towards the side being examined. If the pulse disappears or is significantly diminished, that is a positive. Auscultation should be used to determine whether a bruit is present. The manoeuvre may reproduce the patient's symptoms which is probably more significant, although not part of the original description of the test.

For the hyperabduction test the examiner holds both wrists of the patient in such a way that the radial pulses can be felt. The arms are put into a position of abduction high above the head. Abolition or significant diminution of the pulse is a positive test.

The costoclavicular test is done by holding the patient's wrist and gently pulling the arm down into a position of extension whilst the patient protrudes the chest. Changes in the pulse or paraesthesia are significant.

All these tests have a quite high incidence of positive results in the asymptomatic normal population.[3] This makes their interpretation difficult and the tests must be interpreted with caution and in the light of the patient's symptoms.

Power measurement

This should be carried out because most of the standard scoring systems include some assessment of power. It is, however, the most controversial aspect. The simplest method is to use a spring balance. This method was made popular by Constant, whose functional score is the current European standard. The patient is asked to hold a spring balance with the arm abducted so that it is parallel to the floor. A steady pull is applied to the other end of the spring balance and a reading is taken of the maximum, up to 25 lbs, which the patient can resist. Normal power diminishes with age and should be taken into account. It is most important to compare the normal with the abnormal side.

Recording

It is essential to record accurately the results of the clinical examination. The easiest way to do this is to use a standard proforma. This also ensures that no part of the examination is forgotten.

REFERENCES

1. Gerber, C. & Krushell, R.J. (1991) Isolated rupture of the tendon of the subscapularis muscle. *J. Bone Joint Surg.* **73B:** 389–394.
2. Neer, C.S. & Walsh, R.P. (1977) The shoulder in sports. *Orthop. Clin. North Am.* **8:** 583–591.
3. Rayan, G.M. & Jensen, C. (1995) Thoracic outlet syndrome: provocative examination manouevres in a typical population. *J. Shoulder Elbow Surg.* **4:** 113–117.

Surgical Anatomy and Approaches

A Carr and D Wallace

ANATOMY

The shoulder mechanism consists of three joints in series which connect the upper limb to the thorax and enable the hand to be positioned accurately in space. Most of the great range of motion of the shoulder occurs at the glenohumeral joint, which will be discussed here. The acromioclavicular and sternoclavicular articulations are considered elsewhere.

Osteology

The clavicle and scapula together suspend the upper limb from the trunk. The scapula is sited over the second to seventh ribs and is embedded in muscle. The scapula has three important processes: the acromion, the coracoid and the spine (Figure 2.1). The spine of the scapula provides for the insertion of the trapezium muscle and latissimus dorsi. The acromion process is a continuation of the spine of the scapula and curves forward anteriorly from the spine to cover the humeral head. The acromion provides a platform for the powerful deltoid muscle and increases the mechanical advantage of that muscle allowing powerful abduction of the shoulder. When the muscle is released from the bone during surgery it is therefore important that a secure reattachment is achieved to prevent subsequent weakness.

The construction process of the scapula is an important landmark in the shoulder region and provides the attachment of the short head of biceps, coracobrachialis and pectoralis minor muscles.

The humeral head has a greater tuberosity posterolaterally where the supraspinatus, infraspinatus and teres minor muscles of the rotator cuff insert. The lesser tuberosity, where the subscapularis muscle inserts, lies anteriorly and is separated from the greater tuberosity by the groove formed by the long head of biceps. The head of the humerus articulates with the glenoid of the scapula. The humeral head is retroverted an average of $30°$ on the shaft of the humerus although this varies considerably from individual to individual ($10–55°$ in some series). The glenoid is anteverted in a reciprocal manner to face the humeral head.

Arthrology

The glenohumeral joint has a wide range of motion and is therefore prone to instability. Both static (capsular/ligamentous) and dynamic (muscular) mechanisms are important in providing stability. The joint capsule (Figure 2.2) is attached to the glenoid labrum and is firmly anchored to the periosteum of the glenoid neck. The capsule has discrete thickenings anteriorly known as the superior, middle and inferior glenohumeral ligaments. These ligaments are wound up in abduction and external rotation of the humerus and resist anterior displacement. The articular surfaces of the glenohumeral joint are congruent because of thickening of the articular cartilage of the glenoid towards the periphery, which effectively deepens the shallow socket. The socket is further deepened by a thick fibrocartilaginous labrum. The long head of biceps which inserts into the superior aspect of the labrum and the rotator cuff of muscles further contribute to joint stability.

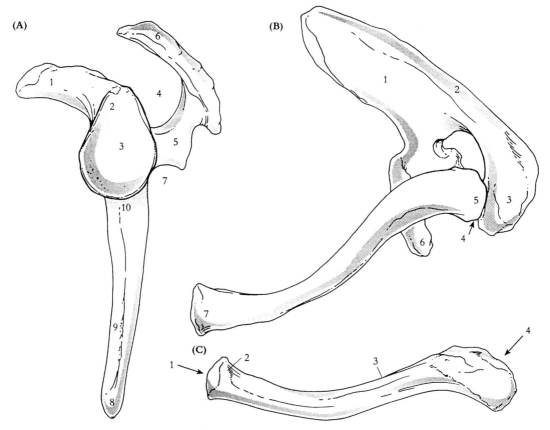

Fig. 2.1 (A) Left scapula from the lateral side. 1, Coracoid process; 2, supraglenoid tubercle; 3, glenoid cavity; 4, supraspinous fossa; 5, spine; 6, acromion; 7, infraspinous fossa; 8, inferior angle; 9, lateral border; 10, infraglenoid tubercle. (B) Articulation of left scapula and clavicle from above. 1, Supraspinous fossa; 2, spine of scapula; 3, acromion; 4, acromioclavicular joint; 5, acromial end of clavicle; 6, coracoid process; 7, sternal end of clavicle. The sternal end of the clavicle is bulbous; the acromial end is flattened. The shaft is convex anteriorly in its medial two-thirds, and the groove for the subclavius muscle is on the inferior surface. (C) Left clavicle from below. 1, Sternal end with articular surface (arrow); 2, impression for costoclavicular ligament; 3, groove for subclavius muscle; 4, acromial end with articular surface (arrow).

The superior joint capsule in the interval between supraspinatus and subscapularis is reinforced by the coracohumeral ligament which runs from the base of the coracoid process. This ligament is also taut in external rotation and is implicated in the restriction of movement seen in capsulitis of the shoulder.

The coracoacromial ligament fans upward from the base of the coracoid and has a broad insertion on the undersurface of the acromion. This structure completes the arch of the acromion anteriorly and may therefore contribute to impingement.

Muscles of the shoulder (Figure 2.3)

The muscles acting on the shoulder lie in two layers, and each layer has different functions. The superficial layer consists of a number of separate groups of muscles. The trapezium, rhomboids, levator scapulae, subclavius and seratus anterior stabilize the scapula on the spine and chest wall, and the pectorals, latissimus dorsi, deltoid and teres major provide power for movement of the glenohumeral joint.

The inner layer of muscles, the rotator cuff, consists of the muscles linking the scapula to the

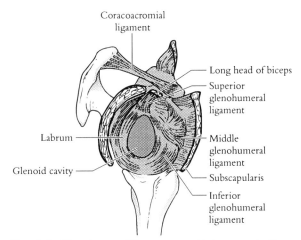

Fig. 2.2 Glenohumeral ligaments and joint capsular ligaments.

Coracoacromial ligament

Long head of biceps

Superior glenohumeral ligament

Labrum

Middle glenohumeral ligament

Glenoid cavity

Subscapularis

Inferior glenohumeral ligament

head of the humerus, namely subscapularis, supraspinatus, infraspinatus and teres minor. These muscles function like guy ropes to centre the head of the humerus in the glenoid during motion and contribute to the dynamic stability of the glenohumeral joint. During elevation of the arm, the rotator cuff and in particular the supraspinatus acts to depress the humeral head and counteracts the upwards pull of the deltoid. The supraspinatus and infraspinatus muscles run in the space betweeen the arch of the acromion and head of the humerus before inserting into the greatert tuberosity and are therefore vulnerable to impingement on the undersurface of the acromion. An imbalance in

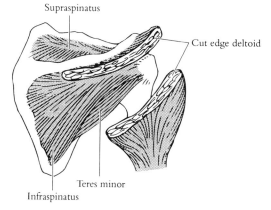

Supraspinatus

Cut edge deltoid

Teres minor

Infraspinatus

Fig. 2.3 Shoulder muscles from the posterior aspect with deltoid detached revealing the rotator cuff.

the action of the cuff muscles and the powerful deltoid may contribute to impingement of the cuff.

Blood supply (Figure 2.4)

The subclavian artery arises from the brachiocephalic trunk on the right and direct from the aorta on the left. The thyrocervical trunk arises from the subclavian artery in the neck and contributes the suprascapular artery to the anastomoses around the scapula. The subclavian artery crosses the first rib and becomes the axillary artery. The pectoralis minor divides the artery conveniently into three parts: the first medial to it, the second under it and the third lateral to it. The first part gives off one branch, the supreme thoracic artery, which runs medially to supply the seratus anterior and pectoral muscles. The second part of the axillary artery gives off two branches: the thoracoacromial artery which supplies the deltoid, pectorals and glenohumeral joint and the lateral thoracic artery which runs down to supply the seratus anterior. The third portion of the axillary artery produces three branches: the subscapular, anterior circumflex humeral and posterior circumflex humeral. The subscapular artery branches into a thoracodorsal and a circumflex scapular branch which anastomoses with the suprascapular artery. The circumflex humeral vessels wind around the neck of the humerus to supply the humeral head and surrounding soft tissues.

A knowledge of the position of the circumflex humeral and suprascapular arteries is of particular importance since they are vulnerable during anterior and posterior approaches to the shoulder respectively. Venous tributaries follow the arterial branches. An important landmark in the shoulder is the cephalic vein which lies superficially as it runs up between the deltoid and pectoralis major muscles in the anterior shoulder region. The humeral head blood supply is derived mostly from the ascending branch of the anterior cicumflex humeral artery which arises at the lower border of the subscapularis and follows a horizontal course in the bicipital groove.[1] The ascending branch runs on the lateral border of the groove to enter

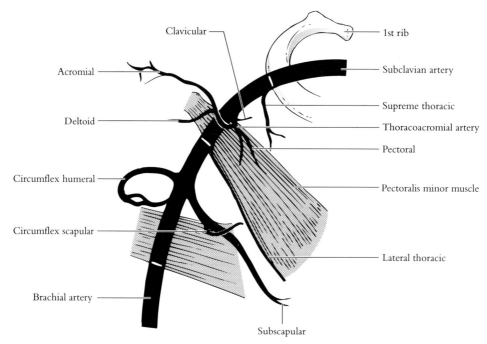

Fig. 2.4 Arterial supply to shoulder including anastomoses around scapula.

the head at the level of the greater tuberosity. This termination is known as the arcuate artery of the head. Anastomoses exist between the arcuate artery and a group of small vessels from the posterior circumflex humeral artery which enter the head posteromedially and a central artery from the humeral metaphysis. Blood also enters the humeral head through the soft tissue attachments of the rotator cuff at the greater and lesser tuberosities. This rich anastomosis allows perfusion of the head even if the arcuate artery is divided at its insertion into the head. When the anastomotic vessels are disrupted in four-part humeral head fractures, however, the head is deprived of a blood supply and avascular necrosis frequently results.

The rich blood supply to the shoulder from the suprascapular, subscapular, circumflex humeral and thoracoacromial arteries and their frequent anastomoses around the scapula makes surgery on the shoulder potentially bloody and, in combination with the muscular thickness of the athletic individual, can make surgical access and good visualization a challenge.

Innervation (Figure 2.5)

The brachial plexus arises from the anterior primary rami of C5 to T1. It lies deep to the clavicle and runs from the scalenus anterior down into the axilla. The structure of the plexus will not be considered in detail. Clinically important branches innervate the rotator cuff and large external muscles of the shoulder. These nerves are at risk during dissection around the shoulder. The axillary nerve which supplies the deltoid and teres minor muscles is vulnerable as it winds posteriorly around the neck of the humerus and continues anteriorly on the undersurface of the deltoid. It is the most commonly injured nerve in operations about the shoulder. With the shoulder abducted and internally rotated the axillary nerve lies against the inferior glenohumeral joint capsule and may be damaged when the joint is incised anteriorly. After winding posteriorly around the humerus, the nerve and its branches are at risk when the deltoid is split for a distance of more than 5 cm from its origin.

The musculocutaneous nerve pierces the bi-

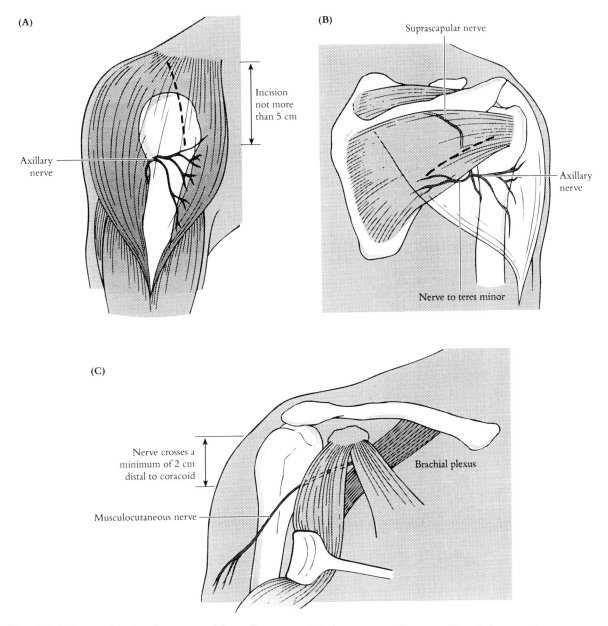

Fig. 2.5　Diagram showing the course of the axillary nerve (A), the suprascapular nerve (B) and the musculocutaneous nerve (C).

ceps and coracobrachialis muscles a variable distance of between 2 and 9 cm below the coracoid. It may be damaged by excessive retraction of these muscles during an anterior exposure.

The suprascapular nerve passes under the transverse ligament of the suprascapular notch and supplies the supraspinatus muscle. It then winds around the lateral border of the neck of the scapula to supply the infraspinatus muscle. At both sites it may become compressed and may also be damaged during a posterior approach to the glenohumeral joint.

SURGICAL APPROACHES TO THE SHOULDER JOINT

The aim of the various surgical approaches to the shoulder is of course whenever possible to dissect between the neurovascular planes and thereby minimize the potential for bleeding and injury to nerves and their branches. This ideal may have to be compromised in the pursuit of adequate access and cosmesis. The optimum direction for a cosmetic skin incision is determined by the direction of the relaxed skin tension lines observed at operation when the skin is pinched. For optimum cosmesis the skin incision may need to be orientated differently from the underlying dissection since the skin tension lines may lie at right angles to the underlying muscle fibres, which should be split rather than divided whenever possible.

Patient positioning

For anterior surgery the patient should be positioned supine towards the edge of the operating table with the head placed on a neurosurgical ring support and with the table broken (the beach chair or deck chair position; Figure 2.6). Alternatively and preferably a modified table is used with a movable attachment designed specifically for shoulder surgery. The arm is draped free, and can be rested on an arm support in slight abduc-

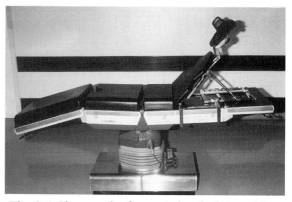

Fig. 2.6 Photograph of set up in beach chair position.

tion. A sandbag beneath the scapula will push the shoulder forward and allow easier access. Assistants can stand both on the contralateral side of the patient and at the ipsilateral head end.

For posterior approaches the patient is placed in the lateral decubitus position with the trunk well padded and supported. The arm is draped free. An alternative position is with the patient prone although it is not easy to manipulate the arm in such a position. This may, however, be appropriate for surgery to scapula fractures or for scapulothoracic fusion.

Deltopectoral approach (Figure 2.7)

The anterior deltopectoral approach of Henry[2] is the utility approach to the shoulder, and the

(A)

(B)

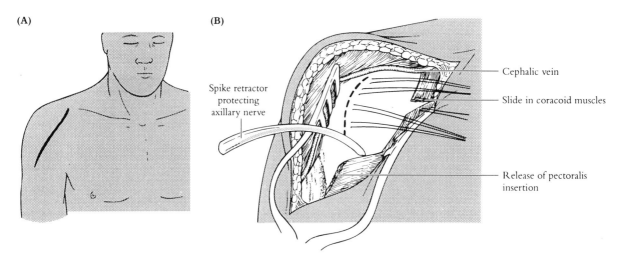

Spike retractor protecting axillary nerve

Cephalic vein

Slide in coracoid muscles

Release of pectoralis insertion

Fig. 2.7 Deltopectoral approach to the shoulder.

majority of shoulder procedures may be carried out through this route. The approach is particularly suitable for total shoulder replacement and internal fixation of fractures as well as anterior stabilization. The incision is extensile between the neurovascular planes of the pectoral and axillary neurovascular bundles, and part or all of the approach may be utilized.

Positioning

The patient is placed in the beach chair position with a sandbag under the operated shoulder.

Procedure

The skin incision runs from the clavicle in a line just lateral to the coracoid along the medial border of the deltoid towards the lateral border of the axillary fold. After the incision in the deep fascia in the line of the skin incision, the key to the approach is to identify the deltopectoral groove marked by the cephalic vein. The vein may be difficult to find in some patients. The interval between deltoid and pectoralis major is then developed by blunt finger dissection. The cephalic vein can be injured during this dissection and some would advocate routinely ligating it at the outset. Postoperative swelling and oedema of the arm is very unusual following such a manouevre but it is probably better to preserve the vein if possible. The vein receives tributaries predominantly from the lateral side and it is therefore easier to mobilize it laterally toward the deltoid. When carrying out total shoulder replacement through this approach it is usually better to mobilize the vein and retract it medially to avoid damaging it during preparation of the humerus and glenoid. The deltoid and pectoralis are then separated by a self-retaining retractor. The clavipectoral fascia is incised in line with the lateral border of the coracoid to reveal the coracoid muscles. These muscles are retracted medially by deepening the self-retaining retractor. In most cases and especially in muscular individuals, it is necessary to release the lateral one-third of the coracoid muscles no more than 1 cm from their origin after first placing a stay suture inferiorly to

facilitate reattachment. The coracoid muscles should not be completely divided since damage to the musculocutaneous nerve may result from subsequent traction on the reflected muscle.

The inferior border of the subscapularis is next identified and the axillary nerve is protected by placing a ring-handled spike retractor inferiorly. The superficial branches of the anterior circumflex humeral vessels may need to be coagulated. The rotator interval (between subscapularis and supraspinatus) is then identified and two or three stay sutures are placed in the subscapularis tendon 1–2 cm medial to its humeral insertion.

The subscapularis can then be incised vertically to expose the underlying glenohumeral joint capsule. In joint replacement surgery where the subscapularis is contracted, the muscle may be incised with an oblique incision to permit lengthening. In instability surgery great care must be taken incising the subscapularis when developing the plane between the subscapularis and the capsule. The two layers are often adherent particularly in the superior part of the incision.

A periosteal elevator can be used to sweep the muscle from the underlying capsule. For some procedures it is not necessary to detach the whole of the subscapularis and the inferior border of the muscle may be left in continuity to provide further inferior protection for the axillary nerve and to facilitate reattachment.

After placement of stay sutures, the joint capsule can be opened laterally 1–2 cm from its humeral insertion through a T-shaped incision or medially through a medially based incision at the glenoid rim. Closure of the capsule and subscapularis is carried out depending on the type of procedure performed. As mentioned above the anterior structures may need to be lengthened in joint replacement and shortened sometimes in cases of instability.

Extensions

To gain better access inferiorly the pectoralis major muscle can be released at the superior third of its insertion and the medial deltoid can be released from the clavicle superiorly. The incision can also be extended down the lateral shaft of the humerus for difficult fractures or revision arthroplasty surgery.

Superior extension is sometimes necessary for tumour resection and can be accomplished by detachment of the deltoid from the acromion and even osteotomy of the clavicle.

Detaching the tip of the coracoid insertion by osteotomy is not recommended although the exposure is improved, because of the risk of a traction injury to the musculocutaneous nerve and the risk of screw misplacement on reattachment.

The brachial plexus can be exposed through the interval between the short head of biceps and the coracobrachialis muscle.

Structures at risk

The axillary nerve is vulnerable in the inferior part of the wound during incision of the inferior capsule, and caution is advised when inserting retractors inferiorly to expose the inferior capsule. The musculocutaneous nerve is at risk when the coracoid muscles are retracted. The nerve usually pierces the short head of biceps at least 5 cm from its origin but the course is very variable and may run within 2 cm of the coracoid. A release of the coracoid musculature should therefore be carried out within 2 cm of the coracoid and the muscle should not be completely detached or retracted too enthusiastically.

Advantages/disadvantages

The main advantage of this incision over other incisions is the potential for extension both proximally and distally. The exposure is excellent for most procedures and the approach is between muscle planes and therefore there is relatively little bleeding from the wound (provided that the cephalic vein is not violated).

The disadvantages of this approach include difficulty in exposing the glenoid for total joint replacement in a muscular individual and difficulty in getting to a displaced greater tuberosity fragment in fracture fixation. These difficulties can usually be overcome by good retraction and releasing the soft tissues proximally and distally.

Modifications

Low anterior approach (Figure 2.8). A cosmetic skin incision is made in the line of the anterior axillary skin fold. The line of the incision is made

(A)   (B)

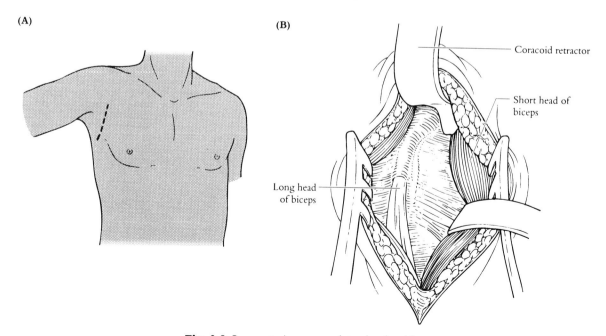

Fig. 2.8 Low anterior approach to the shoulder.

by adducting the shoulder and identifying the apex of the most prominent lateral skin fold then continuing the incision distally for 6 cm into the axilla with the arm abducted slightly. The skin edges are undermined and the approach is then continued through the deltopectoral groove in the usual way. Exposure of the glenohumeral joint requires the use of a coracoid retractor to lever the skin and deltoid superiorly. For this reason this approach works best in young women with elastic tissues and without bulky muscles.

Diagrams of standard deltopectoral app to show slide in coracoid muscles and retraction.

Superior approaches

The anterosuperior approach (Figure 2.9)

This approach was recently described by Mackenzie[3] and developed by Neviaser for glenoid replacement[4].

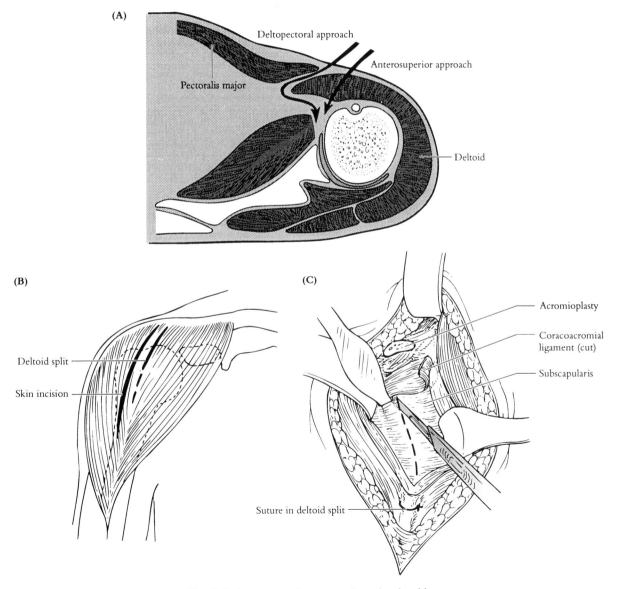

Fig. 2.9 Anterosuperior approach to the shoulder.

Indications. The indications for this approach include total shoulder replacement, rotator cuff repair and small isolated greater tuberosity fractures.

Position. The patient is placed in the semi-sitting beach chair position with the arm draped free and a sand bag under the scapula as for the deltopectoral approach.

Procedure. The skin incision extends from just posteriorly to the acromioclavicular joint distally for a distance of 9 cm in line with the lateral border of the biceps. The acromioclavicular joint is identified and the deltoid fibres are split for a distance of not more than 5 cm. To ensure that the deltoid split does not propagate further distally during the rest of the operation and damage the axillary nerve, a stay suture is placed at the apex of the split. The stay suture should be checked throughout the procedure and replaced if it becomes dislodged. Strong inferior traction by zealous assistants on the soft tissues should be avoided. The deltoid is next detatched from the anterior part of the acromion with an osteo-periosteal flap to aid reattachment. An anterior acromioplasty is carried out and if access to the humerus is still restricted, the lateral 1 cm of the clavicle can be resected. The fascia next to the coracoid muscles is incised and the coracoacromial ligament is split. The coracoid muscles are retracted medially with a self-retaining retractor to expose the subscapularis muscle. After insertion of stay sutures the subscapularis is divided 1.5 cm from its insertion into the lesser tuberosity. Branches of the anterior circumflex humeral vessels are divided and the subscapularis is elevated from the underlying capsule by periosteal elevator and sharp dissection. As with the deltopectoral approach it is not always necessary to divide all the subscapularis, and a few inferior fibres may be left to help protect the axillary artery and facilitate reattachment. The capsule is incised through a T-shaped incision and the humeral head is dislocated by external rotation and extension. After resection of the humeral head, the glenoid is exposed by inserting a Fukuda ring retractor behind its posterior rim, which depresses the humerus, and a Carter Rowe spike anteriorly to reflect the soft tissues medially.

During closure the subscapularis may be reattached to the lateral capsular remnant to gain length and encourage external rotation. Holding the limb in 30° of flexion helps when repairing the deltoid split with interrupted absorbable sutures.

Advantages/disadvantages. Advantages of this approach include good visualization of the glenoid for total joint replacement with minimal retraction of the soft tissues because of a more face on approach. It also allows more posterior access to a greater tuberosity fracture. Other advantages in total joint replacement surgery are the shorter incision and the ease of access to the acromioclavicular joint which may require concomitant surgery. The major drawback of this approach is that it cannot be extended distally for more than 5 cm because of the risk to the axillary nerve. This approach is therefore unsuitable for operations which necessitate exposure of the shaft of the humerus, e.g. three-part fractures and tumour resection. It is also contraindicated in congenitally deformed humeri where the axillary nerve may run close to the acromion due to an abnormally short proximal humerus.

Shoulder strap approach (Figure 2.10)

Indications. This approach is particularly suited to open acromioplasty and rotator cuff repair. It can also be used for fixing small avulsion fractures of the greater tuberosity.

Position. The patient is positioned supine in the beach chair position with the arm draped free to allow rotation of the humeral head and consequently visualization of the entire rotator cuff.

Procedure. A sagittal incision is made in the direction of a shoulder strap starting midway between the lateral tip of the acromion and the acromioclavicular joint and running anteriorly for 6 cm. The skin flaps are undermined and the surface of the underlying acromion is identified.

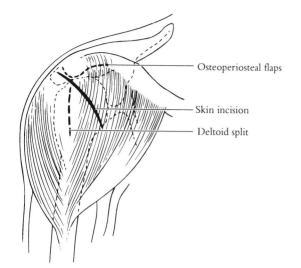

— Osteoperiosteal flaps

— Skin incision

— Deltoid split

Fig. 2.10 Shoulder strap approach: skin incision and deep development.

Osteoperiosteal flaps are then raised from the surface of the acromion using a sharp osteotome. The deltoid is split in the line of its fibres at the junction of the anterior and middle thirds of the muscle where the muscle changes from a multipennate to a unipennate structure. This allows the deltoid to be split in a relatively blood-free plane. A self-retaining retractor is used to expose the underlying cuff. Further exposure is achieved by excision of the coracoacromial ligament and an anterior acromioplasty with a sharp osteotome or oscillating saw. The whole surface of the rotator cuff can usually be visualized by rotating and abducting the humerus. If better visualization is required the osteoperiosteal flaps on the acromion can be extended posteriorly and as far as the acromioclavicular joint and clavicle anteriorly allowing detachment of the deltoid.

As little deltoid as possible should be detached while still permitting adequate access. When the deltoid is detached great care must be taken with reattachment to prevent postoperative retraction of the muscle which may result in unsightly weakness of the shoulder. During closure it is advisable to secure the osteoperiosteal flaps to bone. The deltoid should not be split for more than 5 cm distal to its insertion since the axillary nerve and its branches are at risk inferiorly and damage will result in loss of anterior deltoid function.

Structures at risk. The main structure at risk with this approach is the axillary nerve if the deltoid is split too far distally.

Advantages / disadvantages. The advantage of this approach is that it provides good superior exposure and can be extended posteriorly for cuff access. The scar is well sited and is cosmetically acceptable in women, being covered by a bra strap. The main disadvantage is the poor distal access due to limitations imposed by the axillary nerve and the fact that poor reattachment of the deltoid may lead to defunctioning of the muscle and an unsightly contour to the shoulder.

Transacromial approach (Figure 2.11)

Indications. This approach was described by Kessel & Watson in 1977 for rotator cuff surgery.[5] In addition, it can be utilized for isolated fractures of the greater tuberosity.

Positioning. As with other anterior and superior approaches the patient is positioned supine in the beach chair position with the arm draped free to permit rotation of the humeral head.

Procedure. The incision runs in the coronal plane across the middle of the acromion just posterior to the acromioclavicular joint. The line of incision is identified by placing the index finger in the supraspinous fossa and feeling the back of the clavicle and spine of scapula. The incision then extends along the line of the finger from 3 cm proximal to and 5 cm distal to the outer acromion. The deltoid and trapezius muscles are split in the line of their fibres and osteoperiosteal flaps are raised from the acromion in continuity with the muscles. Beneath the deltoid lies the subacromial bursa and beneath the trapezium is a fat pad separating the incision from the underlying supraspinatus. The acromion is next divided with a saw or sharp osteotome, and a self-retaining retractor is inserted to separate the two halves of the bone. The subacromial bursa is then opened to expose the underlying rotator cuff. The entire cuff can be visualized by internal and external rotation of the arm.

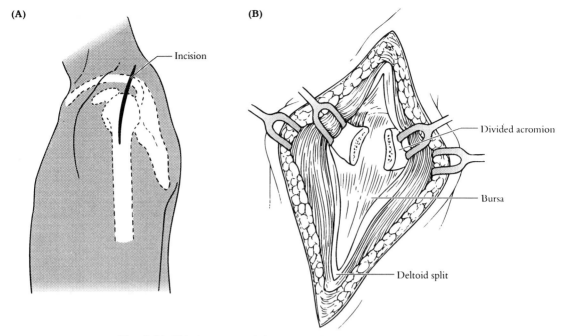

Fig. 2.11 Skin incision and dissection of the transacromial approach.

Closure is facilitated by use of a towel clip to oppose the two halves of the acromion whilst the osteoperiosteal flaps are secured with interrupted sutures. The trapezium and deltoid are also tacked together with a few interrupted sutures.

Structures at risk. The axillary nerve is at risk with excessive inferior extension or retraction. Other complications include the possibility of a non-union of the acromion osteotomy.

Advantages/disadvantages. The advantage of this approach is the wide exposure of the rotator cuff which allows good access for mobilization of a massive cuff tear. The scar is not as cosmetically pleasing as the shoulder strap incision and the other main disadvantage is the possibility of a non-union as mentioned above.

Posterior approaches (Figure 2.12)

Indications

Posterior approaches are primarily indicated for stabilization of posterior instability of the gleno-

humeral joint. Other indications include fixation of scapula and glenoid fractures and tumour surgery.

Postioning

The patient may be positioned either in the lateral decubitus position with operated shoulder uppermost or prone.

Procedure (Kocher or Rowe approach)

A vertical incision is made in the line of the relaxed skin tension lines centred 2 cm inferomedially to the posterior corner of the acromion (the site of the posterior entry portal for arthroscopy). The skin and subcutaneous flaps are raised to allow access to the deltoid muscle. The fascia overlying the posterior deltoid is split and the underlying deltoid muscle is split in the line of its fibres. A layer of fascia lies deep to the deltoid and this must be split to allow access to the infraspinatus and teres minor muscles beneath. The deltoid split is not continued further distally than the teres major to prevent risk of damage to the axillary

(A)

(B)

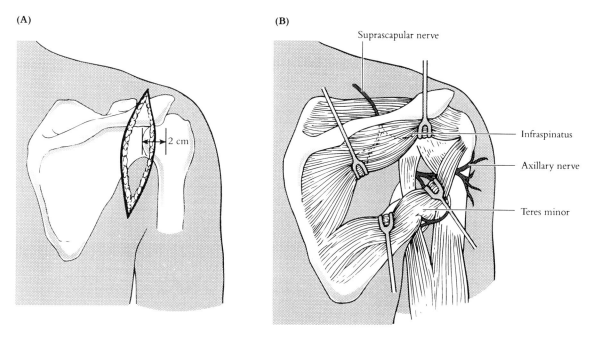

Fig. 2.12 Posterior approach to the shoulder.

nerve. Additional exposure can be gained proximally by detaching the deltoid with an osteoperiosteal flap from the scapula.

The interval between the infraspinatus (suprascapular nerve) and teres minor (axillary nerve) muscles is then looked for. It is often easier to identify the interval at the medial bulkier part of the muscles rather than at their lateral tendinous portions where the structures blend to form the rotator cuff. It may, however, be difficult to identify this interval and the disssection should be kept well lateral to the glenoid to avoid injury to the suprascapular nerve as it winds around the neck of the scapula. The separated muscles can be held with a self-retaining retractor and the posterior glenohumeral joint capsule can be opened to expose the joint. If the interval between the infraspinatus and teres minor is too low or the interval cannot be identified with certainty, then it may be necessary to split the infraspinatus muscle, although this risks denervation of the inferior portion of the muscle.

Structures at risk

As well as the suprascapular nerve and artery the axillary nerve is at risk in the lower lateral part of the wound.

Variations

The skin incision may be made along the spine of the scapula to avoid the need for raising flaps at the expense of poorer cosmesis. The glenohumeral joint can be exposed by dividing the infraspinatus tendon close to its insertion on the humeral head and reflecting the muscle medially rather than splitting the muscle or splitting the interval between infraspinatus and teres minor. If the muscle is divided, then this allows the muscle to be tightened during closure as with an anterior Putti-Platt type of procedure.

Posterior approach to scapula

Indications. This approach is indicated for scapulothoracic fusion and fixation of some scapula fractures.

Position. The patient is positioned prone with the arms by their side and to allow adequate ventilation during the procedure.

Procedure. A vertical incision is made along the medial border of the scapula 8–10 cm in length. The approach is deepened through the subcutaneous fascia and the trapezium muscle is incised to expose the medial scapula border. The infraspinatus is then elevated from the infraspinous fossa using a periosteal elevator.

Subdeltoid approach (Martini⁶)

This approach gives excellent access to the humeral metaphysis at the expense of a poor cosmetic scar. The indications include surgery for complex fractures, infections and tumours of the metaphysis.

Positioning: lateral decubitus. The incision consists of anterior and posterior arms which converge on the deltoid insertion into the humerus. The deltopectoral groove is identified anteriorly and the deltoid is separated from the long and lateral heads of triceps posteriorly. The deltoid is mobilized and when both incisions have been completed the deltoid tendon is divided and the muscle is reflected superiorly in an avascular plane. The proximal humerus is widely exposed and the axillary nerve is seen on the upturned surface of the deltoid and is therefore protected. A modification of the approach is to detach the deltoid insertion by removing a small block of bone from the humerus to aid reattachment.

Disadvantages include poor visualization of the glenoid and potential weakness of deltoid unless reattachment is secure. The resulting scar is not pretty.

REFERENCES

1. Brooks, C.H., Revell, W.J. & Heatley, F.W. (1993) Vascularity of humeral head after proximal humeral fractures. *J. Bone Joint Surg.* **75B:** 132–136.
2. Henry, A.K. (1995) *Extensile Exposure*, 3rd edn. Edinburgh: Churchill-Livingstone.
3. Mackenzie (1993) The anterosuperior exposure for total shoulder replacement. *Orthop. Traumatol* **2:** 71–77.
4. Copeland, S.A. (1995) Surgical approaches to the shoulder. In *Operative Shoulder Surgery*. Edinburgh: Churchill-Livingstone.
5. Kessel, L. & Watson, M. (1977) The transacromial approach to the shoulder for rupture of the rotator cuff. *Int. Orthop.* **1:** 153–154.
6. Martini, M. (1976) Subdeltoid approach to the metaphyseal region of the humerus. *J. Bone Joint Surg.* **58A:** 377–379.

3

The Biomechanics of the Shoulder Joint Complex

A Carr and V Conboy

INTRODUCTION

The forelimb of the quadruped is articulated to the body by a joint which carries mainly compressive loads. This has therefore developed into a stable joint where a degree of mobility has been sacrificed to achieve stability. By contrast the forelimb of the tree-hanging primate needs to act as a fully movable linkage where the ability to withstand compressive loads is of less importance than the need for a large range of motion.

These two examples form the extremes of a spectrum of which *Homo sapiens* stands roughly at the centre. Thus the shoulder complex of man demonstrates a fine balance between mobility and stability. This causes difficulties in studying its mechanics: the mobility of the joint means that the mechanics may change significantly with the different positions attained by the upper limb during function. The need for stability leads to the scapula developing the role of a supporting platform for the humerus during elevation. The interplay of the two in different functions adds to the complexity.

Despite the difficulties, it is important to understand how the component articulations of the shoulder joint complex work. The clinical problems facing the orthopaedic surgeon are intimately concerned with joint mechanics. What factors predispose to instability and what are the consequences of its surgical treatment? What is the optimal design of a replacement arthroplasty? Why do some arthroplasties fail?

The purpose of this chapter is to outline some of the accepted knowledge regarding shoulder function in both health and disease and to explain the principles necessary for a simple mechanical analysis of the glenohumeral joint.

THE SHOULDER JOINT COMPLEX

The shoulder girdle complex comprises the scapulothoracic articulation, the acromioclavicular joint, the sternoclavicular joint and the glenohumeral joint. These articulations act in concert to position the upper limb relative to the thorax.

The clavicle and related joints

The sternoclavicular joint

The sternoclavicular joint is a synovial joint, the surfaces of which are saddle-shaped and reciprocally concavoconvex. The surfaces often do not have identical curvature and congruence is provided by a meniscus which divides the joint into two cavities. The geometry of the articular surfaces essentially limits motion to rotation about two axes: one parallel with the concavity of the clavicular surface and the other parallel to the concavity of the sternocostal surface. The constraints to motion comprise the costoclavicular ligament, running from the undersurface of the clavicle to the first costal cartilage, the sternoclavicular ligament, passing from the upper border of the sternal end of the clavicle to the superior surface of the manubrium, and the subclavius muscle which originates at the costochondral junction of the first rib and inserts into the subclavian groove on the inferior surface of the clavicle. Clavicular motion may occur both in the horizontal plane and the frontal plane. In the former, motion is limited anteriorly by tension in the costoclavicular ligament and capsule and posteriorly by the costoclavicular and capsule. In the latter, motion is limited by tension in the costoclavicular ligament and subclavius muscle when the clavicle is raised and by tension in the superior capsule and by joint contact when the clavicle is lowered. Approximately 30° of axial rotation of the clavicle is permitted by laxity in the constraining ligaments.

The acromioclavicular joint

The acromioclavicular joint is a plane synovial joint between the flat lateral end of the clavicle and the acromion. Constraints to motion are supplied by the conoid and trapezoid ligaments which lie in planes approximately at right angles to each other. These run from the coracoid process of the scapula to the under-surface of the clavicle. The strong acromioclavicular ligament strengthens the joint capsule on its superior surface. Motion at the acromioclavicular joint comprises: (a) forward rotation of the clavicle relative to the scapula (opening the axial angle between the two bones), constrained by tension in the conoid ligament; (b) backward rotation of the clavicle, constrained by tension in the trapezoid ligament; (c) axial rotation of the clavicle, limited by tension in both ligaments.[1]

The scapulothoracic articulation

The articulation of the scapula with the thorax is not a true joint but a muscular linkage. The muscles affecting the movement of the scapula are broadly divided into two groups: axioscapular and scapulohumeral. Activity in the axioscapular muscles causes movement of the scapula relative to the chest wall. The scapula has three basic patterns of movement: protraction/retraction around the chest wall, rotation and elevation/depression.

The important movers of the scapula comprise the following.

1. The trapezius is a fan-like muscle, the upper and lower fibres of which, contracting in opposing directions on insertions at either end of the scapular spine, rotate the scapula in the plane of its blade, so that the glenoid points upwards.
2. The serratus anterior originates on the antero-lateral aspects of the middle ribs and inserts on the medial border of the internal surface of the scapula. Serratus draws the scapula forward around the chest wall, and stabilizes it during upper limb activity by fixing the medial border, preventing winging of the scapula.
3. The rhomboids and levator scapulae arise from the spinous processes of C7–T5 and posterior tubercles of C1–4 respectively. They insert as a continuous sheet down the medial border of the scapula and rotate the scapula so that the glenoid points downwards, opposing the action of the trapezius. Combined action of the trapezius and the rhomboids does not rotate but retracts the scapula around the chest wall, a concerted activity opposing the function of the serratus.

The constraints to scapular movement are its articulations with the clavicle and the humerus, and tension in the axioscapular and scapulo-humeral musculature. Abnormal scapular motion patterns have been implicated in shoulder instability and impingement. This illustrates the close relationship between scapular and humeral motion as problems with one may lead to pathology affecting the other.[2]

The glenohumeral joint

The glenohumeral joint is a synovial joint which is often described as a ball and socket joint, although the area of humeral head covered by the glenoid surface is relatively small. This surface is, however, deepened by a fibrocartilaginous glenoidal labrum. The joint capsule is attached to the scapula proximal to the supraglenoid tubercle (the origin of the long head of biceps) and around the labrum. Distally it is attached around the margins of the humeral articular surface except on the inferior aspect of the joint, where it attaches between 1 and 2 cm below the margin. The tendon of the long head of biceps lies suspended within a fold of synovium as it crosses the joint. The capsule is thickened on its anterior aspect by the superior, middle and inferior glenohumeral ligaments, the last being of considerable importance in joint stability at the extremes of motion.[3] Gaps in the capsule allow synovial continuity with the subscapularis bursa anterior and occasionally the infraspinatus bursa posterior to the joint.

Motion at the glenohumeral joint consists in the main of rotation in three dimensions. The humeral head does, however, glide a little across the surface of the glenoid during movement. This is thought to be accentuated in instability, and in abnormal conditions of the capsule such as tightening after surgery. Combined with scapulothoracic movement, glenohumeral movement gives the shoulder complex the largest range of motion of any joint in the body.

Constraints to glenohumeral movement comprise:

1. articular surface contact;
2. on the superior aspect, the joint capsule, the long head of biceps and the coracoacromial arch;
3. on the anterior aspect, the coracohumeral ligament and glenohumeral ligaments;
4. tension in the rotator cuff muscles around the anterior (infraspinatus), superior (supraspinatus) and posterior (infraspinatus and teres minor) aspects.

SCAPULOHUMERAL RHYTHM

One of the major definers of the way that the different articulations of the shoulder joint complex act together to produce a movement is the scapulohumeral rhythm: the combined motion at the scapulothoracic and glenohumeral articulations. It has long been recognized that the movements at the scapulothoracic and glenohumeral articulations are simultaneous throughout the arc of elevation, the scapulohumeral rhythm being created by the ratio of movement between the two.[4] Inman et al[5], in their classic treatise on the shoulder complex, described an initial 'setting phase' during the first 30–60° of elevation where the relationship between scapular and humeral motion was variable between individuals. Further elevation followed a ratio of 2:1 of glenohumeral to scapulothoracic motion. Poppen and Walker[6] described a ratio of 4:5 after the first 30° of abduction. More recent studies[7–9] using different techniques have produced results compatible with those of both authors, given the differences in methodology employed by each.

Most of the published work on scapulohumeral rhythm concentrates on that occurring during elevation in various planes; it seems likely that the rhythm will change according to the nature of upper limb activity. There is considerable evidence to the effect that the rhythm is altered in pathology affecting either articulation.

GLENOHUMERAL JOINT MECHANICS

Until relatively recently authors studying shoulder complex mechanics concentrated on the motion of the shoulder girdle as a whole, and little was known about the contribution of individual articulations. Codman in 1934 was one of the earliest authors to study shoulder complex motion in detail.[10] He described an interesting observation on the motion of the humerus during elevation, which he termed the 'pivotal paradox'. This was the discovery that the elevated humerus could apparently be proven to be both in internal and in external rotation, depending on the way that it was subsequently lowered. Thus a subject who flexes the elbow to 90° when the arm is fully elevated, so that the forearm is held over the head, then lowers the arm in the sagittal plane without attempting to rotate the humerus, finishes holding the forearm across the body and the humerus is said to be in internal rotation. If the elevated limb is lowered in the coronal plane, again without attempting to rotate the humerus, the forearm is found to be in full external rotation in the finishing position.

In 1944, Inman, Saunders and Abbott published an extensive study[5] on the function of the different aspects of shoulder girdle function. They separated out the different articulations for analysis, looking at each using comparative anatomy, kinematic X-ray analysis and electromyography. In addition to the findings on scapulohumeral rhythm, they also calculated the force requirements for positioning of the upper limb during motion. They concluded that the contact force at the glenohumeral joint reached a maximum of approximately 10.5 times the weight of the extremity at $90°$ of abduction. This was a two-dimensional study and the measurements on which the muscle directions of force were based were not quoted; however, it represented a considerable step forward in the knowledge of shoulder function at the time it was published.

In 1976, Poppen and Walker[6] looked at the kinematics of the glenohumeral joint, again using plain X-ray analysis and a two-dimensional study. They looked at the instant centre of rotation and the contact point of the humeral head on the glenoid. After studying 12 normal subjects and 16 patients with a variety of pathologies they concluded that the centre of rotation remains relatively constant in the normal subjects throughout movement and is located near to the geometric centre of the humeral head. The humeral head was found to glide upwards on the glenoid by about 3 mm during the first $30–60°$ of abduction. These measurements were later used in a kinetic study.[11] Muscle lines of action were calculated from X-rays of cadavers. Electromyographic studies were performed and muscle activity during an arc of motion was used along with cross-sectional area to estimate its relative power. The resultant force acting at the glenohumeral joint was calculated at $0.89 \times$ body weight at $90°$ of abduction. The authors noted that this was twice that calculated by Inman et al[5] (they assumed the weight of the upper limb to be 5.2% of body weight) and that it was explained by the assumption of Inman et al that the line of action of the depressor muscles was parallel to the lateral border of the scapula, whereas it was found in Poppen

and Walker's study to be almost perpendicular to the face of the glenoid. Shear forces were also calculated for the glenohumeral joint and found to peak at $0.42 \times$ body weight at $60°$ abduction.

Dvir and Berme in 1978 constructed a qualitative kinematic model to represent shoulder complex function during elevation.[12] They described the shoulder complex as a two-mechanism system, one of the mechanisms being the skeleton, clavicle and scapula and the other the scapula and humerus. This mechanism was said to act as an optimizing system whereby the movable links positioned the two mechanisms with respect to each other for each specified movement, and the individual mechanisms carried out that movement. This approach carried knowledge of shoulder girdle function forward in that available knowledge of individual parts of the shoulder girdle complex were used to look at the function of the articulation as a whole.

More recent approaches to the study of shoulder girdle function include the construction of further models,[7,13] in which accurate anatomical data regarding muscle origins and insertions and bony geometry were combined with motion studies using implanted tantalum balls and stereo X-rays to produce a biomechanical model. Others have used finite element analysis theory to model the complex.[14]

Although considerable advances have been made in our understanding of the mechanics of the shoulder girdle over the last 50 years, many pertinent clinical questions still remain unanswered. The study of shoulder complex biomechanics is still evolving.

In order to understand the rationale behind research in joint function some knowledge of kinematic description and force analysis is required.

KINEMATIC DESCRIPTORS

In studying the mechanics of any joint the researcher will find that calculation of joint kinematics (motion) and kinetics (forces) is much simpler in two dimensions. This becomes a particular problem with the shoulder joint complex as its motion is not even approximately constrained to a single plane. Thus, for any accurate analysis, a system must be found which describes accurately the motion of the body segments involved in three dimensions.

Most mathematical analyses of kinematics depend for their definition upon the assignment of an axis system particularly to the joint segments under study. For the glenohumeral joint these are the scapula and humerus. The axis system is usually a mutually perpendicular set of three axes (x, y and z) known as a Cartesian axis system. The co-ordinates of certain points on the segments with respect to their axis systems and to a global or laboratory Cartesian axis system form the base of standard motion analysis. Once the co-ordinates are known, there are a variety of ways to describe how one joint segment moves in relation to the opposing segment. For a joint that is not constrained to planar or purely rotational motion, the three-dimensional co-ordinates of at least three points on each segment are required.

The output of kinematic analysis generally takes the form of the magnitude and direction of translation and rotation of the distal segment with respect to the proximal. Translations in three-dimensional space are easily expressed in terms of simple vector algebra; rotations are much more difficult to describe. The surgeon will know that if a number of surgical procedures are available to treat the same condition, it is usually because they all have faults: the same may be said of systems for the description of joint rotation in three dimensions!

Euler/Cardan angles

Euler/Cardan angles describe the pathway through which a joint segment moves from one position to another in terms of three independent rotations, taken in order, about the axes of a selected Cartesian co-ordinate system. These angles are used to describe the attitude (orientation) of the second position with respect to the first. The term 'Euler angles' is used to describe the situation where the first and last axes about which the rotation takes place are the same (e.g. rotation

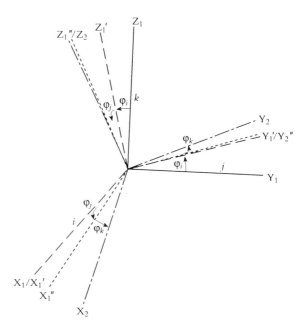

Fig. 3.1 Sequential rotations ϕ_i, ϕ_j and ϕ_k about the axes i, j and k from the starting Cartesian co-ordinate system x_1, y_1, z_1 to obtain the orientation of the finishing co-ordinate system x_2, y_2, z_2.

about x, y, x'). When all three axes are different the term 'Cardan angles' is used. Cardan angles are more frequently used in biomechanics, but some literature sources use the term Euler angles to describe both.

Figure 3.1 shows sequential rotations from the starting co-ordinate system to a finishing position. The problem faced by researchers using this system is that the order in which the rotations are taken is important: consider rolling a six-sided die (Figure 3.2). The die has three axes, through the 1–6 faces, the 2–5 faces and the 3–4 faces. Starting from position A, where face 1 faces you, roll the die clockwise once about the 1–6 axis, and once about the 2–5 axis. It finishes with the 3 facing. Now rotate clockwise about 2–5, then 1–6. Now the die finishes with the 2 facing. The researcher must select the sequence of rotation so that errors are minimized.

Although this may seem like a gross inaccuracy, the mathematics is reflecting conditions that do occur, especially in shoulder motion. The non-commutative nature of rotation sequences is one of the explanations of Codman's paradox.

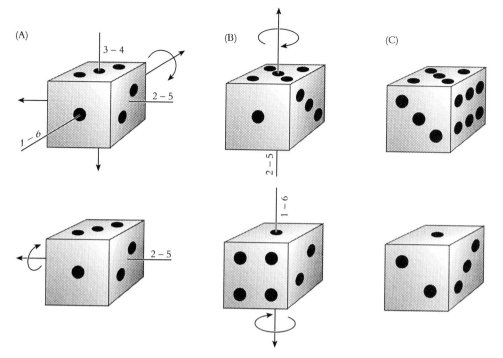

Fig. 3.2 Rotation sequences. (See text)

The joint co-ordinate system

The joint co-ordinate system is a development from Euler/Cardan angles. Rather than use an axis system for the laboratory and for each segment under study, the joint co-ordinate system describes a single co-ordinate system common to the two segments cither side of the joint, with axes e1, e2 and e3 where the e1 axis is 'embedded in' or related to the proximal segment, the e3 axis is embedded in the distal segment, and the e2 axis is derived from mathematical manipulation of the e1 and e3 axes such that it is perpendicular to the plane which they define. The e1 and e3 axes in this system are not necessarily perpendicular. There are two major advantages to this system: first, the sequence of rotations using the joint co-ordinate system is unimportant. This, however, is only because the results are different depending upon which axis of each segment is chosen to construct the joint co-ordinate system. Second, the rotations occurring about the axes of the joint co-ordinate system may be considered to be occurring truly in relation to the joint itself, rather

than in relation to the laboratory axis, or the coronal and sagittal planes of the body.

Unfortunately, in the study of the shoulder joint complex the joint co-ordinate system has one major defect. The calculation of the e2 axis is dependent upon vector multiplication, which is not commutative ($a \times b = -1(b \times a)$). When the rotation of the distal segment about the proximal exceeds 90°, the direction in which the e2 axis points reverses and the calculated rotation angle jumps through 180°. This is known as 'gimbal-lock'. The problems it creates can in part be circumvented by judicious choice of e1 and e3 axes and by using certain corrective techniques.[15]

Helical screw axis

This has developed from the two-dimensional concept of the centre of rotation of a joint. In three dimensions there can be no single point about which the segments move; in the gleno-humeral joint for example, the humeral head glides across the glenoid surface as rotation takes place. Thus movement in three dimensions, caught at a single moment in time, can be seen to be occurring about an axis rather than a point. As the segment rotates around the axis, it also travels along it. This helical movement parallels that of a screw thread, hence the helical screw axis.

The helical screw axis is the most accurate definer of joint motion available. The motion described is that of a single rigid body from one position to another. During an arc of movement the position and orientation of the axis will change, and the path followed by the axis completely defines the arc of movement. There are two main problems with screw axes: first, small inaccuracies in measurement tend to be magnified in the calculation, and for small movements the errors can be large. This can be minimized using various mathematical optimization techniques. Second, and perhaps more importantly, the screw axis does not lend itself easily to clinical interpretation, and is therefore of less use to the clinician.

KINETIC ANALYSIS

Having performed the kinematic analysis, the next step is to consider the kinetics, i.e. the forces acting across the joint. For simplicity here kinetic analysis will be considered only in two dimensions. Some knowledge of basic physics is necessary.

Force

What is a force? Newton's first law states that a body remains in a uniform state of motion (i.e. at rest) if acted upon by zero net external force. This introduces also the concept of equilibrium: that a single force does not act in isolation. Newton's third law also has a bearing on this, as will become apparent.

If the net external force is not zero then the body will move. In order to move from a standing position it must accelerate. Two factors combine to determine how great is the acceleration: the amount of force required (imagine pushing a car)

and the mass of the object to which the force is being applied (the car is full of people). Newton's second law states that the acceleration of a body is proportional to the (unbalanced) force acting upon it and inversely proportional to its mass. Simply, the acceleration produced may be calculated by dividing the force by the mass. The force necessary to produce an acceleration then is given by:

$$\text{Force} = \text{mass} \times \text{acceleration}.$$

Newton's third law is a little less obvious: for every action there is an equal and opposite reaction. This is also a proof of the first law: suppose you are trying to move a wardrobe by pushing it. If the wardrobe is very heavy it may be impossible for you to move. What do you feel? The sensation is as if the wardrobe is pushing back. In terms of the physics of force, it is.

Force is appropriately measured in Newtons (N). A Newton is the force required to accelerate a 1 kg object 1 m per second per second. Mass is measured in kg and acceleration in m per second per second (or $m\ s^{-2}$).

The following example illustrates how force can be calculated. Nigel is a tree surgeon who uses a sit harness while operating in high branches. If he is static while he works on the tree, and his body weight is 70 kg and he carries a chainsaw which weighs 15 kg, discounting the effects of the waist and chest loops, what is the force applied to the thighs by the harness (Figure 3.3)?

In order to solve this we need to construct a diagram of the forces involved. The mass of the body produces a downward force because of the effects of gravity, which wants to accelerate it downwards at $9.81\ m\ s^{-2}$. This force, according to Newton's second law, is $(70 + 15) \times 9.81 = 833.85$ N. Because Nigel is stationary this force must be countered by the tension in the rope to which the sit harness is applied in order to satisfy Newton's first and third laws. Thus the tension in the rope = 833.85 N and this is transmitted to Nigel via the thigh loops. The force therefore applied by each thigh loop is $833.85/2 = 416.925$ N.

Nigel is not a very clever tree surgeon. He applies his chainsaw to the branch to which his

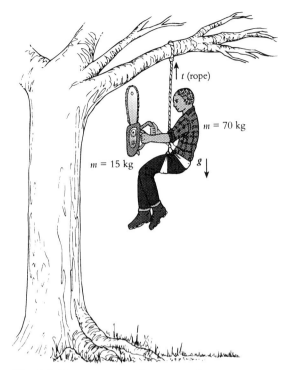

t (rope)

m = 70 kg

m = 15 kg

g

Fig. 3.3 Demonstrating the centre of mass concept.

rope is tied. On cutting through the branch he is no longer supported and starts to fall to the ground. This happens because the gravitational force trying to accelerate him downwards is no longer countered by an upwards force. He will accelerate towards the ground at $9.81 \, \mathrm{m \, s^{-2}}$ whatever he weighs.

Resolving forces

The forces we have been looking at are also vectors. A vector is an entity which has not only magnitude but also direction. It is obvious that we need to know in which direction a force is acting so that we can predict its effects. A box cannot be lifted by applying a force perpendicular to its side: the force must, at least in part, be directed upwards. The concept of force vectors also helps us to understand the effects when several forces are applied to a body.

Example. Imagine trying to move a wardrobe by pushing it. As you lean forwards to apply your weight to the wardrobe you will apply a force to

the wardrobe which is inclined upwards from the horizontal. What is the force acting to push the wardrobe horizontally?

This problem is solved using basic trigonometry (Figure 3.4). Construct a right-angled triangle where the length of the hypotenuse represents the force applied by your body (F) and the angle θ represents the angle between the direction of application of the force (i.e. the inclination of your body) and the floor. The horizontal force (hf) is represented by the length of the horizontal side of the triangle such that:

$$hf = F \cos \theta$$

This shows that the horizontal force is related to, but less than, the total force applied. The vertical component of the total force can also be calculated from the same triangle by $vf = F \sin \theta$. Thus a single force can be divided into two component forces at right angles to each other. Conversely, it is possible to resolve several forces in this way, by dividing each into forces at right angles to each other and then adding or subtracting forces.

Moments

Forces may be applied, not only to discrete objects, but to bodies which behave like levers, such as limb segments. Clearly if a body is constrained at one end by a hinge or a joint then it will turn rather than move to a different place when an unbalanced force is applied. The effect of a force on this type of body depends on where it is applied. The further from the turning point a force is applied, the smaller the force required to produce a given movement. A rusty nut is easier to turn with a long spanner than with a short one, or, as Archimedes more elegantly put it, 'give me a place to stand and I will move the world'. This turning effect is known as a moment. The moment is calculated from the product of the force applied and the perpendicular distance from the point of application of the force to the turning point. This distance is known as the lever arm. Moments are measured in Newton metres (Nm).

Note that the distance measured for the calculation of a moment should always be perpendicular. In the case of a force not applied

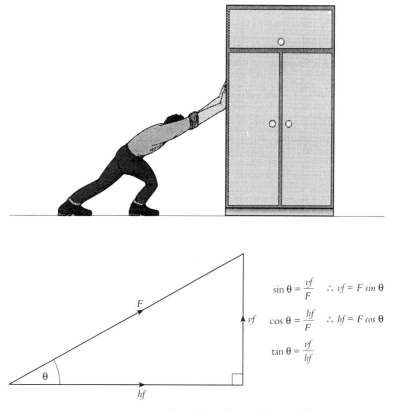

$$\sin \theta = \frac{vf}{F} \quad \therefore vf = F \sin \theta$$

$$\cos \theta = \frac{hf}{F} \quad \therefore hf = F \cos \theta$$

$$\tan \theta = \frac{vf}{hf}$$

Fig. 3.4 Concept of resolving forces. (See text)

perpendicularly, the component of the force which is acting perpendicular to the lever can be calculated using right-angled triangles, as described above.

Example. Joe Bloggs holds his elbow at right angles with the forearm parallel to the floor. He holds in his hand a 2 kg weight. If the distance from the centre of mass of the object to the centre of rotation of the elbow is 30 cm (Figure 3.5), and assuming the weight of the forearm to be zero, what is the moment being applied to the elbow?

Moment tending to extend the elbow = (2 × 9.81)★ × 0.3 = 5.886 Nm

(★N.B. force = mass × acceleration.)

If the elbow does not extend then it follows that this moment is resisted by contracting the elbow flexors.

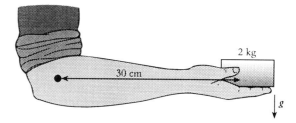

Fig. 3.5 Concepts of moment. (See text)

One or two more concepts need to be understood before we can calculate joint forces.

Centre of mass

The positions of the centre of mass of a limb segment or of a human body, representing the point of application of a force, is necessary to estimate the effects of gravitational forces and to calculate moments at joints. Centre of mass of limb segments can be calculated indirectly by a variety of means; a review of methods and estimates of limb segment parameters were made by Contini and Drillis and co-workers[16,17] studying young fit subjects at New York University. These limb segment estimations will be used in this chapter. Figure 3.6 illustrates the centre of mass concept. Centres of mass may change their position if a segment changes shape: for example, when standing in the anatomical position, the centre of mass of the human body is located roughly in front of the spinal column at the level of S2. However, if sitting with the arms and legs stretched out in front of the body, the centre of mass will be found somewhere outside the body.

The free body diagram

When calculating the effects of forces on a limb segment, it is necessary to separate out that segment in order to make the analysis possible. The segment of interest (the limb segment distal to the joint under study) is drawn, along with its centre of mass and all forces acting upon it. This is known as a free body diagram. The important thing about the free body diagram is that the body in question is assumed to be in equilibrium: this means that all of the forces and all the moments acting upon it are assumed to add up to zero. When using a free body diagram it simplifies calculations to resolve forces into horizontal and vertical components and summate all of these forces.

Example. An orthopaedic house officer of height 1.6 m and weight 60 kg stands upright with her elbow flexed to 40°. In her hand she holds a 5 kg traction weight. Assuming the humerus to be vertical and the only elbow flexor to be biceps which is inserted 5 cm from the elbow joint centre and acts parallel to the humerus, what is the tension generated in the biceps? The mass, length and centre of mass of the forearm calculated from the data of Contini and Drillis are 1.44 kg, 40.64 cm and 17.07 cm from the elbow joint respectively (Figure 3.7). First calculate the forces acting at the centre of mass.

$$A = 1.44 \times 9.81 \quad \text{(mass} \quad \times \quad \text{acceleration)} \quad = \quad 14.13 \text{ N}$$

$$B = 5 \times 9.81 = 49.05 \text{ N}.$$

These two forces will be counteracted, for equilibrium, by the tension in the biceps. The forces act on the elbow as moments. In order to calculate these, the perpendicular distance of each force from the elbow centre needs to be calculated. This is done using right-angled triangles (Figure 3.7). Force A acts 17.07 cm from the elbow centre and the forearm is flexed to 40°. Thus a right-angled triangle can be constructed with a hypotenuse of

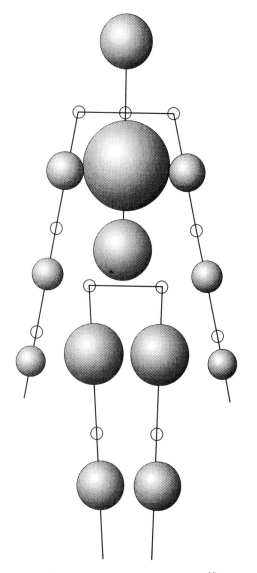

Fig. 3.6 Centre of mass diagram.[18]

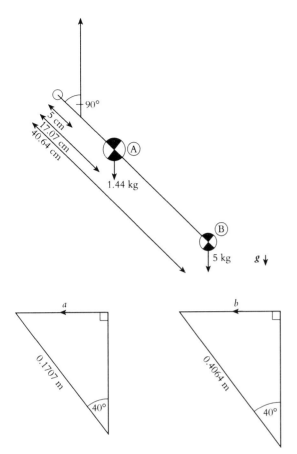

Fig. 3.7 $a=$ perpendicular distance of force A from elbow centre. $b=$ perpendicular distance of force B from elbow centre.

17.07 cm. The distance to be calculated is the side of the triangle opposite the $40°$ angle. Thus the distance is:

$$0.1707 \sin 40° = 0.1097 \text{ m or } 10.97 \text{ cm}$$

Similarly, the perpendicular distance of force B from the elbow centre is given by $0.4064 \sin 40° = 0.2612$ m or 26.12 cm.

The moments tending to extend the elbow may be summated:

$$\text{Moment } A = 14.13 \times 0.1097 = 1.55 \text{ Nm}$$

$$\text{Moment } B = 49.05 \times 0.2612 = 12.81 \text{ Nm}$$

$$A + B = 14.36 \text{ Nm}.$$

These will be counteracted by the moment generated by tension in the biceps acting at $40°$

to the forearm. To calculate the perpendicular force, divide by the distance from the elbow centre in metres: $14.36/0.05 = 287.2$ N. If this is the perpendicular force then the tension in the biceps is calculated by constructing a right-angled triangle of side 287.20 and opposite angle $40°$. The force generated by the biceps is the hypotenuse of this triangle and is calculated by $287.20 \sin 40° = 446.80$ N.

To recap, the concepts so far discussed have been: force, Newton's laws of motion, vectors, moment, mass and centre of mass, the free body diagram. Using this it should be possible to make a simple calculation of joint forces.

CALCULATION OF JOINT FORCES

For the purpose of orthopaedic practice, it would be advantageous to be able to predict where the largest contact forces will be felt, and the direction of their action, given basic information regarding the structure of an individual's joint. An understanding of basic mechanical principles can be allied to a knowledge of the structures involved in calculating approximate forces acting across the glenohumeral joint.

Let us use as an example a patient attempting the power component of the Constant–Murley shoulder assessment. This is defined as the ability to resist a downwards pull of 25 kg with the shoulder at $90°$ of abduction and the elbow straight.[19] The patient is a man of height 1.8 m and weight 85 kg. Assume that the teres minor/pectoralis group of muscles are inactive, and the inferior glenohumeral ligament, passing from approximately the centre of the anterior aspect of the glenoid to the inferior margin of the humeral articular surface, is not acting to stabilize the joint and is therefore not under tension. The deltoid is inserted 8.8 cm from the joint centre and acts at $10°$ to the long axis of the humerus in this position. The rotator cuff, if active, has a combined line of action passing through the centre of rotation of the joint which is located at the geometric centre of the humeral head. Owing to scapular rotation in elevation the glenoid faces $30°$

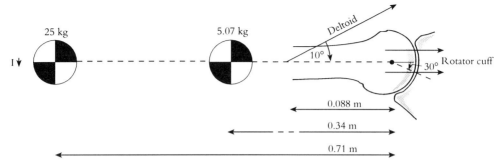

Fig. 3.8 Resultant forces in deltoid in the loaded arm.

upwards (Figure 3.8). From Drillis and Contini, the length of the upper limb is 0.79 m, the centre of mass is 0.34 m from the centre of rotation of the shoulder and the mass of the limb is 5.07 kg. Assume the tips of the fingers are 8 cm from the centre of hand grip.

1. Moments tending to pull the humerus down: 25 kg mass acting at 0.71 m from the centre of the shoulder centre (half of the length of the hand has been subtracted from the limb length to allow for grip):

$$(25 \times 9.81) \times 0.71 = 174 \text{ Nm}$$

Mass of upper limb with centre at 34 cm from the shoulder centre:

$$(5.07 \times 9.81) \times 0.34 = 16.91 \text{ Nm}$$

Total moment producing downwards rotation of humerus $= 174 + 16.91 = 190.91$ Nm.

2. Moments tending to pull the humerus up: Action of the deltoid (d) at 10° to the humerus produces an upwards force of $d \sin 10°$ acting at 8.8 cm from the joint centre:

$$d \times 0.1736 \times 0.088 = 0.01528d \text{ Nm}$$

The deltoid and rotator cuff forces in line with the joint do not tend to move the humerus either up or down but are important when it comes to calculation of joint forces. Assume equilibrium: moments up = moments down:

$$190.91 = 0.01528d$$

Therefore tension in the deltoid $= 12\,494.11$ N.

Given that this is acting upwards, it tends to pull the humeral head upwards on the glenoid. The resultant force points 10° upwards from the geometric centre of the humeral head. Given that the glenoid covers a relatively small area of the humeral head it is possible that this resultant force does not pass through the glenoid articular surface. In order to know if the joint is stable in this position we have to work out the cover of the humeral head (Figure 3.9). From Iannotti et al[20] we know that the mean dimension of the glenoid in the coronal plane is 39 ± 3.5 mm and the mean radius of curvature of the humeral head in the coronal plane is 24 ± 2.1 mm. Measured from the geometric centre of the humeral head the angle θ between the centre of the glenoid and its edge is

$$\theta = \tan^{-1}\left(\frac{1.95}{2.4}\right) = 39.09°.$$

If the glenoid is angled upwards by 30° then the angle between the horizontal and the glenoid edge in this example is 9.09°. Therefore the resultant force at the shoulder joint, acting at 10°

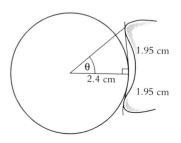

Fig. 3.9 Cover for the humeral head in neutral.

to the horizontal, renders the joint unstable unless the rotator cuff is active. The force generated by the rotator cuff must be sufficient to move the resultant force downwards by at least $0.91°$. This is solved by constructing two right-angled triangles of which the small angles are $10°$ and $9.09°$ respectively. We know that the only upwards force is provided by the deltoid. From the first triangle, given that the tension in the deltoid is 12 494.11 N and the angle of action $10°$ from the horizontal, the vertical force is 12 494.11 sin $10°$ = 2169.58 N. The horizontal force of deltoid is 12 494.11 cos $10°$ = 12 304.30 N. From the second triangle the vertical force remains the same. The horizontal force is calculated by:

$$\left(\frac{2169.58}{\tan 9.09°}\right) = 13\,560.03 \text{ N}$$

This force represents the horizontal component of the deltoid force plus the rotator cuff force. Thus the rotator cuff force = 13 560.03 − 12 304.30 = 1255.73 N.

This brings the resultant force to the edge of the glenoid. It is likely that a greater force would be necessary to render the joint fully stable.

The total joint force (*tjf*) is the hypotenuse of this second triangle, calculated by Pythagoras:

$$tjf = \sqrt{(2169.58^2 + 13\,560.03^2)} = 13\,732.50 \text{ N}$$

acting at the superior edge of the glenoid.

Problems with calculation of mechanics

You will see from the above problem that the calculation of joint forces is not easy, even in two dimensions, and involves making many assumptions. Without making assumptions, the calculation would be impossible, as the algorithms would contain more unknowns than equations, a problem known as indeterminacy. This is the rationale behind constructing complex models of the joint: areas of indeterminacy can be solved.

BIOMECHANICS IN DISEASE

This is the area of particular interest to the orthopaedic surgeon. Knowledge of the me-

chanics of the joint may help us to understand the changes occurring in disease and consequently to influence these changes with surgical intervention.

It will be seen from the previous calculations that the anatomical structures governing movement and joint forces at the glenohumeral interface are in balance, and that a disease process is likely to change this balance, resulting in abnormal function of the joint. It is clear that function is significantly deranged in shoulder pathologies and the pathology may drive the abnormal pattern of motion and force transmission by virtue of destruction of the joint surfaces themselves or by destruction of the constraints. Following on from this, changes occurring as a result of surgery should ideally correct or compensate for abnormality by restoring the joint mechanics. Knowledge of the best ways of restoring normal mechanics should dictate the optimum design of prostheses and methods of surgical implantation. Unfortunately, although a great deal is known, the picture is far from complete.

NORMAL AND ABNORMAL KINEMATICS OF THE SHOULDER JOINT COMPLEX

Before it is possible to calculate joint forces it is necessary to plot the positions attained by the different limb segments during motion, so that moment arms and muscle lines of force can be calculated. In some joints this is relatively easy, as they have an essentially uniplanar movement (for example, knee and elbow). In the shoulder complex this becomes very difficult indeed, as the potential positions obtained by the humerus with respect to the glenoid are numerous, and there is no 'typical' motion of the upper limb which can be studied. This contrasts with the lower limb for which gait is the obvious choice. This problem has been addressed by some who have studied the kinematics (motion) at the shoulder using different activities of daily living as a reference.

Pearl and co-workers[21] looked at the relative positions of the humerus and thorax in nine normal subjects in activities of daily living using a magnetic tracking sensor (Polhemus[TM]). They recorded a maximal elevation of $148 \pm 11°$. An elevation of $112 \pm 10°$ was necessary for combing hair, and the total arc of rotation about the body was approximately $190°$ from the perineum ($-86°$) to the opposite axilla ($104°$). Generally it was found that important functional movements such as eating and hair-combing occurred in a plane approximately $60°$ anterior to the coronal plane ($+30°$ plane) with $33°$ of humeral internal rotation; interestingly this approximated to the plane of maximal elevation. Figures for patients with shoulder complex pathologies are given by some authors looking at the results of arthroplasty. Fenlin et al[22] quote maximal forward elevation (maximal elevation in the $0°$ plane according to Pearl et al) of mean $107°$ for patients with osteoarthritis and $90.6°$ for those with rheumatoid arthritis. Mean internal and external humeral rotation (IR and ER respectively) for these two groups respectively were IR to L5, IR to L4, ER $23.5°$ and $33.0°$. Pollock et al[23] recorded pre-operative movement in 26 shoulders of patients with rotator cuff deficiency. The mean values were $67°$ for active forward elevation (in the plane of the scapula or the $+45–60°$ plane according to Pearl et al[21]), $109°$ passive elevation, $24°$ external rotation. Internal rotation was said to be severely limited but the values were not recorded. It is unfortunate that, as yet, there is no literature describing scapulohumeral motion (as opposed to thoracohumeral motion) in subjects with pathology. It is therefore difficult to infer anything about the mechanics of the complex in pathology from these published data. Attempts have been made to ascertain more clearly how the different segments involved in shoulder motion move in disease.[24]

Joint function in instability

Glenohumeral joint instability does not have one but several patterns: important factors in biomechanics include the degree to which capsular laxity and increased humeral head glide contribute to dislocation, and the effects of abnormal mechanics on joint structure (increased incidence of arthropathy after stabilization).

A number of studies have been performed which look at the changing relationships at the joint surface with pathology. Poppen and Walker[6] used two-dimensional radiography to look at the motion of the scapula and humerus in normal and pathological individuals. Of the pathological subjects only two had instability; these showed a significant shift in the instant centre of rotation and a reduced ratio of glenohumeral to scapulothoracic motion. Ozaki[25], using a similar technique in subjects with multidirectional instability, again found that scapular motion was abnormal, with decreased scapular elevation and protraction, and that the humeral head showed progressive translation during elevation. As these were two-dimensional studies, the true direction of glide could not be ascertained. Similar studies performed using a similar technique in the horizontal plane[26,27] indicated that anterior glide of the humeral head occurred during arm movement in patients with anterior instability. As elsewhere noted, there are difficulties in making accurate inferences for these data, given that different movements were being studied in two dimensions in patients with different pathologies. The precise pattern of humeral head glide related to joint laxity or instability is yet to be elucidated. Lippitt and Matsen,[3] in a theoretical review of the mechanisms of instability, noted that the effective depth of the glenoid is an important factor in limiting humeral head glide, and concluded that damage to the structural constraints to glide (glenoid articular surface and labrum) decreased stability. They believe that damage to the capsule and ligaments are of lesser importance, these constraints to movement being active only at the extremes of range. They also described 'scapulo-humeral balance' the mechanism whereby motion of the scapula acts to position the glenohumeral joint such that the resultant force of activity is directed into the glenoid. This corroborates the finding that imbalance of muscular function is a primary factor in multidirectional instability.

Joint function in rotator cuff dysfunction

The rotator cuff muscles are known to be active in elevation and rotation of the humerus, and to act by centring the humeral head in the glenoid during movement. The precise function of each muscle, however, is less well defined. Electromyographic studies have been performed by several authors, but the results are variable. This group of muscles is a difficult one to assess electromyographically because of the atypical shape of the muscles and the problems attending needle placement. It would appear from *in vitro* mechanical studies that all are involved in elevation, particularly in its early stages, and the infraspinatus and teres minor may be able to compensate for the loss of supraspinatus.[9] Otis et al[28] looked at the changes in the moment arms of the muscles acting around the shoulder and again found that the infraspinatus and subscapularis may contribute to elevation as well as to rotation of the humerus, concluding that dysfunction of the supraspinatus need not preclude good elevation.

If the rotator cuff is important in centring the humeral head on the glenoid during movement, it follows that, if the cuff is incomplete, motion at the glenohumeral joint is likely to be abnormal. Poppen and Walker,[6] looking at the shift of the centre of rotation of the humerus during elevation, found a variety of different patterns of motion, with some subjects having a marked shift in the centre of rotation or humeral glide, and a number with results comparable with the normal. The range of elevation in all of these abnormal shoulders was reduced and the inconclusive nature of these results may be attributed to variations in the pattern of cuff damage, which were not stated in the paper. Leroux et al[29] used the Elite motion analysis system to look at the displacement of the centre of rotation during abduction and found that it was abnormal in patients with capsulitis and with cuff tears, and that it was not possible to differentiate between the two simply by looking at the motion analysis results. After rehabilitation of the patients with cuff tears, however, their results became comparable with the normal. These results are compatible with the belief that loss of the supraspinatus can be compensated for.

Biomechanics of arthroplasty

We have looked so far at the alterations in kinematics which have been recorded in certain shoulder pathologies. One area of particular interest to the orthopaedic surgeon is the behaviour of the glenohumeral joint before and after hemiarthroplasty or total joint replacement for degenerative or rheumatoid arthritis. The issues of current interest are the question of whether a total joint replacement or hemiarthroplasty is the treatment of choice in patients with abnormal rotator cuff function or significant bone loss, and the design of the joint components themselves.

Total or hemiarthroplasty?

It is accepted by some that total shoulder arthroplasty in patients with large defects in the rotator cuff with upward migration of the humeral head is associated with early loosening of the glenoid component. Franklin et al[30] performed a retrospective review of 50 cases of total shoulder arthroplasty carried out over 10 years, with average follow–up of 2–6 years. They identified seven cases where the glenoid was significantly loose after 1–4 years. In all of these cases a large rotator cuff tear was found. They hypothesized that upward migration of the humeral head in the presence of a large rotator cuff tear was responsible for the loosening by eccentrically loading the glenoid, causing it to tip upwards, an appearance they termed 'rocking-horse glenoid'. Boyd et al[31] in a similar, more extensive study, failed to find an association between rotator cuff tear and glenoid loosening, and concluded that total shoulder replacement was the procedure of choice in all cases where there was sufficient bone stock to support a glenoid component, unless the condition requiring the arthroplasty was not associated with any structural abnormality of the glenoid, in which case hemiarthroplasty was recommended. They made the relevant point that the presence or absence of part of the rotator cuff does not necessarily lead to abnormal function of the joint. This being the case, it is difficult to make clear predictions regarding the contraindication of total joint replacement, certainly without much larger numbers. Many recently published studies on results after arthroplasty illustrate this point, with inadequate numbers or length of follow-up to justify the authors' recommendations.

Joint component design

There was a gap of 60 years between the first recorded shoulder replacement (in 1893) and Neer's description of the prosthesis which made routine shoulder arthroplasty a viable proposition. Neer's original design was an unconstrained hemiarthroplasty. He continued to use this throughout the 1960s, while other authors were experimenting with types of constrained arthroplasty. Many of these were later abandoned because of problems with early loosening. In the early 1970s the original Neer design was improved with the addition of a glenoid component. It is currently used as the basis for newer designs which differ in various ways. The congruency of the glenoid and the humeral head has been altered in some; others are modular to allow for changes in the humeral head offset, theoretically to improve range of motion by altering the joint axis of rotation. Such is the nature of research into joint replacement survivorship that, as yet, there are no long-term results, the best available having shorter than 10 years' follow-up. Joint designers must still use their theoretical knowledge of glenohumeral mechanics and the research literature to guide them. Issues of current importance include the relative radii of curvature of the glenoid and humeral components, and the shape of the glenoid keel.

Radii of curvature of the glenoid and humeral head in prosthetic shoulders

The importance of humeral head glide to shoulder motion has been mentioned earlier. It has been postulated that this may be a contributing factor to loosening of the glenoid component in total shoulder arthroplasty. It is thought that excessive pressure occurs towards the edge of the glenoid at extremes of motion due to physiological humeral head glide. Further, in patients with

significant bone loss or irreparable rotator cuff tear, glide is expected to increase, exacerbating the problem. This problem has been addressed in some cases by alteration in the design of the shoulder joint prosthesis to render the two components slightly incongruent, with a greater radius of curvature in the glenoid than the humeral component. The effects of this have been investigated by Severt and co-workers.[32] They studied a variety of prostheses with different characteristics regarding constraint (degree of humeral head cover provided by the glenoid) and conformity (ratio of radii of curvature of the two components). Forces acting on the humeral head during translation across the glenoid component were measured. It was found that the more constrained and more conforming prostheses developed greater forces during humeral head translation. The same group[33] extended this concept in a cadaveric model using a purely kinematic assessment. Similar degrees of translation were found to occur with conforming and non-conforming prostheses, implying that greater forces would be applied at the periphery of the glenoid component in the conforming prosthesis.

The conclusions that may be drawn from these findings are that, even in shoulders that are anatomically intact after arthroplasty, humeral head glide may cause increased loading at the periphery of the glenoid component in completely congruent prostheses. In the shoulder with glenoid bone loss or irreparable rotator cuff tear, this increased loading is likely to be so great as to jeopardize the fixation of the glenoid component.

Design of the glenoid keel

Apart from the radius of curvature, the glenoid component is of interest biomechanically in terms of its fixation to the scapula. The limited bone stock of the scapula makes keel design difficult. Should loosening occur and revision be required, the bone stock is further depleted. It is therefore in the designer's interest to consider carefully the possibility of component loosening and failure.

A number of different keel designs are available. The classic Neer design has a triangular or trapezoidal shape, whereas others have opted for implantation with screws. The different types have been tested with regard to both pull-out strength and resistance to shear forces.[34] They found that stability was increased by increasing glenoid curvature and careful placement of the component relative to the humeral head. They also noted that pull-out strength of the screw-insert designs were significantly higher. Friedman et al[35] performed finite element analysis of different keel designs and found that stair-stepped and wedged glenoid keels provided a more physiological stress distribution than screw-insert designs. Clearly further studies, supported by clinical results for survivorship, would be desirable if design is to be further advanced.

SUMMARY

A knowledge of the mechanics of the shoulder joint complex is valuable to the surgeon, that he or she may understand how the joint behaves in disease, and how abnormalities may be corrected. However, as yet the mechanics of the shoulder joint complex are incompletely understood. Much has been discovered in recent years but this is an area where many discoveries are yet to be made. Further biomechanical research may help to elucidate factors governing the stability of the joint and the changes in function with disease, but these need to be allied to clinical studies before the complete picture can be drawn. Areas where further research would be particularly valuable to the surgeon include a fuller understanding of the roll-and-glide mechanism and the optimum position for the axis of rotation of the joint in three dimensions. Long-term follow-up after arthroplasty, both in terms of function and failure, and with particular reference to the geometry of the components, would be invaluable. A study of the mechanics of the shoulder joint complex provides more questions than answers, and these can only be addressed by correlating existing knowledge with clinical assessment of outcomes.

REFERENCES

1. Kapandji, I.A. (1970) *The Physiology of the Joints*. Edinburgh: E&S Livingsone.
2. Warner, J.J.P., Micheli, L.J., Arslanian, L.E., Kennedy, J. & Kennedy, R. (1992) Scapulothoracic motion in normal shoulders and shoulders with glenohumeral instability and impingement syndrome. *Clin. Orthop. Rel. Res.* **285:** 191–199.
3. Lippitt, S. & Matsen, F. (1993) Mechanisms of glenohumeral joint stability. *Clin. Orthop. Rel. Res.* **291:** 20–27.
4. Cathcart, C.W. (1884) Movements of the shoulder girdle involved in those of the arm on the trunk. *J. Anat. Physiol.* **18:** 210–218.
5. Inman, V.T., Saunders, J.B.D.M. & Abbott, L.C. (1944) Observations on the function of the shoulder joint. *J. Bone Joint Surg.* **26:** 1–30.
6. Poppen, N.K. & Walker, P.S. (1976) Normal and abnormal motion of the shoulder. *J. Bone Joint Surg.* **58A:** 165–170.
7. Hogfors, C., Peterson, B., Sigholm, G. & Herberts, P. (1991) Biomechanical model of the human shoulder – II. The shoulder rhythm. *J. Biomech.* **24:** 699–709.
8. Johnson, G.R., Fyfe, N.C.M. & Heward, M. (1991) Ranges of movement at the shoulder complex using an electromagnetic movement sensor. *Ann. Rheum. Dis.* **50:** 824–827.
9. Sharkey, N.A., Marder, R.A. & Hanson, P.B. (1994) The entire rotator cuff contributes to the elevation of the arm. *J. Orthop. Res.* **12:** 699.
10. Codman, E. (1934) *The Shoulder*. Malaba, FL: Robert E. Kreiger.
11. Poppen, N.K. & Walker, P.S. (1978) Forces at the glenohumeral joint in abduction. *Clin. Orthop. Rel. Res.* **135:** 165–170.
12. Dvir, Z. & Berme, N. (1978) The shoulder complex in elevation of the arm: a mechanism approach. *J. Biomech.* **11:** 219–225.
13. Hogfors, C., Sigholm, G. & Herberts, P. (1987) Biomechanical model of the human shoulder – I. Elements. *J. Biomech.* **20:** 157–166.
14. Van der Helm, F.C.T. (1994) A finite element musculoskeletal model of the shoulder mechanism. *J. Biomech.* **27:** 551–569.
15. Cole, G.K., Nigg, B.M., Ronsky, J.L. & Yeadon, M.R. (1983) Application of the joint co-ordinate system to three-dimensional joint attitude and movement representation: a standardisation proposal. *J. Biomech. Eng.* **115:** 344–349.
16. Drillis, R., Contini, R. & Bluestein, M. (1964) Body Segment Parameters. A survey of measurement techniques. *Artificial Limbs* **8:** 44.
17. Contini, R. (1972) Body Segment Parameters, Part II. *Artificial Limbs* **16:** 1.

18. Harless, J. (1860) The static moments of human limbs. In *Treatises of the Royal Academic Society of Bavaria*, vol. 8, pp. 69–96, 257–294.

19. Constant, C.R. & Murley, A.H.G. (1987) A clinical method of functional assessment of the shoulder. *Clin. Orthop. Rel. Res.* **214:** 160–164.

20. Iannotti, J.P., Gabriel, J.P., Schneck, S.L., Evans, B.G. & Misra, S. (1992) The normal glenohumeral relationships. *J. Bone Joint Surg.* **74A:** 491–499.

21. Pearl, M.L., Harris, S.L., Lippitt, S.B., Sidles, J.L., Harryman, D.T. & Matsen, F.A. (1992) A system for describing positions of the humerus relative to the thorax and its use in the presentation of several functionally important arm positions. *J. Shoulder Elbow Surg.* **1:** 113–118.

22. Fenlin, J., Ramsey, M.L., Allardyce, T.J. and Frieman, B.G. (1994) Modular total shoulder replacement: Design rationale, indications, and results. *Clin. Orthop. Rel. Res.* **307:** 37.

23. Pollock, R., Deliz, E.D., McIlveen, S.J., Flatow, E.L. & Bigliani, L.U. (1992) Prosthetic replacement in rotator cuff-deficient shoulders. *J. Shoulder Elbow Surg.* **1:** 173.

24. Conboy, V.B., Williams, J.R. & Carr, A.J. (1996) Motion analysis of the upper limb: application of the joint co-ordinate system. *J. Bone Joint Surg. B* (Suppl.) In Press.

25. Ozaki, J. (1989) Glenohumeral movements of the involuntary inferior and multidirectional instability. *Clin. Orthop. Rel. Res.* **238:** 107.

26. Howell, S.M., Galinat, B.J., Renzi, A.J. & Marone, P.J. (1988) Normal and abnormal mechanics of the glenohumeral joint in the horizontal plane. *J. Bone Joint Surg.* **70A:** 227–232.

27. Howell, S.M. & Kraft, T.A. (1991) The role of the supraspinatus and infraspinatus muscles in glenohumeral kinematics of anterior shoulder instability. *Clin. Orthop. Rel. Res.* **263:** 128–134.

28. Otis, J.C., Wickiewicz, T.L., Peterson, M.E., Warren, R.F. & Santner, T.J. (1994) Changes in the moment arms of the rotator cuff and deltoid muscles with abduction and rotation. *J. Bone Joint Surg.* **76A:** 667.

29. Leroux, J.L., Micallef, J.P., Bonnel, F. & Blotman, F. (1992) Rotation-abduction analysis in 10 normal and 20 pathologic shoulders. Elite system application. *Surg. Radiol. Anat.* **14:** 307–313.

30. Franklin, J.L., Barrett, W.P., Jackins, S.E. & Matsen, F.A. (1988) Glenoid loosening in total shoulder arthroplasty: Association with rotator cuff deficiency. *J. Arthroplasty* **3:** 39–46.

31. Boyd, A.D., Thomas, W.H., Scott, R.D., Sledge, C.B. & Thornhill, T.S. (1990) Total shoulder arthroplasty versus hemiarthroplasty: indications for glenoid resurfacing. *J. Arthroplasty* **5:** 329–336.

32. Severt, R., Tsenter, M.J., Amstutz, H.C. & Kabo, J.M. (1993) The influence of conformity and constraint on translational forces and frictional torque in total shoulder arthroplasty. *Clin. Orthop. Rel. Res.* **292:** 151.

33. Harryman, D.T., Sidles, J.A., Harris, S.L., Lippitt, S.B. & Matsen, F.A. (1995) The effect of articular conformity and the size of the humeral head component on laxity and motion after glenohumeral arthroplasty. *J. Bone Joint Surg.* **77A:** 556–563.

34. Fukuda, K., Chen, C.-M., Cofield, R.H. & Chao, E.Y.S. (1988) Biomechanical analysis of stability and fixation strength of total shoulder prostheses. *Orthopedics* **11:** 141–149.

35. Friedman, R., LaBerge, M., Dooley, R.L. & O'Hara, A.L. (1992) Finite element modeling of the glenoid component: effect of design parameters on stress distribution. *J. Shoulder Elbow Surg.* **1:** 261.

4

Imaging

MJ Simmons

This chapter restricts itself to discussing the role of imaging the shoulder joint in two clinical areas: shoulder pain; the unstable shoulder. There is overlap of these two areas.

The expansion of imaging techniques has undoubtedly been contributory to the understanding of shoulder pathology over the past decade.

THE PAINFUL SHOULDER

This is probably the third most common complaint in general practice, and to many non-specialists there is difficulty in locating the pain, as evidenced by the number of requests for 'cervical spine and shoulder and acromioclavicular X-rays'.

The imaging methods include plain X-rays, ultrasound, arthrography, computerized tomography (CT), with or without arthrography, and magnetic resonance imaging (MRI), with or without contrast material injected intra-articularly. This section assumes that tumours and infection are not under consideration.

Plain X-rays

These are mandatory and frequently very informative. Calcification in the rotator cuff may be the end result of disease – a visual gravestone – but one-third to a half of these patients will have signs of impingement. Softer calcification may be associated with acute pain. It can disappear if it ruptures into the glenohumeral joint or subacromial bursa, or if it becomes infected during steroid injection treatment; it is important to

appreciate calcification before arthrography or MRI where recognition is difficult.

The axial view is essential. One-fifth of significant pathology is shown only on this view.

The diagnosis of impingement is essentially clinical. However, there are plain film signs so that radiologists can suggest the diagnosis to those less familiar with it.[1]

1. Two-thirds of patients will have bony spurs on the undersurface of the acromion.
2. Two-thirds will have osteoarthritis of the acromioclavicular joint of which half will have inferior osteophytes that compromise the supraspinatus outlet.
3. Two-thirds will have sclerosis of the greater tuberosity, due to failure of teres minor and subscapularis to depress the humeral head below the coracoacromial arch.
4. A quarter or less will have calcific lines in the tendon of supraspinatus.
5. The supraspinatus outlet can be assessed using outlet views. The shape and angle can be measured. In general, the more horizontal and more hooked acromia have a higher incidence of impingement.
6. Other X-ray clues include failure of fusion of the acromial ossification centres – the os acromiale. Movement at this fibrous union may allow impingement.[2] Post-traumatic ossification of the coracoclavicular ligaments and coracoacromial ligaments are also associated with impingement. Examination of the acromioclavicular joint will exclude post-traumatic or stress osteolysis of the lateral end of the clavicle.

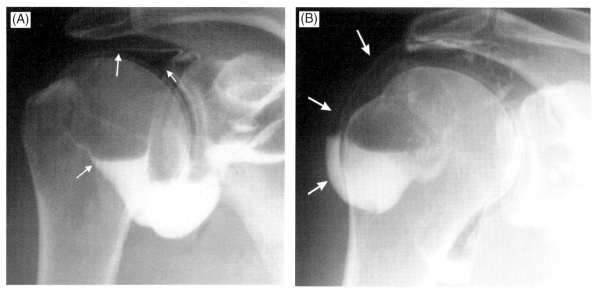

Fig. 4.1 (A) Normal arthrogram. Contrast and air outline superior joint space on undersurface of cuff (medium sized arrows). No contrast is seen between this and the acromion. Lateral limits of joint are around humeral neck (large arrow). Intra-articular part of the long head of biceps is shown (small arrow). (B) Full-thickness cuff tear. Contrast and air in subdeltoid bursa (arrows). The portion of supraspinatus that is not torn can be seen. It is not retracted.

There are also clues as to the integrity of the rotator cuff.

1. Degeneration can be inferred from saucer-like depressions giving ring areas of sclerosis around the insertion of the cuff.
2. Half the patients with subacromial spurs will have a full-thickness tear at the time of presentation.
3. Reduction of the humeral acromion distance to below 7 mm is a very strong indicator of a full-thickness tear. The 4% that progress to 'cuff tear arthropathy' have instability, atrophy of the glenohumeral cartilage, osteoporosis and finally collapse of the humeral head.

Double-contrast arthrography

This is a simple and cost-effective method of determining the presence and size of a full-thickness tear. In a normal arthrogram the contrast will not pass beyond the confines of the capsule. None is seen above the joint line over the humeral head. The long head of biceps can be seen as it runs through the bicipital groove to the superior labrum. When there is a full-thickness tear, air

and contrast enter the subacromial/subdeltoid bursa (Figure 4.1). The amount in the bursa reflects the degree of inflammation of the bursa not the size of the tear. Obtaining tomograms in the erect position either anteroposterior (AP) or lateral will give a good estimation of the size of the tear and the state of the cuff (Figure 4.2).[3] Most series achieve accuracies of about 90%[4] and many would say that certainly for the older population this may still be a satisfactory examination.

Partial-thickness tears will only show as contrast within the tear if the tear is on the undersurface of the cuff. Bursal surface tears will not show. The other downside to arthrography is the increase in shoulder discomfort for a couple of days.

Ultrasound

This has the advantage of being cheap. It has the disadvantage of requiring the expertise of a dedicated radiologist or ultrasonographer. It has a long learning curve. The individual muscles and tendons are identified deep to the deltoid; defects in the tendon or complete absence can be identified (Figure 4.3). It can be done in real time so that the muscles can be seen in action. Its proponents

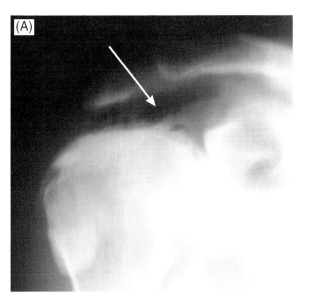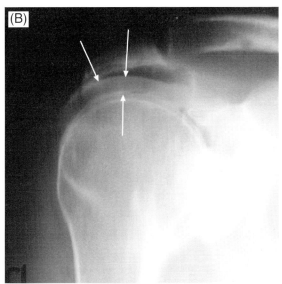

Fig. 4.2 (A) AP tomogram of large full-thickness tear. The tatty edge of the retracted supraspinatus tendon is shown (arrow). (B) AP tomogram of small full-thickness tear. Air and contrast outline a normal-thickness cuff (arrows).

claim sensitivities of around 90% and specificities of between 75 and 95%.[5]

MRI

MRI depends on the hydrogen atom resonating in a strong magnetic field. Hydrogen in the body is largely in the form of water. Fluids, for instance joint fluid, will have high signal in what are called T2-weighted images. High signal is white. Mus-

cle, containing some fluid, will be intermediate signal, i.e. grey. Tendons contain little free water; they return very little signal and will be black.

T1-weighted scans show the anatomy well. T2-weighted scans by highlighting fluid show pathology well.

Supraspinatus is best seen on the coronal oblique scans (Figure 4.4). Teres minor, infraspinatus and subscapularis are best seen on the sagittal and axial scans.

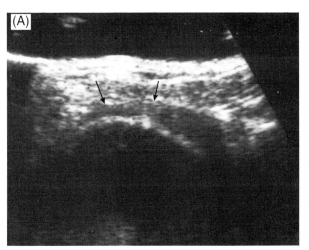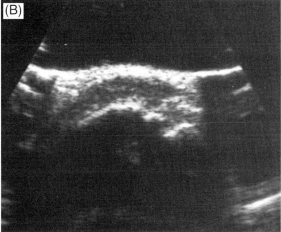

Fig. 4.3 (A) Ultrasound of normal rotator cuff, showing the cuff (arrows) deep to the deltoid. (B) Large full-thickness tear, showing absence of cuff deep to the deltoid.

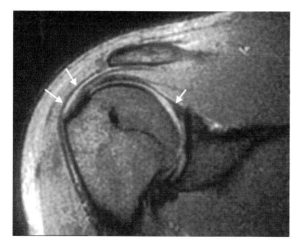

Fig. 4.4 Normal MRI. Coronal oblique T2-weighted image. Normal fat plane (white) separating supraspinatus tendon (arrows) from acromion. The normal tendon may contain some intermediate, but not high, signal. Normal superior labrum (single arrow).

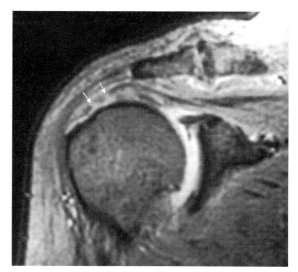

Fig. 4.6 Small-thickness cuff tears. Small high signal defects across the whole width of the tendon (arrows).

Tears will be seen as fluid signal, i.e. white, in the tendon on the T2-weighted scans. If this signal extends from the glenohumeral joint to the subacromial/subdeltoid space, it is a full-thickness tear (Figures 4.5 and 4.6). There is an accuracy of over 90% in this assessment. Increased signal that does not extend right across the tendon may be due to partial-thickness tear or tendonitis. Accuracy in this assessment is about 80%.[6] The size of the tear, the degree of muscle retraction and atrophy can all be determined. Supraspinatus is the commonest tendon involved, as an end stage of impingement under the coracoacromial arch. Infraspinatus and teres minor are also involved in large tears. Isolated tears of subscapularis occur in a small percentage of all tears; they may involve the transverse ligament and allow subluxation of the long head of biceps (Figure 4.7).

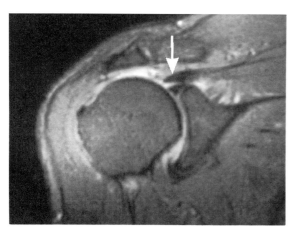

Fig. 4.5 Large full-thickness cuff tear. Fluid is seen in the subacromial/subdeltoid bursa (white). The retracted supraspinatus (arrow) is seen under the acromioclavicular joint.

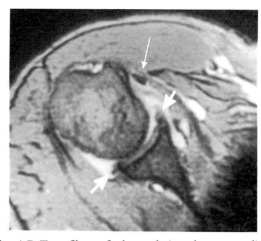

Fig. 4.7 Torn fibres of subscapularis and transverse ligament, allowing long head of biceps to dislocate out of the groove into the torn tendon (arrow). Note also abnormal labra (large arrows) and stripped capsule.

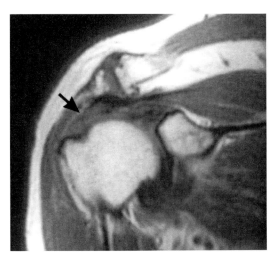

Fig. 4.8 Impingement. Large clavicular osteophytes indent supraspinatus which is swollen distally (arrow). T1-weighted scan.

The coronal views are best for showing acromioclavicular joint osteophytes (Figure 4.8) and acromial spurs, and their associated effect on the tendon. The sagittal views show the supraspinatus outlet, the coracoacromial ligament and the intra-articular long head of the biceps. Tendonitis of the long head of biceps is shown as high signal in a swollen tendon, and a complete tear as absence. The axial views show subscapularis well and are the most useful for showing subcoracoid impingement.

MRI would seem to be the best imaging method. However, it should be pointed out that high signal has been demonstrated in the tendons of many asymptomatic volunteers.[6] There is also intra- and inter-observer variation in its interpretation. These are reduced and the accuracy increased by the use of intra-articular gadolinium.[7] This is, however, invasive, more expensive and often logistically difficult.

These difficulties in interpretation, together with 'managed care' impetus have led some departments to reassess their attitudes to shoulder arthrography and ultrasound. If the decision to explore has been made clinically, and the surgical requirement question is 'Is there a full-thickness tear?' to decide between open operation or arthroscopy, then ultrasound or arthrography should be adequate to answer this.

To add to the clinical difficulties, and muddy the waters, recent papers have demonstrated not only high signal in asymptomatic cuffs but frank full-thickness tears also.[8]

THE UNSTABLE SHOULDER

This is a subject that seems to get more complex with each month's journals. Its separation from painful shoulder is rather artificial since, in the elderly, rotator cuff tears may reduce the humeral head support and thus produce instability; and conversely, the athlete who can externally rotate more than the normal population remodels the soft tissues around the shoulder producing considerable laxity of the anterior and posterior structures to allow impingement, and this is due to the failure of the cuff to depress the humeral head on abduction. Such athletes include those involved in throwing sports, e.g. javelin throwers, but also cricketers, baseball players, gymnasts and swimmers.[9,10]

Plain X-rays

The anterior subcoracoid dislocation and the rare subluxio erecta are usually obvious on plain films. The 3% of dislocations that are posterior are not always so obvious. There are three signs:

1. loss of congruity between head and glenoid;
2. internal rotation producing a round lollipop head – the 'light bulb sign';
3. a vertical dense line down the humeral head produced by an impaction fracture against the posterior glenoid lip, which like the anterior 'Hill–Sachs' lesion can be produced by a single episode.

After the first anterior dislocation, half the patients will have an impaction fracture or 'Hill–Sachs notch' on plain X-rays. One-sixth of them will have glenoid defects visible, and one-sixth will have persistent subluxation.

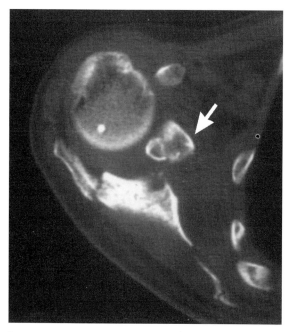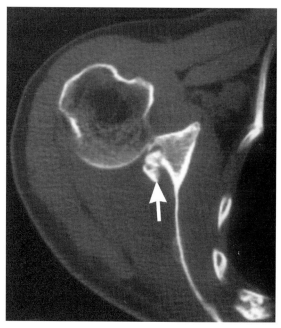

Fig. 4.9 Posterior dislocation of the shoulder with posterior glenoid fracture (white arrow) and scapular fractures. Reduction is prevented by fractured fragment of coracoid (arrow).

CT

This provides axial information without overlapping of the bones, demonstrates the relationship of fracture fragments and whether any are preventing reduction (Figure 4.9), and later can be used in assessing post-traumatic ossification.

Double-contrast arthrography and CT

This provides information on the labra, capsule, joint surface, long head of biceps, synovium and glenohumeral ligaments. It is an excellent method of demonstrating the various combinations of labral and capsular tears, capsular stripping, glenoid fractures and glenohumeral ligament tears. A wrong surgical approach can lead to failure.

Indications include:

1. before surgery to assess joint damage;
2. patients with bizarre and unsubstantiated histories;
3. 'dead arm' syndrome;
4. patients with persistent problems in whom other investigations have been negative;
5. possible long head of biceps subluxation.

The procedure involves the injection of 3 ml of contrast and 12 ml of air and plain X-radiography to see whether there is a full-thickness cuff tear. CT is then performed promptly in a comfortable degree of external rotation (prone sections can also be obtained to show the posterior part of the joint better).

The normal anterior labrum is triangular in shape in cross-section. The tip is pointed. The posterior labrum is more rounded. Both merge smoothly into the articular surface (Figure 4.10). Torn labra are seen as an abnormal shape, or as lines of contrast within the labrum, or as complete avulsion. Some labra appear hypertrophied probably due to a covering of thickened synovium. The subscapularis bursa is seen draped over the muscle. The anterior capsule is inserted a variable amount along the neck of the glenoid. It is normally separated from the cortex by a thin soft tissue line of periosteum and capsule. If this is not present it has been stripped off (Figure 4.11).

The posterior capsule is inserted into the base of the labrum. It does not extend down the posterior glenoid neck (Figure 4.10).

The superior glenohumeral ligament is seen as a

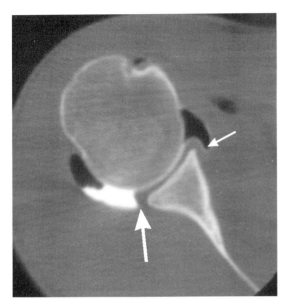

Fig. 4.10 Normal CT arthrogram. Note soft tissue between the joint capsule and the neck of the glenoid anteriorly (white arrow). The posterior capsule inserts into the base of the labrum (large arrow).

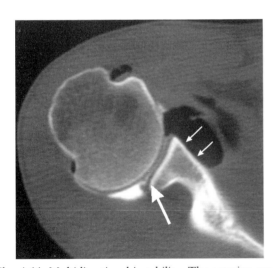

Fig. 4.11 Multidirectional instability. The anterior capsule is stripped off the glenoid (white arrows). The posterior labrum is torn (large arrow).

thin line crossing the top of the joint at the level of the coracoid. The middle and inferior ligaments can sometimes be identified below the coracoid.

The bony parts should be examined; small glenoid rim fractures can be readily imaged, and loose bodies, for example labral fragments, fall

back into the contrast and are seen as filling defects. Humeral head defects are seen more easily on CT than on plain X-rays.

Abnormalities may be confined to the anterior or posterior parts of the joint, but, if both are involved, multidirectional instability can be inferred and surgical approaches planned. A single approach may not be adequate.

Long head of biceps is readily seen in its groove, and complete rupture can be diagnosed when it is not seen. Damage to the intra-articular tendon together with superior labral damage is best seen on MRI.

Labral abnormalities are seen in 75% of operations for instability and capsular abnormalities in 85%. CT arthrography has a high degree of surgical correlation.[11,12] In our own series, accuracy was above 85% and a definite contribution to the surgical approach was made in about 50% of patients with recurrent subluxation who came to surgery.

MRI

This provides the flexibility of imaging in any plane, and of assessing the rotator cuff, as well as the labra and the capsule. It gives the advantage of clarifying the damage in athletes with unstable shoulders presenting with impingement, and in the elderly with large cuff tears presenting with instability. The images differ from CT arthrograms.

The labra being fibrocartilage are low signal and like the menisci in the knee are therefore black triangles sitting on, but often separated from, the glenoid articular cartilage by a fine high signal line (Figure 4.12). There are variations in their attachments so that sometimes they appear perched on the edge.[13] Abnormalities similar to those found in the knee menisci are seen. Tears can be identified as high signal lines across the fibrocartilage (Figure 4.13); they may be truncated or completely avulsed. Care must be taken to identify the middle glenohumeral ligament and trace it laterally as this can simulate a tear.[14]

The superior labrum is well seen on the coronal views. Superior labrum anterior to posterior (SLAP) injuries are due to avulsion of the superior

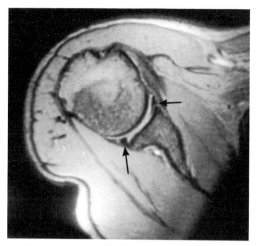

Fig. 4.12 Normal axial MRI. Triangular labra sitting on articular cartilage (arrows).

labral attachment as the result of violent biceps contraction. Patients present with pain and clicking and, unless they involve a large segment, the injuries are not associated with instability. The normal attachment is loose, and care must be taken in this interpretation. The intra-articular portion of the long head of biceps is well visualized on sagittal and axial scans, and tendonitis and subluxations can be diagnosed with considerable accuracy.[15]

Correlation of arthroscopic findings and MRI appearances has been reported in 91% for the anterior labrum, 75% for the superior labrum, 40% for the inferior labrum and a surprisingly low accuracy for the posterior labrum.[16] This can be increased by the use of intra-articular gadolinium (Figure 4.14). Moreover the main stabilizing glenohumeral ligaments can also be visualized.

So, which investigation is best? MRI without distension gives limited information. In Reading we still largely use CT arthrography at present to assess stability. MR arthrography is at least twice as expensive and it has not yet been shown that the small amount of additional information gained justifies this expense.

It can be seen that the variety of imaging methods for the shoulder is wide. It is changing yearly. The optimum examination depends not only on the question to be answered, but also the imaging equipment and expertise and enthusiasm available, together with the rapport between the orthopaedic and radiology departments.

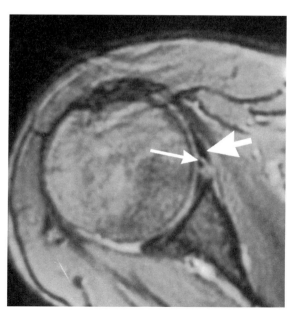

Fig. 4.13 Torn anterior labrum. Tip is separated from base (white arrow). The middle glenohumeral ligament is seen deep to subscapularis (large arrow).

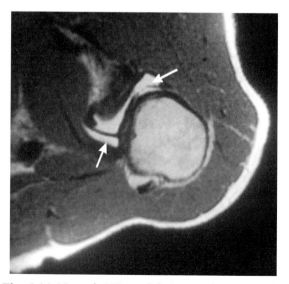

Fig. 4.14 Normal MR gadolinium arthrogram. The glenohumeral ligaments are clearly shown. Even the inferior glenohumeral ligaments are clearly demonstrated (arrows).

REFERENCES

1. Hardy, D.C., Vogler, J.B. & White, R.H. (1986) Shoulder impingement syndrome and correlation with response to therapy. *Am. J. Roentgenol.* **147:** 557–561.

2. Park, J.G., Lee, J.K. & Phelps, C.T. (1994) Os acromiale associated with rotator cuff impingement. MR of the shoulder. *Radiology* **193:** 255–257.

3. Kilcoyne, R.F. & Matsen, F.A. (1983) Rotator cuff tear measurement by erect arthropneumotomography. *Am. J. Roentgenol.* **140:** 315–319.

4. Stiles, R.G. & Offe, M.T. (1993) Imaging the shoulder. *Radiology* **188:** 603–613.

5. Weiner, S.N. & Seitz, W.H. (1993) Sonography of the shoulder in patients with tears of the rotator cuff: accuracy and value. *Am. J. Roentgenol.* **160:** 103–107.

6. Neumann, C.H., Holt, R.G., Steinbach, L.S. et al (1992) MR imaging of the shoulder: appearance of the supraspinatus tendon in normal volunteers. *Am. J. Roentgenol.* **158:** 1281–1287.

7. Hodler, J., Kursunglu-Brahme, S., Shyder, S. et al (1992) MR arthrography versus standard MR imaging in 36 patients with arthroscopic confirmation. *Radiology* **182:** 431–436.

8. Sher, J.S., Uribe, J.W. et al (1995) Abnormal findings on magnetic resonance images of asymptomatic shoulders. *J. Bone Joint Surg.* **77A:** 10–15.

9. Rafi, M., Firoozma, H., Bonamo, J. et al (1987) Athlete shoulder injuries: CT arthrographic findings. *Radiology* **162:** 559–564.

10. Shapiro, M.S. & Finerman, G.A.M. (1992) Traumatic and over use injuries of the shoulder. In L.L. Seeger (ed.), *Diagnostic Imaging of the Shoulder*, pp. 142. Baltimore: Williams and Wilkins.

11. Wilson, A.J., Totty, W.G., Murphy, W.A. et al (1989) Shoulder joint: arthrographic CT and long term follow up, with surgical correlation. *Radiology* **173:** 329–333.

12. Neuman, C.H., Petersen, S.A. & Jahnke, A.H. (1992) MR imaging of the labral-capsular complex: normal variations. *Am. J. Roentgenol.* **157:** 1015–1021.

13. Kaplan, P.A., Bryans, K.C., Dowick, J.P. et al (1992) MR imaging of the normal shoulder: variants and pitfalls. *Radiology* **184:** 519–524.

14. Tuckman, G. (1994) Abnormalities of the long head of biceps tendon of the shoulder: MR findings. *Am. J. Roentgenol.* **163:** 1183–1188.

15. Legan, J.M., Buekhard, T.K., Goff, W.B. et al (1991) Tears of the glenoid labrum: MR imaging of 88 arthroscopically confirmed cases. *Radiology* **179:** 241–246.

16. Palmer, W.E., Brown, J.H. & Rosenthal, D.I. (1994) Labral ligamentous complex of the shoulder: evaluation with MR arthrography. *Radiology* **194:** 645–653.

5

Assessment of Shoulder Function

CR Constant

INTRODUCTION AND HISTORICAL BACKGROUND

Historically, surgeons have assessed the outcome of treatment in orthopaedic surgery by clinical assessment and radiology. The concept of functional recovery after treatment is a relatively recent one. The idea of a clinical method of functional assessment of the shoulder to examine and determine the results of treatment for shoulder problems began in the early 1980s with the development of the Constant score.[1] This score was originally developed in order to assess the functional recovery after injury in groups of patients of different ages and with different kinds of injuries. The method was first published in 1987 and subsequently has been used by its author in the assessment of nearly 5000 patients over a period of 15 years. Many centres found the method of assessment described by Constant as being useful to their needs and in 1990 it was accepted by the European Society for Shoulder and Elbow Surgery, as their standard method of assessment for use in publications and at the Society's meetings. Since the development of the Constant score a number of other countries have attempted to develop and advocate their own scoring systems.[2] The Japanese Shoulder Society produced a scoring system similar to that of Constant although it is apparent that the majority of shoulder surgeons in Japan use the Constant score. Similarly,[3] in the United States, a committee has recently advocated the use of a scoring system which is yet to receive acceptance. In the United States many authors use the Constant score in the presentation of their work, particularly of course if that work is to be presented in Europe.

WHY A FUNCTIONAL SCORE?

In considering this question it should be remembered that the diagnostic assessment of shoulder problems is well established.[4] This involves history taking, physical examination and elicitation of specific physical signs, radiological and sometimes haematological investigation and special investigations including single- or double-contrast radiography[5] and computerized axial tomography[6] as well as magnetic resonance image (MRI) scanning and possibly arthroscopy. The result of these diagnostic investigations produces an anatomical, physiological and pathological determination of the problems. It does not, however, give an indication of the level of function of the affected shoulder. The use of a method whereby an allocation of points towards specific physical findings[7,8] combined with points for investigative results, including perhaps X-ray appearances, in order to obtain a functional level is not a suitable one. Authors have assessed function in this way in the past.[9] In using such an assessment, it is implied that the more abnormal the physical findings, the less is the functional ability of the shoulder. There is, however, no evidence to suggest that there is such a relationship between the presence of physical signs and the level of shoulder function. An extreme example is the paralysed shoulder where signs may be few, and include only wasting and paralysis, in which passive motion is normal, but function is nil. Therefore assessment of shoulder function by assessment of diagnostic criteria is inappropriate and unsuitable for all forms of study into the functional recovery of the shoulder in disease and after treatment.

The use of a functional score which is separate from a diagnostic assessment will allow the meaningful assessment of results of treatment, together with appropriate assessment of ongoing progress after treatment. Comparable evaluation of results and comparison of treatment effectiveness can also be judged. In a world of increasing scientific communication, a functional score will allow uniformity, and a worthwhile exchange between surgeons. Furthermore functional assessment when used in large numbers of patients will allow prediction of the results of treatment in such patient groups.

Lack of function results in disability. An assessment of functional ability, or its lack, can be extrapolated by the use of a disability quantification table into a reasonably accurate assessment of disability. The level of disability brought about by a specific functional loss will depend on the degree of functional loss and the normal activity level of the person being assessed. It is clear that a high-level athlete will be severely disabled by only a small functional loss, while a similar functional loss in a sedentary or retired individual will cause significantly less disability. The Disability Quantification Table (Table 5.1) shows the relationship between functional loss and degree of disability in athletes, active and retired individuals. The use of the terms 'mild, moderate and severe' disability are approximate terms and only give a broad indication of the level of disability in each group.

Table 5.1. Disability quantification

Severity of disability	Activity level (points deficit)		
	Athlete	Active	Retired
Mild	0–10	0–20	0–30
Moderate	10–20	20–30	30–40
Severe	20–30	30–40	40–50
Total	30+	40+	50+

It is very clear that diagnostic assessment and functional assessment are indeed separate entities and should be assessed individually. The European Society for Surgery of the Shoulder and Elbow have endorsed this important point of keeping the two assessments separate.

CRITERIA NECESSARY FOR A FUNCTIONAL SCORE

If a functional score is to be of any value it has to be used in all cases. Intermittent use of a score makes it valueless when using it to study outcomes. If repeated and universal use of a scoring system is to be achieved, it must be simple and quick to perform, inexpensive and reliable, include functional parameters while excluding specifically diagnostic parameters, and it must be independent of the individual diagnosis involving the shoulder in which the assessment is taking place. Clearly it must also be applicable in a clinical setting as the majority of our patients are treated in this way rather than by application of research tools in the laboratory. Interobserver error must be low and it should be possible for anyone involved in the ongoing care of the patient with shoulder problems to be able to undertake this assessment with minimal training. A simple manually completed form of the kind seen in Table 5.2 must be available to complete the assessment. It may be used to computerize the assessment.

FUNCTIONAL PARAMETERS

Numerous parameters may be used when assessing a patient's shoulders. In considering the question of shoulder function, however, only those parameters that contribute to the usefulness of the shoulder in activities of everyday life can be considered functional. Diagnostic parameters should clearly be excluded. Since most persons and patients do many thousands of individual activities throughout the day and night, it is necessary for the sake of simplicity to establish a

Table 5.2. Form for use with Constant score

Parameter	Right		Left	
	Description	*Score*	*Description*	*Score*
Pain				
ADL: Work				
ADL: Recreation				
ADL: Sleep				
ADL: Position				
Range: Flexion				
Range: Abductn.				
Range: Ext Rot.				
Range: Int Rot.				
Power				
Total				

ADL, activities of daily living.

limited number of parameters, specifically important to shoulder function, to be assessed in each case. Some methods of functional assessment of the shoulder include individual specific activities of daily living, allocating points for each ability and denying points to patients who are unable to perform individual tasks. In the Constant score, parameters are limited to four general groups, and in the case of activities of daily living are related to work, recreation and sleep. There is no evidence to suggest that the individualization of activities throughout daily life gives a more accurate result, when assessing overall shoulder function, than the use of general parameters such as the ability to work, enjoy recreational activities or sleep. After studying the various parameters, the Constant score has chosen to include four groups of parameters within the assessment it performs: (1) pain; (2) activities of daily living; (3) range of motion; (4) power. Each are given points as shown in Table 5.3.

Table 5.3. Functional parameters in the Constant score

Parameter	Points
Pain	15
Activities of daily living	20
Range of motion	40
Power	25
Total	100

The overall scoring system consists of a 100 point score, with points unequally allocated to the various parameters as is indicated below. Note that in describing the method, I will use the masculine gender for simplicity.

Pain

Clearly the presence of pain diminishes shoulder function. The pure assessment of pain is undertaken as part of the assessment, although the presence of pain limits other parameters throughout the assessment and therefore is reflected throughout the scoring system. The assessment of pain is based on the patient's description of his pain during normal activities of daily living. A maximum of 15 points out of the total of 100 is available to the patient who has no pain during normal activities of daily living (Table 5.4). The patient is first asked to state whether he has pain, and if no pain is present during normal activities

Table 5.4. Scores for pain

Severity of pain	Points
No pain	15
Mild pain	10
Moderate pain	5
Severe pain	0

15 points are awarded. If the patient experiences pain, he is asked to state the severity, particularly as to whether it is mild, moderate or severe, during ordinary activities. If the patient describes the pain as mild then 10 points are awarded, if the pain is moderate then 5 points are awarded and if the pain is severe then no points are given (Table 5.4). In order to increase the accuracy of the pain assessment, a further test is undertaken. The patient is asked to state what he would consider is his level of pain on a linear scale between 0 and 15 (0 being no pain and 15 being severe pain). On the basis that more points are given for less pain in the scoring system, the patient's own subjective assessment of his numerical degree of pain is subtracted from 15 to give the pain assessment score for this part. For example, if a patient says his pain is 5 on the linear scale between 0 and 15 then he is awarded 10 points in this part of the assessment. The average between this score and the score on the basis of his verbal assessment of degree of pain in the earlier part of the assessment is the final subjective score for pain. While the use of a linear visual analogue type scale (used in reverse) is a useful addition, it is not by any means essential and many people use the pain assessment score merely on the basis of the patient's description of the pain. It is after all a subjective assessment by the patient as to his degree of pain that is being considered, and in tests to see whether there is a significant difference between those patients asked to assess their severity in one or both ways, there was little difference noted.

Activities of daily living

The assessment of activities of daily living is awarded a total of 20 points if normal. This is divided into a number of parts: 4 points are awarded for normal working activities (occupation); 4 points are awarded for leisure activities (sports or hobbies) if they are normal; and 2 points are awarded for the ability to sleep undisturbed (Table 5.5). A further 10 points are allocated for the ability to use the arm at varying levels in relation to the trunk from below waist to above head level (Table 5.6). In assessment of the proportion of the 4 points to be given for work

Table 5.5. Scoring for activities of daily living (part one)

Activity	Points
Full work	4
Full recreation	4
Undisturbed sleep	2
Total	10

Table 5.6. Scoring for activities of daily living (part two)

Position	Points
Up to waist level	2
Up to xiphoid process	4
Up to neck level	6
Up to top of head	8
Above head level	10

Note: Maximum total for this section of the assessment of activities of daily living is 10 points.

or recreation, the patient is asked to state how much of his occupation or leisure activities are affected by the bad shoulder. Points are allocated as a fraction of 4 in each case depending on the answer. In assessing sleep, the patient with an undisturbed night's sleep is awarded 2 points, while the patient who has a disturbed but reasonable sleep is given 1 point. Those who describe badly affected sleep, as a direct result of their shoulder pain, are given no points for this part of the assessment. The patient is then asked to state at what level he can use his affected arm for painless reasonably strong activities. The level to which he can use his arm comfortably is assessed and given points on a scale from 0 to 10, depending on the level described. Activities possible to below waist level only are given 2 points. From waist to xiphisternal level are allocated 4 points and activities at chest level up to neck level are allocated 6 points. If it is possible for the patient to undertake normal activities between the neck and the top of the head then 8 points are awarded and if above head level activities are possible then 10 points are allocated (Table 5.6). A maximum of 10 points can be given for this part of the assessment, resulting in a total of 20 points for activities of daily living. There are therefore 35 points (out of the total 100 points) for the subjective part of the assessment, already described, combining the level of pain and the ability of the patient to undertake normal activities of daily living.

Range of movement

The useful functional range of movement which is used in this score is only that which is active and painless. Assessment of active painless forward and lateral elevation as well as assessment of functional external and internal rotation are undertaken. Ten points for each assessment are allocated giving a total of 40 points for the normal active painless range of functional shoulder motions (Table 5.7).

When assessing forward and lateral elevation, 10 points each are allocated for 180° of forward and lateral elevation, as assessed with the goniometer. Proportionally fewer points are allocated for less motion as indicated in Table 5.8. Equal points are allocated similarly for both forward and lateral

elevation. It is important to take care, when assessing the degree of motion in this way, that the patient does not tilt his trunk in order to achieve a greater result. This substitution of spinal movement for active painless motion of the shoulder is not an advantage to shoulder function. It should also be noted that it is the overall movement, rather than separate glenohumeral and scapulothoracic movement, that is being assessed in this part of the functional assessment as the patient achieves no greater functional ability by dividing these two motions individually during activities of daily living.

Assessment of *functional external rotation* for which a total of 10 points is allocated is undertaken by assessing the ability of the patient to put his hand behind and above his head with his elbow held forward and backwards. This assesses a combination of forward elevation, external rotation and abduction which constitutes the functional external rotation manoeuvre being considered. Two points each are allocated for the four manoeuvres of having the hand above and behind the elbow with the elbow forward and backwards. A further 2 points are allocated for full elevation of the arm giving a total of 10 points for full functional external rotation (Table 5.9).

In examining *functional internal rotation* the ability of the patient to place his hand behind his trunk is assessed. This is effectively a combination of extension, adduction and internal rotation which is being assessed in this movement. The ability to place the dorsum of the hand at the level of the lateral aspect of the thigh gets 0 points while increasing ability to put the hand up to the interscapular area gets an inrreasing number of

Table 5.7. Score for motion ranges in the Constant score

Motion	Points
Forward flexion	10
Abduction	10
Functional external rotation	10
Functional internal rotation	10
Total	40

Table 5.8. Points for each of forward elevation and abduction

Motion range	Points
0–30°	0
31–60°	2
61–90°	4
91–120°	6
121–150°	8
151–180°	10

Table 5.9. Assessment of functional external rotation

Action	Points
Hand behind head with elbow held forward	2
Hand behind head with elbow held back	2
Hand on top of head with elbow held forward	2
Hand on top of head with elbow held back	2
Full elevation from on top of the head	2
Total maximum	10

Table 5.10. Assessment of functional internal rotation

Activity	Points
Dorsum of hand to lateral thigh	0
Dorsum of hand to buttock	2
Dorsum of hand to lumbosacral junction	4
Dorsum of hand to waist (3rd lumbar vertebra)	6
Dorsum of hand to 12th dorsal vertebra	8
Dorsum of hand to interscapular level (7th dorsal vertebra)	10

points as shown in Table 5.10. The full 10 points for functional internal rotation are achieved if the patient can place the dorsum of his hand painlessly between his shoulder blades.

Power

In assessing shoulder power, 25 points are allocated to normal shoulder power. Normal shoulder power is defined as the power of the normal male 25-year-old adult. In assessing power it is the general strength of the shoulder that is being assessed. Individual muscle groups are not being tested, endurance of the shoulder is not being tested and fatiguability of the shoulder is also not being assessed. Where assessment of individual muscles is required, that is separate from the assessment of function.

The assessment within the Constant score is based on the patient's ability to resist a downward pull on his arm while actively abducting the arm against this resistance. The use of a spring balance is advocated. Various authors have advocated the use of other equipment such as an Isobex (Gerber), while other attempts have been made to standardize the assessment of power by more sophisticated means using repeated testing, time testing and combinations of both. The method advocated by Constant is a simple one. A spring balance is attached to the arm by means of a piece of Tubigrip or other cuff-like structure and the patient is asked to elevate his arm in the plane of the scapula to a maximum of 90° (horizontal level) or to whatever level below 90° is possible without pain. The patient is asked to maintain elevation against the pull of the spring balance and

the maximum power exerted is measured in pounds or kg. The patient is asked to maintain this resisted elevation for a period of 5 s and the test is repeated three times. The average resisted pull in pounds or kg is noted over the three tests and it is the quantitative average value of the three results that is accepted as shoulder power; 25 points are given for a maximum of 25 pounds pull (or 12 kg). A conversion factor of 2.2 easily converts pounds to kg when considering the points to be given. The fatiguability of the shoulder in repeated testing is an important diagnostic sign but is not a specific functional test, and it is the average of the three tests that is used in assessing general shoulder power as part of the overall assessment of shoulder function.

The assessment of shoulder strength has given rise to considerable controversy over the years in which the Constant functional scoring system has been used. It should be remembered that it is a general test of strength which should be uniformly performed by a simple method. The use of a spring balance is both cheap and easy while the use of an Isobex dynamometer is expensive. It is, according to Emery et al,[10] probably no less sensitive to use a spring balance. Uniformity is the key to successful use of the assessment.

CONSTANT FUNCTIONAL SCORE

Once the method has been undertaken, a record is kept on paper or computer. An example of a Constant score is included in Table 5.11. Bilateral assessments are always undertaken, and individual parameters can be assessed in terms of progress with time. Overall function can be assessed by addition of the scores obtained for each parameter as part of 100 point score.

COMPLETION OF THE ASSESSMENT

The assessment is now complete. There should now be a completed form which indicates: (1)

Table 5.11. Example of a completed shoulder functional assessment in a patient with osteoarthritis of the right shoulder using the Constant score

Parameter	Right		Left	
	Description	*Score*	*Description*	*Score*
Pain	Moderate	5	None	15
ADL: Work	Full	4	Full	4
ADL: Recreation	Nil	–	Full	4
ADL: Sleep	Poor	1	Unaffected	2
ADL: Position	Top of head	8	Above head	10
Range: Flexion	105°	6	180°	10
Range: Abductn.	90°	4	180°	10
Range: Ext Rot.	Limited	4	Full	10
Range: Int Rot.	LV 5	4	DV 12	10
Power	10 pounds	10	20 pounds	20
Total		46		93

ADL, activities of daily living.

points for pain; (2) activities of daily living in relation to work, recreation and sleep, as well as in positioning of the hand in relation to the trunk; (3) points for active painless ranges of shoulder movements in four directions; (4) shoulder power. The sum of all these is the total Constant shoulder functional score and it cannot exceed 100. Comparison should be made with the opposite side which should be recorded at the same time, an example of which is seen in Table 5.11.

ABSOLUTE VERSUS RELATIVE CONSTANT SCORES

The absolute Constant score is the total numerical value of the assessments mentioned. Early studies using the Constant score have indicated that the normal shoulder function deteriorates with age and this is specific to age and sex. The age- and sex-related deterioration of shoulder function has been plotted and is shown in Table 5.12. These are average values when large numbers of normal shoulders were assessed in different age groups. Some authors prefer to express the shoulder function as a percentage of what is normal for that

patient's age and sex as indicated by table. Other authors prefer to use the normal shoulder on the opposite side as a guide and express the abnormal shoulder function as a ratio of what is normal for that patient. In expressing the shoulder functional score as a ratio, these authors refer to the relative Constant score as against the absolute Constant score. It has become apparent over the past 10 years that the deterioration in function which occurs as a physiological characteristic of ageing

Table 5.12. Normal shoulder function in different decades of life showing physiological age- and sex-related shoulder function

Age (years)	Average shoulder function	
	Males	*Females*
21–30	98	97
31–40	93	90
41–50	92	80
51–60	90	73
61–70	83	70
71–80	75	69
81–90	66	64
91–100	56	52

is not universal for all countries. The figures from studies in this country appear to differ from those obtained in other countries using the Constant score in recent years. The use of a relative Constant score is therefore perhaps best avoided so as to avoid confusion when comparing results between one country's work and another. The relative Constant score can be used, but this has to be clearly stated, and should run in parallel with the absolute Constant score to avoid such confusions.

CONCLUSIONS

Many studies have used the Constant score over the past 5 years or more. Functional recovery has been assessed in numerous situations, after all kinds of surgery, and during the treatment of various diseases. It has proved its usefulness in many countries, and is now probably the most widely used method of scoring shoulder function. It is an essential part of the work of any unit involved in shoulder surgery and the treatment of shoulder disorders, and, with more widespread use, will hopefully one day allow all shoulder surgeons to speak the same language when it comes to discussing treatment, and the results of such treatment, in problems affecting the shoulder.

REFERENCES

1. Constant, C.R. & Murley, A.H.G. (1987) A clinical method of functional assessment of the shoulder. *Clin. Orthop. Rel. Res.* **214:** 160–164.
2. Takagishi, K., Saitoh, A. & Itoman, M. (1995) Assessment of shoulder function using the Japan Orthopaedic Association system. 6th International Congress on Surgery of the Shoulder, Helsinki, June, 1995.
3. Richards, R. (1994) A standardized method for the assessment of shoulder function. *J. Shoulder Elbow Surg.* **3:** 347–352.
4. Moseley, H.F. (1969) *Shoulder Lesions*, 3rd edn, pp. 22–30. Edinburgh: E&S Livingstone.
5. Franji, S.M. & El-Khoury, G.Y. (1981) A new radiographic technique utilizing arthrotomography for studying the shoulder derangements. *Radiol. Technol.* **52:** 384–389.
6. Shuman, W.P., Kilcoyne, R.F., Matsen, F.A. et al (1983) Double contrast computed tomography of the glenoid labrum *Am. J. Roentgenol.* **141:** 581–584.
7. Steward, M.J. & Hundley, J.M. (1955) Fractures of the humerus – a comparative study in methods of treatment. *J. Bone Joint Surg.* **37A:** 681–692.
8. Hawkins, R.J. & Hobeika, P.E. (1983) Impingement syndrome in the athletic shoulder. *Clin. Sports Med.* **2:** 391–405.
9. Knight, R.A. & Mayne, J.A. (1957) Comminuted fractures and fracture dislocations involving the articular surface of the humeral head. *J. Bone Joint Surg.* **39A:** 1343–1355.
10. Emery, R.J.H., Bankes, M.J.K. & Crossman, J.E. (1995) A standard method for strength measurement in the Constant score using a spring balance. 6th International Congress on Surgery of the Shoulder, Helsinki, June, 1995.

6

Examination of the Shoulder under Anaesthesia

SA Copeland

INDICATION

It is often said that examination under anaesthesia (EUA) is not a useful procedure as instability of the shoulder is a dynamic abnormality and EUA can only test the static structures. This is true but it is usually the static restraints that require repair. The examination must be carried out in a systematic and careful manner. The information gained may obviate more expensive and sophisticated investigations. The difference between laxity and instability must be emphasized. Laxity is asymptomatic and instability is symptomatic, such that there may be multidirectional laxity but only unidirectional instability. EUA must be carried out prior to every shoulder stabilization as the information gained may be extremely valuable.[1] It is wise to gain as much information as possible before surgically stabilizing any shoulder. EUA and arthroscopy can delineate the exact cause and type of instability, and the surgery tailored accordingly.

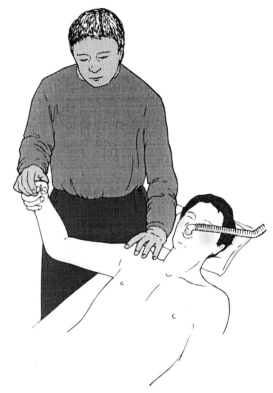

Fig. 6.2 Examination of the right shoulder under anaesthesia. Reproduced, by permission of Churchill-Livingstone, from S. Copeland *Operative Shoulder Surgery*, 1995.

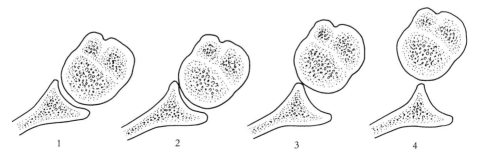

Fig. 6.1 Scoring system for displacement of the joint during examination. Reproduced, by permission of Churchill-Livingstone, from S. Copeland *Operative Shoulder Surgery*, 1995.

(A)

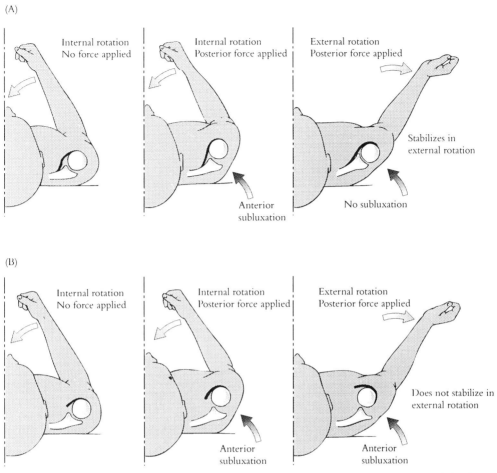

(B)

Fig. 6.3 Demonstration of the difference between ligamentous laxity (A) and incompetence (B) when testing for anterior instability. The lax shoulder stabilizes in external rotation; in the ligamentous incompetent shoulder it does not. Reproduced, by permission of Churchill-Livingstone, from S. Copeland *Operative Shoulder Surgery*, 1995.

TECHNIQUE

With the patient lying supine under general anaesthesia, the abnormal side is compared with the normal opposite side. The variation of laxity in the normal shoulder is extremely wide. The important factor is the difference between the normal and the abnormal side. Under anaesthesia almost any shoulder can be made to sublux. The degree of subluxation must be charted carefully. With experience a reliable scoring system can be used to chart and compare the two shoulders (Figure 6.1). To examine the right shoulder the examiner stands at the head of the table and grasps

the shoulder with the left hand such that the thumb is on the posterior surface of the shoulder and the middle finger on the anterior surface (Figure 6.2). Anterior and posterior translocation forces may now be applied. The right hand grasps the patient's wrist and the shoulder tested in different positions of rotation and abduction. When testing for anterior instability, for example, an attempt is made to sublux the shoulder anteriorly with the shoulder in internal rotation and 20° of abduction. Invariably this can be achieved either partially or totally with the patient under anaesthesia. A note is made of the degree of translocation. With the arm in the same degree of abduction, with full external rotation, the same

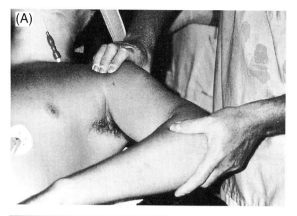

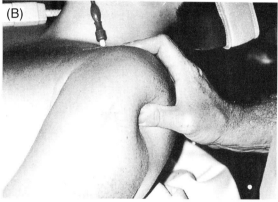

Fig. 6.4 Examination of the 'normal' shoulder for (A) posterior shift in internal rotation and (B) anterior shift.

ligamentous laxity, and, if it is the same as the asymptomatic side, then this must be considered normal. If the examination of the shoulder in external and internal rotation reveals the same degree of translocation, this indicates that the anterior retaining structures are incompetent and there is a major degree of anterior instability. The same procedure is then tried testing for posterior translocation and then inferior translocation with the appropriate force applied, again with varying degrees of rotation. The opposite 'normal' shoulder is then tested in the same manner (Figure 6.4). The opportunity to examine the shoulder under anaesthesia should not be missed as often instability may be part of a problem when the patient presents with a painful shoulder. Presenting symptoms may be those of impingement, but the causation may be instability. With experience, very minor degrees of subtle instability may be recognized more easily, which may be useful to confirm or refute the clinical findings. The EUA is just part of the work-up of investigation of the unstable shoulder. Taking in combination, the history, clinical examination, EUA and arthroscopy, then in all but the minority of cases an adequate diagnosis can be made and the surgery tailored more exactly to the patient's instability.

posterior force is applied. If external rotation completely abolishes the anterior translocation, this indicates that the anterior structures are entirely competent (Figure 6.3). If some degree of translocation is retained, but not as much as in internal rotation, this indicates some degree of

REFERENCES

1. Cofield, R.H., Nessler, J.P. & Weinstabl, R. (1993) Diagnosis of shoulder instability by examination under anaesthesia. *Clin. Orthop. Rel. Res.* **291**: 45–53.

7

Manipulation of the Shoulder under Anaesthesia

SA Copeland

INDICATIONS

The commonest indication for manipulation under anaesthesia (MUA) is the idiopathic frozen shoulder syndrome (see Chapter 9). However, occasionally a shoulder that has been painful for any length of time may have developed secondary stiffness, for example, after a long-term rotator cuff impingement or calcific tendonitis. In these patients the underlying pathology must also be addressed. The ideal time for manipulation of the idiopathic frozen shoulder is at the stage when night pain is decreasing but stiffness has remained static. There is a global loss of movement, with the majority of movement taking place at the scapulothoracic joint and very little at the glenohumeral joint.[1] Physiotherapy at this stage usually tends to make the shoulder more painful but is invaluable immediately after manipulation. Prior to manipulation the patient must be warned that this may be a painful procedure, adequate analgesia must be given and that physiotherapy is an absolute essential to prevent restiffening of the joint.

CONTRAINDICATIONS

Long-standing post-traumatic stiffness involving intra-articular fracture does not respond well to manipulation and is better treated by open techniques. The elderly with osteopenic bone should be treated with caution as possible fracture could be caused by the manipulation. Post-irradiation fibrosis of the shoulder is a contraindication to manipulation as a traction lesion of the scarred brachial plexus may ensue. Insulin-dependent diabetics have a higher incidence of frozen shoulder, but unfortunately may not respond well to manipulation, a high proportion restiffening within 2–3 weeks.

TECHNIQUE

Under general anaesthesia the patient lies supine with the head resting on a head ring. If the patient is being manipulated on a trolley the stretcher pole is removed from the affected side. The surgeon stands at the head of the table with one hand stabilizing the scapula in a resting position. The surgeon's other hand is then placed in the patient's axilla such that the surgeon's forearm is resting against the whole of the inside of the patient's arm to reduce the leverage force on the humerus itself.[2] The range of passive motion without force applied is then tested and recorded. Then with the scapula firmly held down, forceful abduction is made to as near normal movement as possible (Figures 7.1 and 7.2). The scapula must not move at any stage to prevent traction on the brachial plexus.[3] This manoeuvre will rupture the inferior capsule. The shoulder is then forcibly abducted such that the affected elbow is pushed in front of the patient's chin to rupture the posterior capsule. Finally, external rotation and internal rotation are pushed to the limit. Great care is taken during rotation as a spiral fracture of the humerus could be caused if too great a force is applied. Occasionally the range of movements cannot be increased

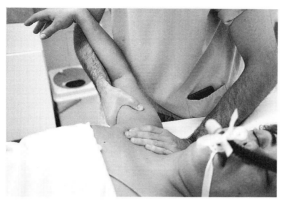

Fig. 7.1 The scapula is held down while the humerus is forcibly abducted.

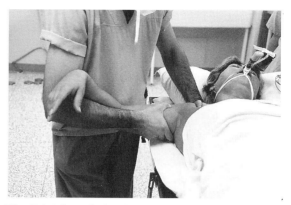

Fig. 7.2 The right hand is held in the patient's axilla and the force exerted through the whole of the operator's forearm on the patient's humerus.

by application of reasonable force. In this case, either open or arthroscopic capsulotomy and division of the coracohumeral ligament may be performed.

POSTOPERATIVE MANAGEMENT

The patient will benefit from injection of a longer-acting local anaesthetic such as bupivacaine 20 ml 0.5% injected into the joint. A steroid may also be added such as Depo-Medrone or triamcinolone to reduce post-operative adhesion formation and swelling. The physiotherapist then sees the patient in the recovery room so that mobilization may be started immediately. It is important that the patient sees the shoulder in the fully abducted or elevated position immediately after surgery so that they realize that this is possible and achievable by physiotherapy thereafter. For the first few days, daily physiotherapy is encouraged and a home exercise programme is begun whereby the patient is asked to stretch the shoulder through maximum range of movements, stretching to extremes at least three times daily. Although the majority of patients undergo physiotherapy as an outpatient,

occasionally a patient may have to be hospitalized for pain control. Although the shoulder may have been manipulated through a full range of movements under anaesthesia, it is rarely gained immediately upon recovery and may take several weeks to regain the range of motion. Recovery from MUA can be extremely variable. If the shoulder 'gives' with one definite snap during the manipulation, then a good result is usually achieved fairly quickly. However, if the shoulder has a plastic 'slow giving way' during manipulation, then this is associated with a less than optimal result.

REFERENCES

1. Neviaser, R.J. & Neviaser, T.J. (1987) The frozen shoulder diagnosis and management. *Clin. Orthop.* **223:** 59–64.
2. Beacon, J.P., Bayley, I., Kernohan, E. & King, R.J. (1985) Manipulation of frozen shoulder. *J. Bone Joint Surg.* **67:** 495.
3. Birch, R., Jessop, J. & Scott, G. (1991) Brachial plexus palsy after manipulation of the shoulder. *J. Bone Joint Surg.* **93:** 172.

8

The Frozen Shoulder

C Kelly

INTRODUCTION

The frozen shoulder is commonly regarded as the enigma of shoulder pathology. Controversy still exists on diagnosis and treatment. The pathophysiology is not clearly defined. Management often depends on the individual doctor's concept of this difficult diagnosis. Treatment options that are strongly defended by shoulder specialists range from skilful neglect to operative release of the soft tissue contractures. This wide diversity of opinion and treatment modalities only goes to illustrate the persistent confusion that still surrounds the diagnosis. Much of this confusion is due to the plethora of terminology used in the literature of the past 50 years. This in turn has meant the study populations have been ill-defined making conclusions on treatment or prognosis difficult or impossible.

DEFINITIONS AND TERMINOLOGY

The term frozen shoulder is probably the most common name used for this condition. Codman[1] is credited with the initial use of the term. Other names include 'adhesive capsulitis' and 'periarthritis'. None of these terms reflect the limited understanding we have of the pathophysiology of the condition. We do know that intra-articular adhesions and arthritis have no place in the primary condition. Whether the condition should be considered a diagnosis or a symptom of

other disease is also controversial. Neer[2] believes that the condition is a symptom just like a headache. Similarly I believe frozen shoulder is the reaction of this joint to an insult occurring in a predisposed patient.

Primary and secondary frozen shoulder are now understood as distinct entities. Primary frozen shoulder is idiopathic and not associated with other pathology such as rotator cuff tears, impingement or significant trauma. Many conditions can contribute to a painful stiff shoulder (Table 8.1) and in these cases we use the term secondary frozen shoulder. However, the harder we look for associated pathology the more we reclassify patients into the latter group.[3] The advent of shoulder arthroscopy and magnetic resonance imaging has allowed identification of

Table 8.1. Some causes of secondary frozen shoulder

Local shoulder disease
Impingement syndrome/subacromial bursitis
Rotator cuff disease
Trauma/fractures
Osteoarthritis
Inflammatory synovitis
Gout/pseudo-gout

Systemic disease
Diabetes mellitus
Thyroid disease
Myocardial infarction
Head injury
Pulmonary tuberculosis
Carcinoma of the lung
Hemiplegia
Drugs, e.g. phenobarbitone

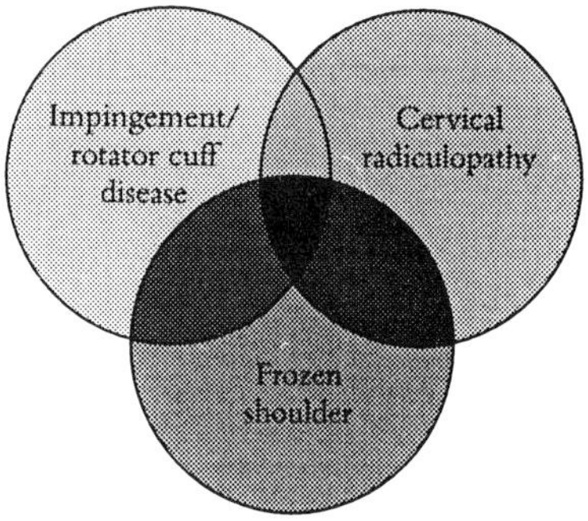

Fig. 8.1 Close association of frozen shoulder with referred neck pain and rotator cuff disease.

Table 8.2. Differential diagnosis of a painful stiff shoulder

Diagnosis	Features
Frozen shoulder	Initially painful, then immobilization, then pain/stiffness
Osteoarthritis	Gradual onset, classical X-ray appearance
Shoulder/hand syndrome	Tenderness, swelling and pain in elbow, wrist and hand. Increased sympathetic activity with redness and sweating
Posterior glenohumeral dislocation	Major trauma or fall. Axillary X-ray shows dislocation. Anteroposterior shows 'light bulb' sign

subtle lesions such as partial undersurface rotator cuff tears so that 'primary' frozen shoulder is now less commonly diagnosed. In a recent study of 935 patients with shoulder pain, only 50 fitted the criteria of primary frozen shoulder.[9] The situation is more confused by the close association of frozen shoulder with referred neck pain and rotator cuff disease. All may occur alone or in combination (Figure 8.1).

EPIDEMIOLOGY AND DIAGNOSIS

Patients with frozen shoulder present with a gradual onset of shoulder pain with subsequent stiffness with restricted active and passive shoulder movement. The condition is more common in women, with a peak age incidence in the sixth decade. It occurs in 2–3% of the population (10–20% in diabetics). Occupation does not seem to play a role and the non-dominant limb may be more commonly affected.

A history of minor trauma direct or indirect is common. This may range from a minor twist while reaching to the back seat of the car to a stumble against a wall. A period of immobilization of the limb to protect against pain follows. Immediate pain is uncommon but patients often identify a sensation of 'something giving way'. The second shoulder can be involved in 10–20% of patients and this usually happens within 5 years. Relapse is extremely rare but some patients do develop other upper limb enthesiopathies such as tennis elbow.

The patient must fulfil the following criteria for a diagnosis of primary frozen shoulder:[4]

1. insidious onset of shoulder pain;
2. restricted active and passive forward elevation and external rotation;
3. normal X-ray appearance;
4. no identifiable cause.

Secondary frozen shoulder has the same clinical features but has a clear causation such as trauma, rotator cuff tear, cervical disc prolapse, myocardial infarct or diabetes mellitus. Other pathologies causing shoulder pain with reduced abduction and external rotation must be excluded (Table 8.2). The differential diagnosis must also include Pancoast tumour, syringomyelia, rheumatoid arthritis and supraspinatus nerve compression. Shoulder pain can be referred from the cervical spine, pleura and the subdiaphragmatic area. These places may harbour benign and malignant tumours. Always question the diagnosis of frozen shoulder made by others.

THEORIES ON PATHOPHYSIOLOGY

Despite 60 years of science applied to the frozen shoulder the pathophysiology is still unclear. In his original report Codman described the problem of the frozen shoulder as 'difficult to define, difficult to treat and difficult to explain from the point of view of pathology'. To some extent this is true today. Neviaser[5] was the first to examine histological specimens after which he coined the term adhesive capsulitis. He described adhesions of the humeral head to the capsule. Since then many authors have failed to confirm these finding at open or arthroscopic surgery.[3,6] However, in many studies it is not clear during which clinical stage these observations were made. Adhesions have also been reported between the rotator cuff and undersurface of the acromial arch.

All the tissues surrounding the glenohumeral joint and subacromial bursa have been implicated at some stage in the pathology of frozen shoulder. These include the biceps and supraspinatus tendons, the subacromial bursa and recently the coracohumeral ligament. Other theories on aetiology suggest the causative factors to include supraspinatus nerve entrapment, reflex sympathetic dystrophy and autoimmune mechanisms.

The restriction of movement in frozen shoulder is due to the tight contracted capsule. Histological examination does not confirm inflammation in the synovium but in the deeper layers.[7] The changes seen may represent the healing phase of connective tissue and increased fibroblastic collagen has been identified.

More recently the area between the biceps tendon and the subscapularis muscle has been implicated in the pathology. Contracture and fibrosis of the coracohumeral ligament may explain the limitation of external rotation and certainly release of contracture in this area can produce immediate improvement in external rotation and forward flexion.[8] The cause of this contracture remains a mystery and certain evidence suggests that the fibrous contracture is analogous to Dupuytren's contracture in the hand. High serum lipids are found in both of these diseases and this may be the common link to such conditions as diabetes, phenobarbitone use and cardiac disease.[9]

THE NATURAL HISTORY OF FROZEN SHOULDER

Frozen shoulder is a self-limiting disease and usually progresses to resolution within 3 years. It starts spontaneously and passes through three phases.

The painful phase

This lasts up to 6 months and features rest pain moderately resistant to simple analgesics and anti-inflammatory drugs. The pain is severe at night and the patient has difficulty lying on that side.

The stiffening (adhesive) phase

Although the severe pain settles, increased stiffness is associated with discomfort at the limits of movement. Problems with personal care and overhead activities occur with variable severity.

The resolution phase

Pain continues to settle as movement improves with stretching exercises. Complete resolution may take 3 years but is often incomplete. Full recovery can occur but many authors now accept that loss of movement is common despite the lack of disability. Reeves[10] in a study of 41 patients over a 5–10-year period has shown that some patients have symptoms up to 10 years later. Twenty-two of 41 patients had detectable loss of movement but only three of these had functional deficit. A short painful stage may be a good prognostic indicator.

PRESENTATION

The typical patient presenting to a shoulder clinic is a lady in her sixth decade with shoulder pain and stiffness lasting weeks to months. She is otherwise fit and well and has no history of shoulder problems in the past. Pain came on a few days after a minor injury as she reached

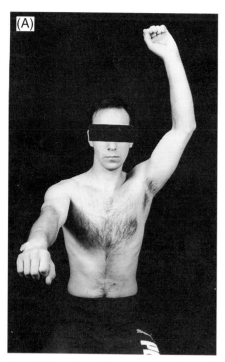
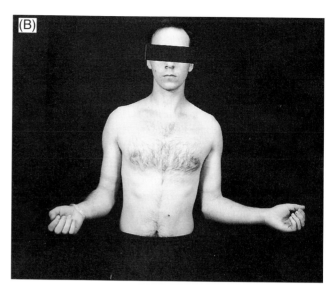

Fig. 8.2 This patient demonstrates reduced forward flexion (A) and external rotation (B) of the right shoulder compared with the unaffected left side.

backwards to catch a falling ornamental vase. Initially the pain was severe and localized to the outer aspect of the shoulder and the deltoid insertion. The patient rested the arm in a sling as advised by the local doctor and took anti-inflammatory medications. Gradually over a period of months the pain improved but there was increased stiffness. Physiotherapy involved ultrasound and passive mobilization but this seemed to exacerbate the condition. After several months the pain improved but the patient now finds difficulty using the arm especially for overhead activities. There is pain at the extremes of movement. On examination there is mild wasting of all shoulder muscles including deltoid and the rotator cuff. Tenderness is diffuse around the neck and shoulder and also in the interscapular area. All passive and active movements are reduced. Specifically forward flexion is less than 90° and external rotation with the arm at the side is 50% of the uninvolved shoulder (Figure 8.2). On examining the range of motion, the patient has excessive scapulothoracic motion and tilts the thoracic spine

to compensate for loss of glenohumeral forward flexion and abduction. Remember restricted external rotation is also a sign of posterior glenohumeral dislocation. Muscle testing within the restricted range of movement does not demonstrate any gross weakness. The patient is now 6 months from the onset of symptoms and although admitting improvement she does have major functional problems affecting her job and dressing. Combing her hair and putting on a bra are particularly difficult. 'Can anything be done doctor?'

INVESTIGATION

The diagnosis of frozen shoulder is a clinical one. Investigations may help to exclude associated disease and classify into primary and secondary problems. Erythrocyte sedimentation rate and bone biochemistry are normal. Routine X-rays are normal for the age group under study. Therefore minor degenerative changes are commonly seen. Prolonged pain and disability may produce diffuse osteoporosis. Calcium deposits are seen in up to 10% of patients and are probably no more common than in an asymptomatic population. Technetium bone scan is usually positive although the cause is not clear. It has not been useful in deciding treatment or predicting prognosis.[11] Shoulder arthrography demonstrates the contracted capsule and reduction in volume and is considered by many the essential element in diagnosis.[12] Despite a typical clinical diagnosis, 10% of patients may have a normal arthrogram. The distension and rupture of the capsule by the introduction of dye under pressure does produce some dramatic relief of symptoms in some patients. This has led several authors to recommend it as a treatment.[13] Magnetic resonance imaging of a primary frozen shoulder is unlikely to be helpful. It may highlight unexpected abnormalities and to date its value in this condition has not been defined.

Blood tests to identify diabetes and thyroid disease are commonly performed. Latent diabetes and subclinical thyroid disease can be detected and in the latter case treatment may improve the shoulder.

Arthroscopy can identify capsular contraction and help rule out other intra-articular and sub-acromial pathology. However, it has also questioned the pathology of frozen shoulder. In a study of 37 patients, Wiley[3] found no evidence of obliteration of the infraglenoid recess.

MANAGEMENT

Frozen shoulder is a self-limiting disease. As the cause is unknown, treatment is symptomatic and directed at relief of pain and improvement in shoulder motion. Progress can be slow, and frustration in patients, doctors and therapists is common. As with any protracted illness psychological factors come into play and may need attention of their own right. It is unlikely that depressive personality types are more prone to this condition.[14] The decision to interfere with

the natural history of resolution should be made with caution as many 'treatments' are now known to be associated with prolongation of the disease. Hazelman[15] showed that a quarter of the population he studied had an exacerbation of symptoms with physiotherapy; this is a common complaint from patients when passive mobilization techniques are administered in the acute painful stage. Associated disease in secondary frozen shoulder, e.g. diabetes, pulmonary tuberculosis, should be treated although this may have no effect on the clinical course of the painful shoulder.

If one searches the literature for advice on treatment there is great confusion because of conflicting reports on efficacy. Many studies are retrospective lacking control groups with inadequate definition of the study population and the clinical stage of the disease. The importance of graduated active stretching exercise programmes in the adhesive and resolution phase is highlighted in most publications. Prophylaxis should involve avoidance of immobilization of the shoulder in those at risk. The management problem arises usually in the second phase when there is an apparent arrest in progress or when the patient is disabled by the reduced shoulder movement. At the end of the resolution phase some patients may have residual stiffness and a few of these have a functional deficit.

There are six broad treatment options: systemic analgesic therapy; use of local and systemic steroids; manipulative therapy; hydraulic capsular distension; surgical release of contracted tissues; miscellaneous.

Systemic analgesic therapy

There is little to choose between the different analgesic and anti-inflammatory medications. They do not alter the course of the disease. Ward et al[16] showed no difference in pain relief between paracetamol and diclofenac. Gastrointestinal sensitivity to anti-inflammatory drugs must be monitored to prevent complications of ulceration and bleeding. Acupuncture and alternative medicines have all had their advocates especially for the painful stage.

Use of steroids, local and systemic

Short courses of oral steroids have been used successfully for pain relief. Once again they have not altered the natural course of the disease. Local steroid injections into the glenohumeral joint and subacromial bursa are commonly given. In the early painful stages they can improve pain and movement.[17] In a small number of cases there is a rapid response when even one injection can 'turn off' the painful process. Up to three glenohumeral joint injections over a 6 week period can be used in the acute stages of frozen shoulder.

Manipulative therapy

There are many conflicting reports on the efficacy of manipulation under anaesthesia. Its value may be in the second (adhesive) stage of disease and is indicated when the loss of movement has not responded to an exercise programme or a plateau phase is reached. It works by tearing of the antero-inferior capsule and coracohumeral ligament and can be combined with local steroid injection for pain. Care should be exercised in the method used avoiding any torsional forces on the humerus especially where there is osteoporosis (Figure 8.3). Only experience will dictate how much force is safe. Complications include fractures of the humerus, shoulder dislocation and rotator cuff tear.

Hydraulic capsular distension

The benefit of arthrograms in frozen shoulder was noticed early on. Rupture of the capsule and leakage of dye was sometimes associated with improved pain and movement. Recently this management has regained popularity as a minimally invasive and safe technique.[13] I have no experience of this technique.

Surgical release of contracted tissues, open and arthroscopic

Open surgical release of the contraction in frozen shoulder is recommended by some surgeons.

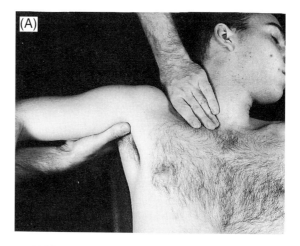

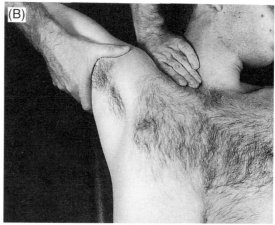

Fig. 8.3 (A) and (B) When manipulating the right shoulder, the surgeon uses his left hand to stabilize the scapula. The surgeon's right forearm is placed along the patient's arm. Placing the hand high in the patient's axilla causes reduction in angulatory forces on the humeral neck and shaft.

Ozaki et al[8] have described open release of the coracohumeral ligament in the recalcitrant case. In a series of 17 cases followed for 6.8 years, 16 had rapid pain relief and full movement at review.

Arthroscopy of the shoulder allows confirmation of the diagnosis and exclusion of other pathology such as impingement lesions in the subacromial bursa. Because of the reduced joint volume, access to the glenohumeral joint may be difficult and the risk of damage to the articular cartilage of the head of the humerus is high. Using diathermy or laser the contracted tissues can be

Table 8.3. A treatment protocol for frozen shoulder

Stage	First line	Second line	Third line
Painful	1. Simple analgesics 2. Anti-inflammatory drugs (One or more of the above + pendulum exercises)	1. Glenohumeral joint steroid injection (no more than three in a 6-week period) 2. Transcutaneous electrical nerve stimulation (TENS) (One or more of the above + pendulum exercises)	1. Acupuncture 2. Ultrasound, laser, interferential local treatment 3. Suprascapular nerve block 4. Stellate ganglion block (One or more of the above + pendulum exercises)
Adhesive	Simple analgesia plus home exercise stretching programme, with physiotherapist monitoring progress	No improvement after 3 months then glenohumeral steroid injection and manipulation under general anaesthetic. Follow-up by physiotherapist with intensive stretching programme	In diabetics and resistant cases, arthroscopy/bursoscopy and capsular release. Follow-up by physiotherapist with intensive stretching programme
Resolution (after 2 years)	Significant loss of motion: if no functional deficit, then no treatment	Significant loss of motion: if definite functional deficit, arthroscopic capsular release plus physiotherapy	Significant loss of motion: if all else fails, consider open release. Guarded prognosis

sequentially divided to improve passive movement. Pollock et al[18] reported satisfactory results in 25 of 30 shoulders treated with manipulation followed by arthroscopic surgical release of the coracohumeral ligament. Results in diabetics were worse and the authors recommend it as a safe and reliable treatment in resistant cases.

Miscellaneous

The following other approaches have been recommended over the years alone or in combination with techniques already mentioned:

1. suprascapular nerve block;[19]
2. stellate ganglion block and sympathectomy;
3. subcutaneous calcitonin injections.

A management protocol for the frozen shoulder is given in Table 8.3. The majority of patients referred to the shoulder clinic do not need manipulation or surgery. Most are satisfied with an explanation of the diagnosis and its natural history. They are encouraged to continue with a home exercise programme and are monitored every 6–12 weeks.

SUMMARY/CONCLUSIONS

The pathophysiology of frozen shoulder remains a puzzle. The clinical course to resolution may take 3 years and may be incomplete. Treatment consists of pain control in the early stages and exercise to maintain and improve movement. Inappropriate or untimely intervention can aggravate symptoms. Manipulation and occasionally surgical release has a role to play in the recalcitrant case. Some patients have little disability despite significant loss of glenohumeral motion.

REFERENCES

1. Codman, E.A. (1934) *Ruptures of the Supraspinatus Tendon and other Lesions in or about the Subacromial Bursa.* Boston: Thomas Todd and Co.

2. Neer, C.S. II. (1990) *Shoulder Reconstruction*. Philadelphia: W.B. Saunders Co.
3. Wiley, A.M. (1991) Arthroscopic appearance of frozen shoulder. *Arthroscopy* **7:** 138–143.
4. Zuckerman, J.D., Coumo, F. & Rokito, S. (1994) Definition and classification of frozen shoulder. *J. Shoulder Elbow Surg.* **3:** Abstract Z.72.
5. Neviaser, J.S. (1945) Adhesive capsulitis of the shoulder. A study of the pathological findings in peri-arthritis of the shoulder. *J. Bone Joint Surg.* **27:** 211–222.
6. Uitvlugt, G., Detrisac, D.A., Johnson, L.L., Austin, M.D. & Johnson, C. (1993) Arthroscopic observation before and after manipulation of frozen shoulder. *Arthroscopy* **9:** 181–185.
7. Lundberg, B.J. (1969) The frozen shoulder. *Acta Orthop. Scand. (Suppl.)* **119:** 1659.
8. Ozaki, J., Nakagawa, Y., Sakurai, G. & Tamai, S. (1989) Recalcitrant chronic adhesive capsulitis of the shoulder. *J. Bone Joint Surg. Am.* **71:** 1511–1515.
9. Bunker, T.D. & Esler, C.N.A. (1995) Lipids and frozen shoulder. A Dupuytren's like disease. *J. Bone Joint Surg.* **77B:** 684–686.
10. Reeves, B. (1975) The natural history of Frozen shoulder syndrome. *Scand. J. Rheumatol.* **4:** 193–196.
11. Binder, A., Bulgen, D. & Hazleman, B. (1984) Frozen shoulder: an arthrographic and radionuclear scan assessment. *Ann. Rheum. Dis.* **43:** 365–369.
12. Neviaser, J.S. (1962) Arthrography of the shoulder joints: study of the findings in adhesive capsulitis of the shoulder. *J. Bone Joint Surg.* **44A:** 1321–1330.
13. Rizk, T.E., Gavant, M.L. & Pinals, R.S. (1994) Treatment of adhesive capsulitis (frozen shoulder) with arthrographic capsular distension and rupture. *Arch. Phys. Med. Rehabil.* **75:** 803–807.
14. Wright, V. & Haq, A. (1976) Peri-arthritis of the shoulder. *Ann. Rheum. Dis.* **35:** 220–226.
15. Hazelman, B.L. (1972) The painful stiff shoulder. *Rheumatol. Rehabil.* **11:** 413.
16. Ward, M., Kirwan, J., Norris, P. & Murray, N. (1986) Paracetamol and diclofenac in the painful shoulder syndrome. *Br. J. Rheumatol.* **25:** 412–420.
17. Bulgen, D.Y., Binder, A.I. & Hazelman, B.L. (1984) Frozen shoulder: prospective clinical study with an evaluation of the treatment regimens. *Ann. Rheum. Dis.* **43:** 353–360.
18. Pollock, R.G., Duralde, X.A., Flatow, E.L. & Bigliani, L.U. (1994) The use of arthroscopy in the treatment of resistant frozen shoulder. *Clin. Orthop.* **304:** 30–36.
19. Wassef, M.R. (1992) Suprascapular nerve block. A new approach for the management of frozen shoulder. *Anaesthesia* **47:** 120–124.

9

Acromioclavicular and Sternoclavicular Joints

R Emery

ACROMIOCLAVICULAR JOINT

Introduction

The acromioclavicular joint is of diarthrodial type comprising a fibrocartilaginous disc which may be complete or meniscoid. The plane and shape of the joint is very variable; Moseley[1] believed that shallow inclination was a predisposing factor to injury. The amount of movement occurring in this joint has always aroused debate. Codman[2] thought that the acromioclavicular joint was only slightly movable. Inman et al[3] demonstrated the potential motion by drilling pins into the clavicles of volunteers; they obtained as much as 20° angulation and 40–50° of rotation. Thus, in theory, overhead elevation could be lost if this movement was prevented by, for example, a coracoclavicular screw. However, in clinical practice it is not uncommon to encounter patients with complete ossification of the coracoclavicular ligaments who retain full elevation.

The stability of the acromioclavicular joint is maintained by the acromioclavicular and coracoclavicular ligaments. The superior acromioclavicular ligaments are relatively weak and blend with the fascia of the deltoid and trapezius muscles. It is the conoid and trapezoid parts of the coracoclavicular ligament that function as the primary supports of the acromioclavicular joint. From these ligaments the upper limb is suspended, which has been quite aptly described by Rockwood as being analogous to the suspension of jet engines on an aircraft wing.

Classification of injuries

The mechanism of injury is usually as a consequence of a fall onto the point of the shoulder in which the force is directed at the posterior aspect of the acromion (Figure 9.1). It is possible that some acromioclavicular joint strains occur due to an upward indirect force. Cadenat's classic experiments reported in 1917 showed that a moderate blow ruptured the acromioclavicular ligaments whereas a heavier blow also ruptured the coraco-

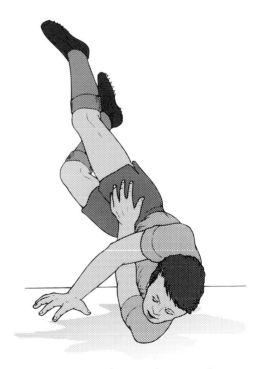

Fig. 9.1 Common mechanism of injury to the acromioclavicular joint.

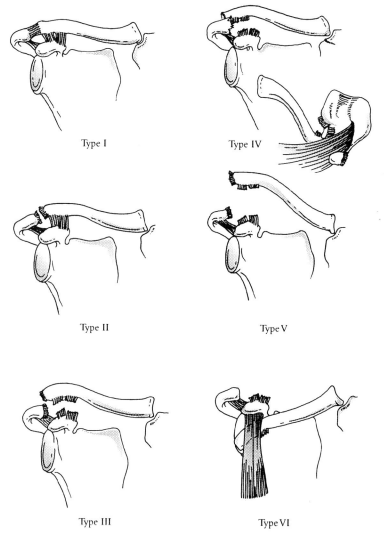

Type I

Type IV

Type II

Type V

Type III

Type VI

Fig. 9.2 The Rockwood classification of acromioclavicular joint injuries.

clavicular ligaments and that both the conoid and trapezoid parts must be divided to produce a full dislocation.[4] In more recent times, Rockwood[5] demonstrated from cadaver studies that horizontal stability was controlled by the acromioclavicular ligaments whereas vertical stability was dependent on the coracoclavicular ligaments.

The original classification of these injuries was made by Tossy et al[6] and Allman.[7] In the Tossy–Allman classification grade I is a sprain of the acromioclavicular ligaments, grade II a subluxation with rupture of the acromioclavicular ligaments and a sprain of the coracoclavicular

ligaments, and grade III is a dislocation. This grade was expanded subsequently by Neviaser[8] to include two other types: 3A a locked separation and 3B when the clavicle buttonholes through the trapezium. Rockwood[9] has stressed that these injuries with tearing of the deltoid and trapezius muscle attachments from the clavicle should be correctly termed scapuloclavicular rather than acromioclavicular separations and defined three other types to the original description (Figure 9.2). In type IV injuries the clavicle is displaced backwards through the trapezius. Rockwood describes an injury in which the scapula remains in the anatomical position and the clavicle is displaced posteriorly. In my experience the scapula is usually forcibly protracted allowing the clavicle to perforate the trapezius. In type V injuries there is greater displacement than in type III; the distinction between type III and V depends on the increase in coracoclavicular interspace, with 25–100% and 100–300% greater than normal respectively. Type VI is rare; the clavicle is driven inferior to either the acromion or the coracoid. Dislocations with a split in the periosteal sleeve in the younger patient are included as type III injuries.

Presentation

These injuries comprise 12% of all dislocations of the shoulder. The patient usually presents with localized pain and cradling the arm. It is best to examine the patient standing, allowing the shoulder girdle to descend if pain allows. This facilitates assessment of the degree of injury. The fascial coverings should be examined as well as feeling for tenderness, both in the vicinity of the lateral end of the clavicle and in the interspace between the clavicle and coracoid. Instability is assessed by observing the displacement in the horizontal and vertical planes. Pressing the outer end of the clavicle downwards may give a feeling similar to depressing a piano key. Particularly in suspected type IV injuries, posterior angulation of the clavicle should be looked for as well as the distance from the medial border of the scapula to the midline. A haematoma overlying the trapezius indicates the degree of additional soft tissue disruption. In the very rare type VI injury an inferior step down may not be noted as the defect is rapidly concealed by the haematoma.

Investigation

Plain radiographs are the essential investigation. It is important to request films of the acromioclavicular joint and not the glenohumeral joint to avoid overpenetration. An axillary view should be requested for assessment of posterior displacement. Other specific views have been described: the Zanca view taken with $10°$ cephalic tilt and

stress views may be of value in distinguishing a type II from a type III injury. This is potentially useful if this distinction changes the management. The stress views compare the coracoclavicular space of the affected with the normal side. The widening of the interspace can be observed by applying weights suspended by loops from the wrists. It is thought that as little as 40% displacement probably reflects some disruption of the coracoclavicular ligaments. The Alexander or lateral dynamic protraction view may be of value in identifying a coracoid fracture, when there may be a dislocation of the acromioclavicular joint but little change in the interspace distance. If the fracture is poorly seen, it is useful to request a Styker notch view which shows the base of the coracoid extremely well.

Treatment

Indications

In order to formulate a plan of management it is necessary to know the natural history and results of conservative treatment. Bergfeld et al[10] reported the results of conservative treatment in type I and II injuries. Of patients with type I injuries, 30% described their disability as a nuisance and 9% as significant. For type II injuries the outcome was 23% and 13% respectively. Many other papers show no difference. A recent paper looked at the natural history of type II and III injuries: 48 cases were reviewed after a mean interval of 12.5 years. There were 24 Tossy II and 24 Tossy III injuries; 69% achieved a good result with no difference between groups. Functionally the Tossy II patients fared marginally worse probably due to the higher incidence of post-traumatic arthritis which was found in 9%.[11] Similar experience has been reported by Taft et al,[12] Glich et al[13] and Dias et al.[14] Furthermore many papers (e.g. Larsen et al[15]) describe a significant complication rate with operative management, including wound infection, osteomyelitis, late arthritis, soft tissue calcification, erosion of clavicle by fixation devices, late fracture through the implant holes, the need for a second procedure to remove the fixation device, pin or wire

Table 9.1. Reasons for and against operative management

For	Against
Young	Older
Athletic	Non-athletic
Manual work	Sedentary occupation
Joint stable	Joint unstable
Irreducible	Reducible
Fascia disrupted	Fascia intact
Prefer a scar	Prefer a bump
Thin patient	Thick subcutaneous fat
Compliant	Non-compliant

complications, metal failure, unsightly scar and fixation failure with recurrent deformity. The decision to operate should therefore be carefully considered and take into account the patient's needs and the balance of advantages and disadvantages as summarized in Table 9.1.

Conservative treatment has been considered, but it is important to specify what is meant by conservative treatment. Usually it consists of 'skilful neglect' with a sling for 1–2 weeks until the patient is comfortable. Alternatively, reduction with a Kenny Howard sling can be attempted and worn for 3 weeks (Figure 9.3). However, this device and others cause problems with skin pressure areas and are uncomfortable. It is interesting to recall that Galen sustained an acromioclavicular dislocation which he treated himself in the manner of Hippocrates with tight bandages to hold the projecting clavicle down while keeping the arm elevated. He reported that it was so uncomfortable that he discontinued it after a few days. There have been many other ingenious devices including crotch loops and stocking and garter straps.

Surgical reconstruction was required in 12.7% of all acromioclavicular separations in the series reported by Morrison & Lemos[16]. There are numerous operations described which can be grouped into four basic types:

1. intra-articular repair;
2. extra-articular repair;
3. excision of distal end of clavicle;
4. dynamic muscle transfer.

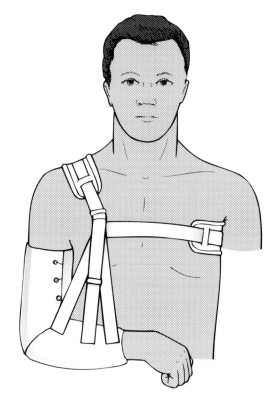

Fig. 9.3 The Kenny Howard sling.

Before discussing the method of intra-articular repair, it is interesting to see the effect of reduction. Sperner et al[17] reported 109 cases treated by reduction with two Kirchner wires and polydioxanone suture (PDS) tension band wiring followed by 3 weeks of immobilization. The wires were removed at 6 weeks; 13% experienced complications, including pin breakage, pin migration and infection associated with PDS sutures. However, of particular note was the poor reduction and acromioclavicular arthrosis requiring revision to a resection of the lateral end of the clavicle. Other authors have also shown a higher incidence of post-traumatic arthritis following surgery than with conservative treatment.[12] The incidence was particularly high in patients treated with transarticular wires rather than coracoclavicular stabilization with a Bosworth screw. In addition to the risk of arthrosis, pin breakage and migration are well recognized. The only time I would advise pins fixation is in the rare acromioclavicular separation associated with a base of coracoid

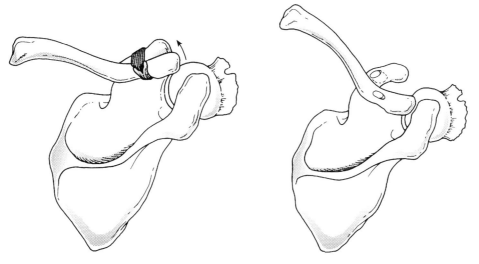

Fig. 9.4 Modified coracoclavicular banding technique described by Morrison and Lemos.

fracture to permit bone union. Another variation of intra–articular repair for cases of symptomatic horizontal instability sometimes seen after excision of the lateral end of the clavicle merits discussion. In this situation the important superior acromioclavicular ligament is deficient[18] and may require reconstruction by transfer of the coracoacromial ligament to the upper surface of the clavicle as described by Julius Neviaser[8] (Figure 9.4).

My personal view favours extra–articular repairs in most instances. The Bosworth operation was originally described as a closed procedure with fluoroscopy under local anaesthesia.[19] The screw was left indefinitely. The procedure is usually modified and often used as a temporary device. However, it can be difficult even as an open procedure. Its use is commended in the description by Gerber & Rockwood[20] for the extremely rare type VI injuries following open reduction. In this situation the reconstruction of the strut of the shoulder girdle allows the severely injured soft tissues to heal and if necessary facilitates late reconstruction and excision of the distal clavicle.

Ligament transfer was originally proposed by Cadenat in 1917.[14] In 1972, Weaver & Dunn[21] reported on 12 acute and three chronic grade III injuries with good results. Once again the techni-

que is often modified but the principle is to transfer the coracoacromial ligament from the acromion to the excised end of the clavicle (Figure 9.5). Probably the most important aspect of the reconstruction is the repair of the trapezius fascia. After the operation a broad arm sling is worn for 4 weeks allowing gentle circumduction exercises. Warren-Smith & Ward[22] have demonstrated that this procedure is equally effective in early and late cases.

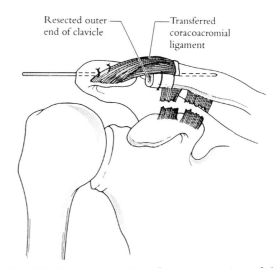

Fig. 9.5 Neviaser procedure for reconstruction of the acromioclavicular joint.

Copeland & Kessel[23] describe a modification gaining length whereby the ligament is transferred with a sliver of bone insertion to the superior surface of the clavicle and held with screw fixation. The major disadvantage of this technique is local discomfort from the bone block and screw. Recently Bigliani (1995, unpublished data) reported a further modification with transfer of the posteromedial band of the coracoacromial ligament alone, in order to preserve the coracoacromial arch.

Occasionally the coracoacromial ligament is not substantial enough to act as a stabilizer, and alternative techniques are required. The coracoclavicular ligaments cannot be repaired reliably but should be apposed to achieve some reconstitution by fibrous scarring. Coracoclavicular banding with either PDS cord or tape are preferable to the use of non-absorbable materials such as Dacron or wire, which may cause erosion and fracture of the bone.

Morrison & Lemos[16] advised passing the loop through drill holes in the base of the coracoid and anterior third of the clavicle, so that when the loop is tightened the clavicle is reduced without the anterior subluxation caused by simple cerclage (Figure 9.5). It is important to recognize that significant damage to the joint cartilage occurs and that the isolated removal of torn meniscus is insufficient to avoid post-traumatic arthritis. Thus primary resection of the joint should be performed in conjunction with coracoclavicular banding.

The Mumford procedure,[24] in which the distal end of the clavicle is excised, is also indicated in type I and type II injuries with persistent pain or secondary post-traumatic arthritis. Originally described for late post-traumatic arthritis, the results of this procedure appear to be equally as effective in the acute and semi-acute stages. Therefore it is difficult to advise how long to wait before excising the lateral end of the clavicle in these cases; 6 weeks is probably too short and 6 months probably too long in making the decision. At surgery, not less than 1.5 cm should be removed and clearance should be assessed on the operating table. Particular care should be taken not to remove too much clavicle or destabilizing

the coracoclavicular ligaments, as well as creating a strong overlying fascial repair.

Late reconstruction of instability is difficult. A Bosworth screw[19] alone is inappropriate and most of these cases can be treated by a coracoacromial ligament transfer. Should this procedure fail, transfer of the coracoid process to the clavicle provides a dynamic stabilizer.[25] In rare circumstances too much clavicle has been excised, presenting a difficult problem of an unstable clavicle and a poor cosmetic appearance. Robert Neviaser (1995, unpublished data) has suggested a coracoid transfer to stabilize and restore the length of the clavicle.

Atraumatic conditions

Symptomatic degenerative arthritis of the acromioclavicular joint is extremely common, and narrowing of the disc space can be considered a normal ageing process after the age of 40.[26,27] Symptomatic cases can be treated by excision of the lateral end of the clavicle together with the adjacent osteophytes.[24] This procedure can also be effectively performed arthroscopically: Ciullo (1995, unpublished data) recently reported the results of 230 resections performed between 1987 and 1994 with complete relief of pain in 91%.

The acromioclavicular joint is often affected in rheumatoid arthritis and can be identified as a major source of pain by lignocaine injection studies even in patients with severe glenohumeral or rotator cuff disease. In these cases the acromioclavicular joint may be the only restraint against upward migration, and a dome-type arthroplasty may be a preferable alternative to conventional excision.

Acromioclavicular joint cysts are usually encountered with both degenerative changes in the joint and underlying rotator cuff tears (Figure 9.6). Simple excision is unpredictable, and resection of the outer end of the clavicle is preferable. Another uncommon condition is osteolysis of the distal clavicle. This is usually seen in men, particularly weight-lifters. It is commonly unilateral and usually resolves with rest and local injections. Curiously the clavicle may even reconstitute itself. The acromioclavicular joint is also a rare site for

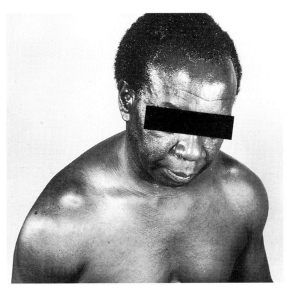

Fig. 9.6 Cyst of the acromioclavicular joint.

septic arthritis, with many case reports describing infection with a variety of organisms.

THE STERNOCLAVICULAR JOINT

Introduction

The sternoclavicular joint is remarkable for its lack of bony congruity and its dependence on the surrounding ligaments for its stability. This saddle

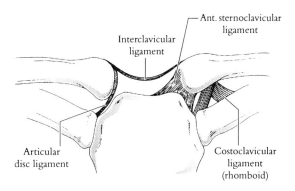

Anatomy of the sternoclavicular joint

Fig. 9.7 Anatomy of the sternoclavicular joint.

type of diarthrodial joint contains the curious intra-articular disc ligament (Figure 9.7). It is covered by the sternoclavicular ligaments within the capsule but the major structural support is derived from the costoclavicular (rhomboid) and interclavicular ligaments.

Direct force causing a posterior dislocation is rare. The commonest mechanism of injury is an indirect force in which either the torso is compressed and rolled backwards causing an ipsilateral anterior dislocation or compressed and rolled forwards causing an ipsilateral posterior dislocation (Figure 9.8). Thus the direction of dislocation is either anterior or posterior. The spectrum of severity ranges from a mild sprain to a moderate

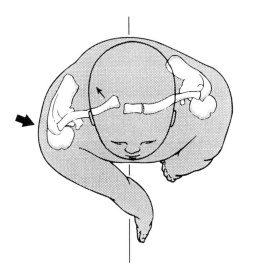
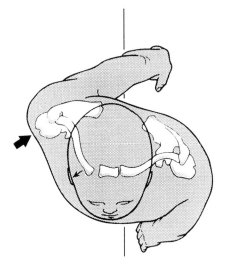

Fig. 9.8 Mechanism of injury to the sternoclavicular joint.

Table 9.2. Classification of conditions affecting the sternoclavicular joint according to aetiology

Traumatic injuries	Atraumatic conditions
Sprain or subluxation	Spontaneous subluxation or dislocation
Acute dislocation	Congenital or developmental
Recurrent dislocation	subluxation or dislocation
Unreduced dislocation	Arthritis
	Osteoarthritis
	Arthropathies
	Condensing osteitis of the medial clavicle
	Sternocostoclavicular hyperostosis
	Post-menopausal arthritis
	Infection
	Tumours

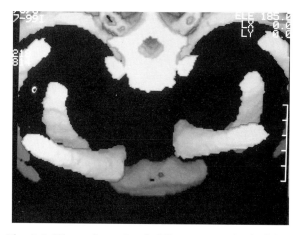

Fig. 9.9 Three-dimensional CT reconstruction of the sternoclavicular joint showing a left-sided posterior dislocation.

sprain or subluxation to a full dislocation. In addition to dislocation of the joint, it is important to consider fracture separations of the epiphysis of the medial clavicle even in young adults. This is the last epiphysis to fuse in the 23–25th year and accounts for a number of pseudo-dislocations in this age group and younger. The vast majority of these injuries occur with road traffic accidents and sports.

Conditions affecting the sternoclavicular joint may be classified according to aetiology (Table 9.2). Anterior dislocations present with fairly significant signs of swelling and deformity, whereas the posterior dislocations may be less obvious. The patient usually presents with more pain and even dysphagia or dyspnoea. Initially the absence of the normal contour of the medial end of the clavicle and the superolateral corner of the manubrium may be palpable. However, these signs are lost once the swelling and haematoma develop. Venous engorgement in the ipsilateral arm may be found in unrecognized cases.

Evaluation of these conditions may be significantly hindered by the difficulties of imaging this joint. The history and clinical findings may be diagnostic, but imaging is often required. For example, not all cases demonstrate the typical appearances of anterior or posterior dislocation and even assessment of the direction of displace-

ment may be difficult. Plain radiology is limited even with special views including the 40° cephalad tilt or 'serendipidity' view advocated by Rockwood. If any doubt persists, either a tomogram or a computed tomography (CT) scan is required. Figure 9.9 shows a three-dimensional CT reconstruction in a case of traumatic posterior dislocation, in which the plain X-rays were interpreted as normal. We have found ultrasound scanning to be a simpler and quicker method of observing displacement (Figure 9.10). MRI scans

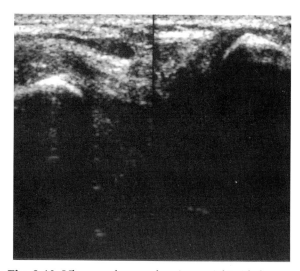

Fig. 9.10 Ultrasound scans showing a right-sided posterior dislocation.

show the intra-articular disc ligament very clearly, and isotope studies are particularly helpful in identifying infection, inflammation and rare tumours.

Treatment of dislocations

Dislocations are relatively rare, with anterior dislocation occurring three times as commonly as posterior dislocations. In principle, every attempt should be made to treat these injuries by closed reduction as most of the complications seen are iatrogenic. Anterior dislocations are treated by applying traction to the arm in 70–90° of abduction with some extension. This can be facilitated by placing a sand bag behind the shoulder blades and applying direct pressure on the medial end of the clavicle. The reduction is quite frequently unstable and may be helped by a figure-of-eight

bandage. Posterior dislocations are treated similarly except that the clavicle is pulled out with finger grip or a towel clip (Figure 9.11). Even with strong counter traction this manoeuvre may fail. The reduction is usually more stable and a sling is adequate for a period of 4 weeks. Whereas chronic anterior dislocations become pain free with time, posterior dislocations should always be reduced because of the risk of mediastinal compression.

Open reduction is potentially dangerous due to the immediate posterior relations of the sternoclavicular joint which include the arch of aorta, superior vena cava, innominate vein, pulmonary and subclavian vessels. Consequently an experienced anaesthetist and a cardiothoracic surgeon should be available. The arm is draped free and the joint approached by a transverse incision. By careful soft tissue dissection and arthrotomy of the capsule, the medial end can be freed and lifted from behind the sternum. The joint can be adequately stabilized by capsular and periosteal repair alone. Anterior physeal injuries can be

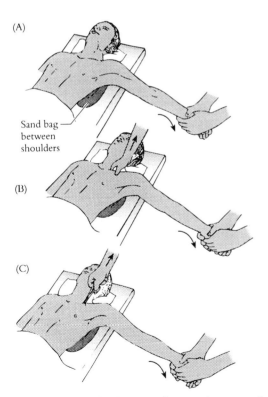

Fig. 9.11 Method of reduction of a posterior sternoclavicular dislocation by (A) traction into abduction and extension combined with anterior traction on the sternoclavicular joint either (B) digitally or (C) following the application of a towel clip.

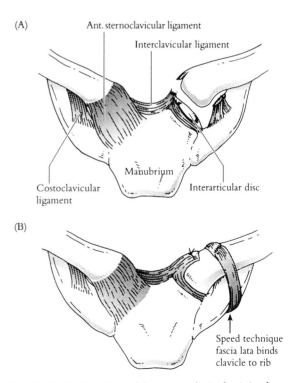

Fig. 9.12 Stabilization of the sternoclavicular joint by a fascia lata loop.

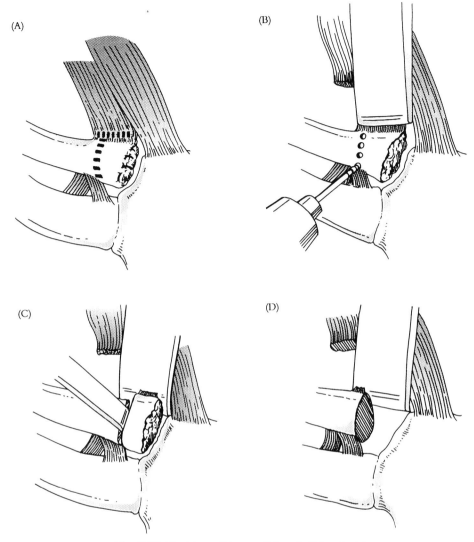

(A)

(B)

(C)

(D)

Fig. 9.13 Excision of the medial end of the clavicle.

treated conservatively with impressive remodelling; however, posterior injuries should be reduced as described.

In the majority of cases recurrent or unreduced anterior dislocation can also be treated non-operatively. Occasionally the symptoms are severe or persist and open stabilization is required. I favour Speed's technique with either a fascia lata strip or a PDS tape looped round the first rib and repair of the intra-articular disc ligament to the periosteum of the clavicle (Figure 9.12). The alternative procedure described by Jackson Burrows[28] is a subclavius tendon transfer. This requires a much longer incision to harvest the tendon. This procedure is combined with a resection of the medial end of the clavicle which also accentuates the poor cosmetic appearance and can result in persistent pain and weakness.[29]

Treatment of atraumatic conditions

Spontaneous subluxation or dislocation is fortunately commonly a self-limiting condition and almost never requires surgery.[30] Arthritis of the sternoclavicular joint may also become asymptomatic with time, and conservative management including a limited number of intra-articular steroid injections should be tried. If surgery is required, the costoclavicular ligaments are intact and excision arthroplasty alone is recommended. Resection of 2 cm of medial clavicle will not compromise the stability. Particular care must be taken when dividing the clavicle; a blunt retractor should be placed behind the clavicle before making a series of drill holes. The osteotomy is completed with an osteotome. The clavicular head of sternomastoid is released and sutured into the space created by the resected clavicle (Figure 9.13).

Condensing osteitis of the medial clavicle, sternocostoclavicular hyperostosis and post-menopausal arthritis are poorly defined conditions with many similar features and little guidance on management from the small numbers of cases reported. Infections are occasionally encountered and culture will reveal a wide range of organisms. Although needle biopsy may help with the diagnosis, anterior arthrotomy is usually required for treatment.

Conclusion

Despite the rarity of these injuries and conditions, the complications associated with surgery to this joint are easily recalled. The use of any type of pin is not only dangerous but also unwarranted; their insertion risks injuring the immediate posterior relations of the joint, and migration of pins is well documented (Figure 9.14). It is depressing that their persistent use still generates ever more bizarre case reports of pins as far away as the liver

and spinal cord. There have been fatal and near-fatal cases, culminating in two German surgeons being charged with manslaughter by negligence. It is worth considering the following understatement when considering surgery on this joint:

'It would seem that complications are common in this rare surgical problem'

Omer 1967

REFERENCES

1. Moseley, H.F. (1959) Athletic injuries to the shoulder region. *Am. J. Surg.* **98**: 401–422.
2. Codman, E.A. (1934) *Ruptures of the Supraspinatus Tendon and other Lesions in or about the Subacromial Bursa.* Boston: Thomas Todd and Co.
3. Inman, U.T., Saunders, B. & Abbott, L.C. (1944) Observation of the function of the shoulder joint. *J. Bone Joint Surg.* **26**: 1–30.
4. Cadenat, F.M. (1917) The treatment of dislocations and fractures of the outer end of the clavicle. *Int. Clin.* **1**: 145–169.
5. Rockwood, C.A. Jr (1984) Injuries to the acromioclavicular joint. In *Fractures in Adults*, 2nd edn, vol. 1, pp. 860–910. Philadelphia: J.B. Lippincott Company.
6. Tossy, J.D., Mead, N.C. & Sigmond, H.M. (1963) Acromiclavicular separations: useful and practical classification for treatment. *Clin. Orthop.* **28**: 111–119.
7. Allman, F.L. Jr (1967) Fractures and ligamentous injuries of the clavicle and its articulation. *J. Bone Joint Surg.* **49A**: 774–784.
8. Neviaser, J.S. (1968) Acromioclavicular dislocation treated by transference of the coracoacromial ligament. *Clin. Orthop.* **58**: 57–68.
9. Rockwood, C.A. Jr. (1975) Dislocations of the sternoclavicular joint. *Instr. Course Lect.* **24**: 144–159.
10. Bergfeld, J.A., Andrish, J.T. & Clancy, W.G. (1978) Evaluation of the acromioclavicular joint following first- and second-degree sprains. *Am. J. Sports Med.* **6**: 153–159.
11. Mau, H., Loew, Schilenwolf, M. (1995) Long-term follow-up of acute AC-separation treated conservatively. 6th International Congress on Surgery of the Shoulder (ICSS), Helsinki/Stockholm, 27th June–4th July, 1995. No. 60.
12. Taft, T.N., Wilson, F.C. & Oglesby, J.W. (1987) Dislocation of the acromioclavicular joint: an end result study. *J. Bone Joint Surg.* **69A**: 1045–1051.
13. Glich, J.M., Mibburn, L.J., Haggerty, J.F. & Nishimoto, D. (1977) Dislocated acromioclavicular joint follow up study of 35 unreduced acromioclavicular dislocations. *Am. J. Sports Med.* **5**: 264–70.

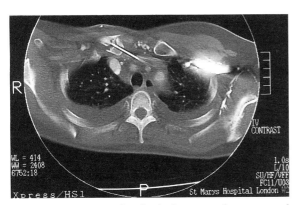

Fig. 9.14 CT scan of a fistula between the aorta and innominate vein.

14. Dias, J.J., Steingold, R.E. & Richardson, R.A. (1987) The conservative treatment of acromioclavicular dislocation. *J. Bone Joint Surg.* **69B:** 719–722.

15. Larsen, E., Bjerg-Nielsen, A. & Christensen, P. (1986) Conservative or surgical treatment of acromioclavicular dislocation. *J. Bone Joint Surg.* **68A:** 552–555.

16. Morrison, D.S. & Lemos, M.J. (1995) Acromioclavicular separation: reconstruction using synthetic loop augmentation. *Am. J. Sports Med.* **23:** 105–110.

17. Sperner, G., Reichkendler, M., Golser, K., Wambacher, M. & Hamberger, A. (1995) Early complications after operative treatment of A-C dislocations. 6th International Congress on Surgery of the Shoulder (ICSS), Helsinki/Stockholm, 27th June–4th July, 1995. No. 62.

18. Fukuda, H., Craig, E.V., An, K. et al (1986) Biomechanical study of this ligamentous system of the acromioclavicular joint. *J. Bone Joint Surg.* **68A:** 434–440.

19. Bosworth, B.M. (1941) Acromioclavicular separation: a new method of repair. *Surg. Gynecol. Obstet.* **73:** 866–871.

20. Gerber, C. & Rockwood, C.A. Jr. (1987) Subcoracoid dislocation of the lateral end of the clavicle: a report of three cases. *J. Bone Joint Surg.* **69A:** 924–927.

21. Weaver, J.K. & Dunn, H.K. (1972) Treatment of acromioclavicular injuries, especially complete acromioclavicular separation. *J. Bone Joint Surg.* **54A:** 1187–1194.

22. Warren-Smith, C.D. & Ward, M.W. (1987) Operation for acromioclavicular dislocation. *J. Bone Joint Surg.* **69B:** 715–718.

23. Copeland, S. & Kessel, L. (1980) Disruption of the acromioclavicular joint: surgical anatomy and biological reconstruction. *Injury* **11:** 208–214.

24. Mumford, E.B. (1941) Acromioclavicular dislocation. *J. Bone Joint Surg.* **23:** 799–802.

25. Dewar, F.P. & Barrington, T.W. (1965) The treatment of chronic acromioclavicular dislocation. *J. Bone Joint Surg.* **47B:** 32–35.

26. De Palma, A.F. (1963) Surgical anatomy of the acromioclavicular and sternoclavicular joints. *Surg. Clin. North Am.* **43:** 1540–1544.

27. Petersson, C.J. (1983) Degeneration of the acromioclavicular joint. *Acta Orthop. Scand.* **54:** 431–433.

28. Burrows, H.J. (1951) Tenodesis of the subclavius in the treatment of recurrent dislocation of the sternoclavicular joint. *J. Bone Joint Surg.* **33B:** 240–243.

29. Eskola, A., Vainionpaa, S., Vastamaki, M., Slatis, P. & Rokkanen, P. (1989) Operation for old sternoclavicular dislocation. *J. Bone Joint Surg.* **71B:** 63–65.

30. Rockwood, C.A. Jr. & Odor, J.M. (1989) Spontaneous atraumatic anterior subluxation of the sternoclavicular joint. *J. Bone Joint Surg.* **71A:** 1280–1288.

10

Winging of the Scapula

R Emery

INTRODUCTION

It is interesting to observe from our clinical practice how commonly the shoulder may preserve near-normal function despite significant tears of the rotator cuff or even nerve palsies of the muscles acting across the glenohumeral joint. By contrast, conditions affecting the scapular stabilizing muscles usually lead to profound loss of function. These muscles are of paramount importance to shoulder function. It is of note that, although we use the terms *protraction*, *retraction* and *winging*, there can be few joints in the human body whose movement is so poorly defined. We do not even have proper terms of reference regarding the range of motion of the scapulothoracic joint. This lack of recognition becomes even more surprising when we observe the remarkable range of movement maintained in patients who have undergone a glenohumeral arthrodesis.

A great deal of emphasis has focused on scapulothoracic rhythm, disturbance of which is a useful finding but usually reflects to pathology arising from the glenohumeral or subacromial articulations. The movements of the scapula are complex because of constraints imposed by the sternoclavicular and acromioclavicular joints: little motion occurs with the first 60° of elevation and the scapula moves around a centre of rotation in the lower part of blade. Subsequently the centre of rotation moves to a point near to the base of the scapular spine. Above 120°, the centre of rotation changes again to a point at the base of the glenoid. This rotation combined with protraction creates an active suspension and fulcrum system for the glenohumeral joint.

This chapter will discuss functional impairment associated with loss of isolated muscles and then with global loss of the scapular stabilizing muscles. In discussing the effects and treatment of these conditions and other causes of winging, it is important to consider the secondary effect on the soft tissues and the nerves around the shoulder.

LOSS OF TRAPEZIUS FUNCTION

In the erect position, the trapezium and levator scapulae supports the entire weight of the upper extremity (Figure 10.1). In addition to their suspensory role they participate in a complicated muscle coupling controlling scapulothoracic movement. Neer[1] likens the action to lifting a suitcase off the ground; the upper fibres of trapezius and levator scapulae pull cephalad, whilst the lower fibres of the trapezius acting with the rhomboids and latissimus dorsi pulls the arm backwards (Figure 10.2) allowing the upper fibres of the trapezius to rotate the scapula.

The major cause of trapezius palsy is injury to the spinal accessory nerve. Although the dangers of iatrogenic injury cannot be overstressed, it is important to appreciate that this palsy is more commonly seen when it is sacrificed intentionally during radical neck dissection for malignant disease. The ensuing disability can be so great that preservation should be encouraged if at all possible. Furthermore, ENT surgeons must be alerted to the risks and need to avoid using the levator

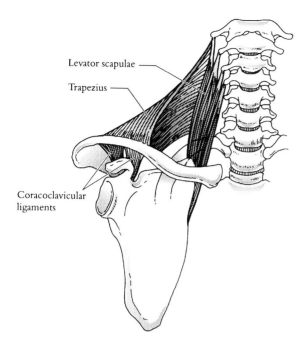

Fig. 10.1 The suspensory mechanism of the scapula.

scapulae muscle to cover the carotid artery during radical neck dissection. Not only is it the only other suspensory muscle but also of great importance in late reconstruction of the shoulder girdle.

The spinal accessory nerve is the major nerve supply to the trapezius. It exits the base of the skull through the jugular foramen and passes obliquely through the sternomastoid muscle in its upper

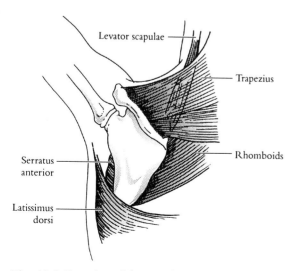

Fig. 10.2 Function of the scapular stabilizing muscles.

third before crossing the posterior triangle of the neck to enter the trapezius. As it lies very superficially, it is vulnerable to injury and is at risk with even the simplest surgical operation in the neck region. The injury is usually not recognized at the time of surgery and the diagnosis is often delayed until the patient describes inability to abduct the arm without pain. Some of the palsies are due to neuropraxia and recover spontaneously. Electromyographic examination may be of help but if there is no recovery by 10 weeks the nerve should be explored. If the nerve is found in continuity lying in scar tissue, neurolysis may be successful, but if there is obvious discontinuity, suture or grafting is necessary. Should the repair be unsuccessful or not possible, surgical reconstruction with muscle transfer should be considered.

Reconstruction is the only option in post-radical neck resection patients. There is a marked contrast in the perception of the condition between the iatrogenic cases and these patients. Many do not wish to consider further surgery and have insufficient disability to require reconstruction. The degree of disability is extremely variable which may be partly due to the dual innervation from C2 and C3 (occasionally C3 and C4) in some patients. Indications are usually not precise and depend on activity level, age and life expectancy of the patient.

The cause of pain in these patients may be uncertain. It is important to try to ascertain the mechanism in order to plan treatment. Pain from neurological denervation and adhesive capsulitis may be a factor in the early phase. Ptosis of the scapula may cause discomfort from brachial plexus traction radiculitis. More commonly the pain appears to be due to fatigue and functional impingement of the supraspinatus within the subacromial space due to failure to rotate and retract the scapula. This impingement can even progress to a rotator cuff tear and thus an additional cause of pain. These causes can be evaluated by the response to the impingement test after local anaesthetic injection into the subacromial bursa. Neer[1] has even suggested that anterior acromioplasty alone may be sufficient in these patients. There is little information to support this and unless there there is a rotator cuff tear requiring

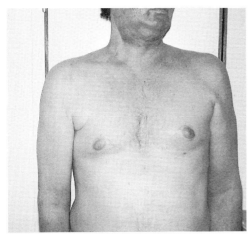

Fig. 10.3 Deformity seen with loss of trapezius function.

repair I favour attempts to improve scapula function by tendon transfer. These reconstructions also improve the deformity which may be severe (Figure 10.3).

The procedures to restore the function of the scapulothoracic articulation must address not only the winging, but also the ptosis due to loss of the scapular suspension mechanism. The complex nature of force couples makes substitution of even one muscle acting in a single plane difficult. The Eden–Lange tendon transfer of levator scapulae and the rhomboids (Figure 10.4A) is probably best for near-normal function.[2,3] These three muscles are used to replace the upper, middle and lower portions of the trapezius respectively. Bigliani, Perez-Sanz and Wolfe[4] described their experience in ten cases; seven had been followed for more than 2 years, of which five had an excellent result.

The alternative procedures, originally used in patients with facial nerve paralysis in which the spinal accessory nerve was used as a motor for the facial muscles, have significant disadvantages. Dewar & Harris[5] transferred the levator scapulae insertion laterally to substitute for the upper trapezius and used a fascial sling in place of middle and lower parts of the trapezius (Figure 10.4B). The slings were passed from the vertebral border of the scapula to the spinous processes of the second and third thoracic vertebrae. Unfortunately these slings stretch with time. If

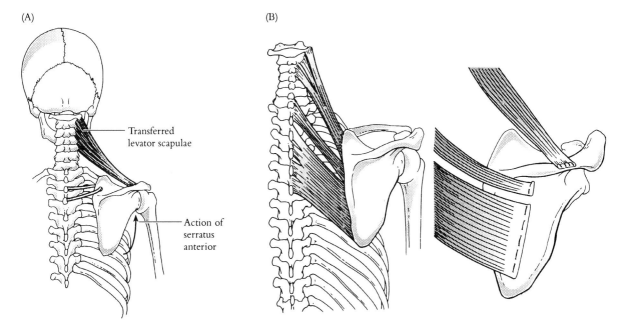

(A)

Transferred
levator scapulae

Action of
serratus
anterior

(B)

Fig. 10.4 The principles of muscle transfer for the loss of trapezius function: (A) Dewar and Harris and (B) Eden–Lange procedures.

soft tissue reconstruction fails the only other option is scapulothoracic fusion. This procedure has also been suggested as a primary procedure in cases where heavy demands are anticipated. Conservative treatment has not been found successful other than treating concomitant adhesive capsulitis.

Eden–Lange procedure

The patient is placed in the lateral decubitus position but allowed to roll slightly prone. The arm is draped free and the head of the table is elevated 15°.

Two incisions are used, allowing sufficient proximal exposure to enable dissection of the levator scapulae muscle in the neck. The initial vertical incision is made midway between the spinous processes and the medial border of the scapula and extends along the length of the scapula. The atrophied trapezius is identified and divided close to the scapula border, taking care to avoid the underlying rhomboids. The borders of the levator scapulae, rhomboideus minor and rhomboideus major are identified and their insertions separated with slings. They can be detached with their bony insertions using an osteotome. These cuts should be made at an angle to avoid the serratus anterior insertion. The rhomboideus major often adheres very tightly at its insertion and must be carefully separated. The levator scapulae and rhomboids are dissected proximally, taking care not to injure the dorsal scapular nerve and transverse cervical artery. It is particularly important to dissect out the levator scapulae sufficiently to allow its new alignment. The infraspinatus is elevated from its fossa and six 4.5 mm drill holes are made approximately 2 cm apart and 5 cm lateral to the medial border of the scapula. No. 5 Ethibond sutures are placed through these holes with a reversed 45 mm Mayo needle. The sutures are then passed through the rhomboids close to their insertion. The scapula is reduced with the arm abducted to 90° when the sutures are tied. The infraspinatus is used to cover the reconstruction. A second incision is made 4 cm medial to the acromion running medially along the scapular spine. The trapezius,

deltoid, lower fibres of the supraspinatus and upper fibres of the infraspinatus are carefully dissected off, being careful to avoid the suprascapular nerve. Three 2.5 mm drill holes are made in the spine of the scapula. A tunnel is made under the atrophied layer of the trapezius so that the levator scapulae can be reattached as far laterally as possible on the spine of the scapula.

After surgery, the arm is placed in an abduction brace at 45° for 6 weeks. It should be checked that the shoulder is not held with the scapula protracted. Some authors use a sling; this is acceptable as long as the muscle reattachment, in particular the levator scapulae, is secure and the protraction deformity is easily and fully corrected.

At 6 weeks a standard three-phase rehabilitation programme is commenced with active assisted (passive), active and finally resisted exercises against therabands. Training of scapular protraction and retraction should also begin at 6 weeks.

Complications include injury to the dorsal scapular nerve and the suprascapular nerve. Neither structure should be at risk if care is taken with the dissection.

Tip: Langenskiold and Ryoppy[3] describe the procedure through a single curved and more laterally based incision. This gives better exposure of the medial border of the scapula but makes proximal dissection of the levator scapulae slightly more difficult.

LOSS OF SERRATUS ANTERIOR FUNCTION

We have seen how the upper fibres of the trapezius rotate the scapula the serratus anterior assists in upward rotation but also rotates the scapula laterally or forwards. It keeps the vertebral border of the scapula in firm apposition with the chest wall in all positions (Figure 10.2). Loss of this muscle may limit active elevation, but more frequently presents as a deformity with fatigue pain on elevation of the arm. The fine tuning of scapula movement is of paramount importance in shoulder performance. The glenohumeral joint has aptly been described as a golf ball on a tee. In many vigorous shoulder activities the scapula is positioned so that the glenoid centre line and axis of the humeral head are closely aligned, for example in a boxer's punch, bench press, throwing action and tennis shot. It is easy to demonstrate the effect of fatigue if the glenoid centre line and humerus are not aligned. Try maintaining the arm or lifting an object with the scapula deliberately retracted. With the scapula correctly protracted, the glenohumeral joint stabilizes with ease, making more muscle action available for power.

Rupture of the serratus anterior is a rare condition associated with severe pain. It is not infrequently diagnosed but rarely proven.[6] When found, it may be in conjunction with a rupture of the rhomboideus major. The treatment is reattachment. This condition has been reported in elderly rheumatoid patients on long-term steroid therapy. In these patients operative treatment is probably unnecessary.

Long thoracic nerve palsy is the major cause of serratus anterior weakness. This nerve is formed from the roots of C5, C6 and C7 immediately after leaving their intervertebral foramina. It runs collaterally to the main brachial plexus and is often spared in traction lesions. The cause of isolated serratus palsy is often difficult to explain, but may follow viral illness, carrying objects on the shoulder, open iatrogenic injury in the axilla, lying on the operating table and following long periods of anaesthesia. It is also described after recumbency for a prolonged period of time and immunization but these causes are rarely encountered in clinical practice. Recently, Kauppila and Vastamaki[7] presented 17 cases of iatrogenic causes. These occurred during seven operations for first rib resection, four mastectomies with axillary clearance, two scalenotomies, two surgical procedures for spontaneous pneumothorax, two infraclavicular plexus anaesthetic blocks, nine post-general anaesthesia and one after spinal anaesthesia. Of these cases only one recovered spontaneously.

Palsies occurring after closed trauma are usually traction lesions, and spontaneous recovery can be anticipated. Recovery is usually seen by 1 year; in

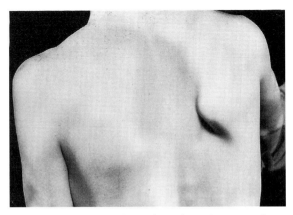

Fig. 10.5 Winging due to long thoracic nerve palsy.

cases persisting beyond a year the prognosis is poor, although some may still recover at 2–3 years.

The major problem is pain with difficulty lifting the arm (Figure 10.5) and discomfort from winging when sitting against a chair back. Lifting weights is difficult. The shoulder may also be painful at rest as a consequence of functional impingement within the subacromial space. There is little useful treatment. Vastamak described the use of a shoulder cap brace, but it is uncomfortable and rarely tolerated. However, it may be of value in selected patients required to lift at work. Many patients learn to live with the disability and thus few come to surgery. There is no place for nerve repair and the only option is tendon transfer. Pectoralis major transfer with a fascia lata graft to the lower pole of the scapula gives satisfactory results (Figure 10.6).[8] Although this procedure is considered to be a dynamic transfer, it is possible that some of the benefits are derived from a tenodesis effect. Pectoralis minor has been used but is probably of insufficient strength to act as an active transfer.

Pectoralis major transfer

The patient is placed in the lateral decubitus position, with a rolled blanket placed under the chest to relieve pressure on the arm underneath. The arm is draped free.

The original description advises a single incision of approximately 17 cm running along the inferior margin of the pectoralis major across the

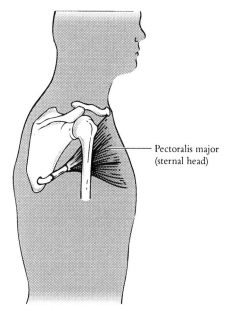

Fig. 10.6 Transfer of pectoralis major with fascia lata graft for serratus anterior palsy.

Pectoralis major
(sternal head)

GLOBAL WEAKNESS OF THE SCAPULAR STABILIZERS

Generalized weakness of the scapular stabilizers is commonly seen with many injuries and conditions affecting the shoulder. Careful examination will often demonstrate minor winging even in the absence of stiffness of the glenohumeral joint. However, if the weakness is severe, the relative strength of the deltoid is much greater. On elevation of the arm, this imbalance allows the deltoid to pull up the scapula causing winging. Duchenne[9] showed this mechanism of winging of the scapula in his treatise *The Physiology of Motion* (Figure 10.7). This is the situation in muscular dystrophies affecting the muscles of the scapula.

Muscle dystrophies should be considered in cases of atraumatic onset of weakness and atrophy

chest to the anterior axillary line and down the lateral margin of the scapula to the inferior angle of the scapula. Alternatively two incisions can be used; the first is a lower deltopectoral approach extended into the axilla as far as the posterior fold and the second is approximately 4 cm in length placed just medial to the lower pole of the scapula. The insertion of the sternal head of the pectoralis major is detached from the humerus and is dissected free from the clavicular head. The pectoralis major is split to form a fish mouth. The split must not be deeper than 6.5 cm to avoid damaging its nerve supply. A rolled or tubulated piece of fascia lata about 10 cm long and 3.5 cm wide is taken and sutured into the split in the pectoralis major. The inferior one-third of the scapula is exposed and a hole made through the scapula about 2 cm from its inferior angle and 1.5 cm medial to its lateral border. A passage is made by blunt dissection under the brachial plexus. The graft is taken through this passage and the hole in the scapula. It is sutured upon itself with slight tension. The incisions are closed in layers.

Wearing of a sling is advised for 8 weeks. A standard rehabilitation regime is employed to regain range of movement and strength.

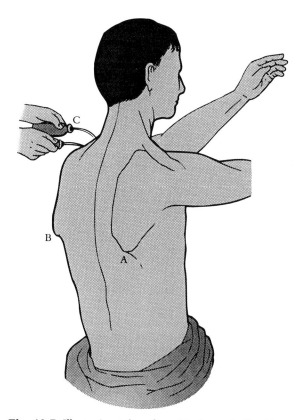

Fig. 10.7 Illustration taken from Duchenne's *Physiology of Motion*[10] showing faradic stimulation creating winging of the scapula.

occurring in the first and second decade. The commonest type is fascioscapulohumeral dystrophy. This is an autosomal recessive condition, and, on questioning, a family history may be elicited. This is a bilateral condition but on presentation it is usually unilateral; the other side may not develop until months or even years later. Involvement of the facial muscle may be detected early with the child's inability to whistle or blow out candles on his or her birthday cake. This condition has a variable muscle involvement and prognosis. There is usually good life expectancy and slow deterioration. The deltoid is spared but loses its stable origin and tilts the scapula rather than raises the humerus. The cosmetic appearance caused by the selective muscle loss is characteristic and may cause difficulty with clothing (Figure 10.8).

In these conditions there is global involvement, therefore there is no suitable muscle transfer. If the disability increases with function of the deltoid muscle, preserved scapulothoracic fusion should be considered. This operation recreates the stable origin by anchoring the scapula to the fourth, fifth and sixth ribs. This procedure was described by Copeland and Howard.[10] There are many technical variations performed but the principles remain the same. The results in 11 shoulders were reported with an average range of 90° flexion and 100° abduction. There was no deterioration with time and the vital capacity was preserved. The most frequent complication reported is stress fracture, which was treated by immobilization in a sling.

Thoracoscapular fusion

The patient is initially placed supine to harvest sufficient corticocancellous bone graft from the iliac crest in the usual manner. The patient is then moved into the prone position with the arm free and supported on an adjustable stool.

An incision is made along the medial border of the scapula. The atrophied muscles on the under and superficial surface are denuded 2 cm laterally. The subjacent three ribs (usually fourth, fifth and sixth) are exposed by subperiosteal dissection. Retractors are placed under the ribs to protect

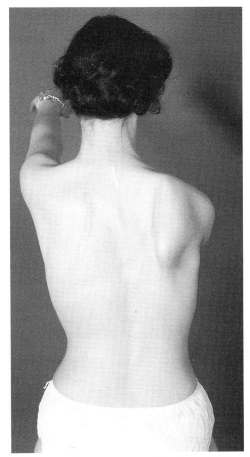

Fig. 10.8 Typical appearance of fascioscapulohumeral dystrophy.

the pleura. Corticocancellous grafts are placed between each rib and the scapula. Three to four screws are inserted taking care that they do not protrude into the pleura. Chips of bone are packed between the grafts. The patient is turned carefully. The shoulder should be immobilized in 50° abduction and 30° forward flexion with sufficient internal rotation to place the hand in front of the mouth.

A spica cast or shoulder brace is worn for 3 months. On removal, the abduction is slowly decreased with wedges.

An alternative method of fixation is with Lucque wires through drill holes in the scapula, possibly incorporating a pelvic reconstruction plate on the posterior surface to increase the strength of fixation. With this method it may be unnecessary to immobilize the shoulder in a sling.

LOSS OF THE SCAPULAR SUSPENSORY MECHANISM

I have already discussed how the upper fibres of the trapezius contribute to the suspensory mechanism. The coracoclavicular ligaments are also important static suspensory structures. They not only prevent the scapula from dropping but also prevent posterior displacement of the clavicle and protraction of the scapula (Figure 10.1).

An injury commonly not recognized is described by Rockwood & Matsen[11] and termed 'scapulothoracic dissociation'. This results from violent lateral displacement of the scapula with fracture of the clavicle and disruption of the soft tissues. Vessel or brachial plexus damage may occur with these injuries. There is also a more discrete type of injury in which there is stretching of the scapular stabilizers usually associated with type IV acromioclavicular joint separations and displaced clavicular fractures, particularly those of the lateral third. The increased distance from the spinous processes to the medial border of the scapula can be appreciated on clinical examination or on the chest radiograph. Similarly protraction of the scapula with soft tissue stretching is seen with malunion and non-union of the clavicle.

Restoration of the skeletal injury even with repair of the disrupted ligaments may be insufficient to correct the deformity and specific rehabilitation of the scapular muscles must be stressed.

PSEUDO OR OBLIGATORY WINGING

Obligatory winging is seen after glenohumeral fusion. This is rarely of significance with the exception of arthrodesis for brachial plexus injury. In some cases of C5 and C6 root avulsion, the upper part of the serratus anterior may be denervated. This should be assessed before surgery.

Injuries to the upper roots of the brachial plexus during childbirth may also cause winging of the scapula. Anterior contracture and capsular tightness develops with posterior subluxation of the humeral head and stretching of the posterior capsule. The glenohumeral joint becomes fixed in abduction, so that, when the shoulder is forced into adduction and external rotation, superior winging due to the contracture occurs known as the scapular sign of Putti.

An abduction contracture of the deltoid may cause secondary winging. This is not so rare with many cases reported and should be looked for in clinical practice.[12] It is often bilateral and usually affects the anterior part of the deltoid. Two types occur: congenital and secondary to multiple intramuscular injections. The treatment is by release of fibrous bands and manipulation. A defect in the deltoid may result and require closure by transfer of the posterior deltoid anteriorly. Displacement of the scapula and pseudo-winging may be seen with large subscapular osteochondromata.

VOLUNTARY WINGING

Rowe[13] describes four patients with voluntary winging. A more common appearance of winging is seen in habitual or voluntary glenohumeral instability. In this situation the ability to sublux the shoulder requires winging of the scapula to destabilize the glenohumeral joint.

REFERENCES

1. Neer, C.S. (1990) *Shoulder Reconstruction.* Philadelphia: W.B. Saunders.
2. Lange, M. (1951) Die Behandlung der irreparablem trapeziuslahmung. *Langenbecks Arch. Klin. Chir.* **270:** 437–439.
3. Langenskiold, A. & Ryoppy, S. (1973) Treatment of paralysis of the trapezius muscle by the Eden–Lange operation. *Acta Orthop. Scand.* **44:** 383–388.
4. Bigliani, L.U., Perez-Sanz, J.R. & Wolfe, I.R. (1985)

Treatment of trapezius paralysis. *J. Bone Joint Surg.* **67A:** 871–876.

5. Dewar, F.P. & Harris, R.I. (1950) Restoration of function of the shoulder following paralysis of the trapezius by fascial sling fixation and transplantation of the levator scapulae. *Ann. Surg.* **132:** 1111–1115.

6. Hayes, J.M. & Zehr, D.J. (1981) Traumatic muscle avulsion causing winging of the scapula. *J. Bone Joint Surg.* **63A:** 495–497.

7. Kauppila, L.I. & Vastamaki, M. (1995) Iatrogenic serratus anterior paralysis: long-term outcome in 26 cases. 6th International Congress on Surgery of the Shoulder, Helsinki, June 1995. Paper no. 199.

8. Marmor, L. and Bechtol, C.O. (1963) Paralysis of the serratus anterior due to electric shock relieved by transplantation of the pectoralis major muscle. A case report. *J. Bone Joint Surg.* **45A:** 156–160.

9. Duchenne, G.B. (1949) *The Physiology of Motion.* Philadelphia: J.B. Lippincott.

10. Copeland, S.A. & Howard, R.C. (1978) Thoracoscapular fusion for fascioscapulohumeral dystrophy. *J. Bone Joint Surg.* **60B:** 547–551.

11. Rockwood, C.R. & Matsen, F.A. (1990) *The Shoulder.* Philadelphia: W.B. Saunders.

12. Mullaji, A. (1992) Idiopathic contracture of deltoid – A report of 3 cases. *J. Orthop. Surg.* **6:** 164–167.

13. Rowe, C.R. (1988) *The Shoulder.* New York: Churchill Livingstone.

11

Classification of Instability

PT Calvert

INTRODUCTION

There is a tendency to regard classification as an exercise in learning for the purpose of examinations. It is true that those classifications that merely serve to perpetuate the name of their originator should be regarded in that light and be deleted from the literature. Classification is important when it aids in determining treatment or prognosis. It is also essential for the purpose of communication. Finally proper classification allows different groups of workers to compare outcomes.

Nowhere is classification more important in all these three aspects than with instability of the shoulder. It follows therefore that there should be common agreement about terminology, that it should be easy to place each 'case' into the appropriate box and that each group should have differences either in their management or prognosis.

In general terms classifications can be based on various parameters which can be broadly divided into clinical, radiological and pathological. With shoulder instability it is the clinical and pathological that are important. Radiological features may be used to help place a particular patient into one or other clinical category but do not provide a classification on their own. This chapter will concentrate on the clinical classification because it is this that is most important for determining both treatment and prognosis. Pathological findings are important and need to be classified but usually patients can be categorized before the precise anatomical abnormality is defined.

INCIDENCE AND PROGNOSIS

The shoulder is the joint that is most commonly dislocated. It accounts for about 45% of all dislocations.[1] It is difficult to determine the precise population incidence. In a study by Kroner et al[2] it was determined that the incidence of glenohumeral dislocation was 17 per 100 000 population per year. When anterior dislocations alone were considered the incidence was 16.5 per 100 000 per year. If only primary dislocations were included the figure fell to 12.3 per 100 000 per year. There were two age-related peaks: one in men between the ages of 21 and 30 years and a second in women between 61 and 80 years. In that study the incidence of associated nerve lesions was 7.4% with a 2.8% incidence of axillary nerve damage. Hovelius[3] in a random sample of the Swedish population between the ages of 18 and 70 years found that the prevalence was 1.7% in the general population and 8% in ice hockey players.

Considering injuries around the shoulder girdle, Nordqvist and Petersson[4] found that in 504 shoulder injuries, fractures of the proximal humerus were most frequent (53%), followed by clavicular fractures (29%) and then primary dislocations of the glenohumeral joint (11%). If one looks at only dislocations around the shoulder girdle then one study found that anterior dislocation of the glenohumeral joint accounted for 84%, the acromioclavicular joint for 12%, the sternoclavicular for 2.5% and only 1.5% were posterior glenohumeral dislocations. It is likely that the incidence of posterior instability is underestimated because approximately 60% of acute posterior dislocations are missed. In addition Gerber and Ganz[5] have shown that, if one looks carefully for posterior instability using appropriate clinical tests, the frequency of diagnosis of the condition rises.

The natural history and prognosis following an initial anterior dislocation has been best studied by Hovelius[6–8] in a prospective study of 257 patients no older than 40 years. These patients were reviewed at 2, 5 and 10 years. Immobilization made no difference to the prognosis. Age was the most important prognostic factor with a recurrence rate of at least 60% for those under 25 years compared with less than 25% for those over 34 years. Interestingly in each group only about half of those who had recurrences had an operation by the time of the 10-year follow-up; of those who had not had an operation, some had stabilized and some were living with their instability. Fracture of the greater tuberosity improved the prognosis for recurrence and a Hill–Sachs lesion made it slightly worse.

HISTORY

Recurrent dislocation of the shoulder was certainly recognized in Egyptian times as evidenced by murals on tombs from several thousand years BC depicting methods of reduction. As is well known Hippocrates in ancient Greece described the method of closed reduction which still bears his name. What is less well known is his description of a method of surgical treatment of recurrent dislocation which involved cauterizing the anterior structures with a hot iron through a subcutaneous approach. This must be the forerunner of arthroscopic laser cauterization! Various methods were described in the 18th century for reduction of the dislocated shoulder but it was not until the late 19th century and early part of this century that the pathology really began to be defined. Although Hill and Sachs are credited with the posterolateral humeral head defect associated with anterior dislocation, it was first described by Flower in 1861. Caird in 1887 described both the humeral head defect and the detached labrum and capsule. Both these lesions were again

described by Broca and Hartman in 1890. Strictly Perthes in 1906 should be credited with the idea that the detached labrum and capsule be surgically reattached to the glenoid rim. It was Blundell Bankart in his classic papers, who brought this procedure to the prominence which it still maintains and as a result bears his name. Thereafter traumatic recurrent anterior dislocation was, except in a few isolated instances, regarded as the only significant shoulder instability until about the middle 1960s. This had the unfortunate consequence that all instabilities were treated in the same manner with inevitable failure in those incorrectly classified.

Carter Rowe published his paper on the prognosis of recurrent instability in 1956.[9] He noted that 98% were anterior and only 2% posterior. He also stated in this paper that dislocations could be grouped as atraumatic and traumatic with 4.4% in the former group. This was really the start of a modern classification of shoulder instability. In 1969 Blazina and Saltzman[10] described recurrent transient subluxation as opposed to dislocation; this was further publicized by Rowe and Zarins in 1981 and 1987.[11,12] Others, such as Rockwood and co-workers[13,14] have emphasized the importance of distinguishing between traumatic and atraumatic instability and have devised specific classifications for subluxation. In 1980 Neer and Foster[15] introduced the concept of multidirectional instability and described the procedure of inferior capsular shift to treat the condition. Subsequently not only has the aetiology and direction been defined but also the degree, frequency, chronicity and volition have all become components of the classification. Further words such as laxity, hyperlaxity and habitual have been added to the various descriptions of instability. This has created some confusion with the terminology. The first task therefore is to define the terms.

DEFINITION OF TERMINOLOGY

Laxity versus instability

It has been suggested that a suitable definition for instability is the inability to maintain the humeral head centred in the glenoid fossa. Instability implies that there is an undesirable component to the problem. A better definition therefore is the symptomatic inability to maintain the humeral head centred in the glenoid fossa.

It is important to distinguish between shoulder joint laxity and instability. Shoulder joint laxity means that the humeral head can be passively translated across the glenoid more than one would expect in the normal individual. This need not be symptomatic and can be associated with perfectly normal function. Matsen's group compared 16 subjects requiring surgery for symptomatic instability with eight normal subjects. The 16 symptomatic subjects included eight with recurrent traumatic instability and eight with an atraumatic aetiology. They found that objective measurements of anterior and posterior draw, sulcus sign, push–pull and fulcrum tests were no different between the groups.[16] Adolescents, in particular, can have asymptomatic laxity.[17]

Shoulders which are quite lax can be completely stable. Conversely shoulders without significant laxity can be symptomatically unstable. The diagnosis of instability depends on identifying the symptomatic problem for the individual patient.

Direction

The concept of anterior and posterior are easy to comprehend. The vast majority of traumatic dislocations are anterior (98%) with a much smaller proportion (2%) being posterior. Even within this fairly straightforward distinction between anterior and posterior the direction of the instability should strictly be defined as either anteroinferior or posteroinferior because in reality that is where the humeral head crosses the glenoid margin and where the pathology is seen.

Multidirectional instability (MDI) is a much more difficult concept to grasp and is a term that is used somewhat loosely. To make a diagnosis of MDI there should be an inferior component to the instability. This implies that there is some degree of shoulder joint laxity and a positive sulcus sign. A shoulder in which the predominant direction of the instability is either anterior or posterior but there is in addition inferior laxity can

be said to exhibit MDI. It is also possible to have a shoulder which is unstable both anteriorly and posteriorly and has inferior laxity; this shoulder certainly has MDI. The shoulder which has instability in both an anterior and posterior direction but without inferior laxity is not really one with MDI. This situation is a rarity but can occur after separate episodes of trauma causing structural damage to both the anterior and posterior structures.

Chronicity

There is no trouble with understanding the term acute dislocation. In this context acute means a single symptomatic episode of instability. If these acute episodes occur more than once then the situation is one of recurrent instability. If a dislocation or subluxation occurs and remains unreduced then this should be termed a chronic dislocation or subluxation.

Degree

Complete separation of the joint surfaces is a dislocation. At least as common in the shoulder is partial separation of the joint surfaces; this is subluxation. The essential point to understand about recurrent subluxation is that it may not present as obvious instability but as pain or as a 'dead arm' with overhead activities; it can be difficult to diagnose.

Volition

It should be easy to avoid confusion with the terms voluntary and involuntary. Unfortunately the term habitual enters into the equation and has been used in some instances as synonymous with voluntary. This should be avoided. Voluntary instability should be reserved to describe those shoulders where the patient actively dislocates or subluxes the shoulder with a deliberate voluntary muscle contraction. Habitual should be used to describe those shoulders where the humeral head dislocates or subluxes every time the shoulder passes through a particular phase of movement. The usual situation is the adolescent with posterior habitual subluxation. This is not necessarily voluntary although the two may coexist.

Involuntary means that the humeral head is unstable without a deliberate voluntary muscle contraction on the part of the patient.

Another conceptual problem which tends to arise once the patient is labelled as having either voluntary or habitual instability is the idea that these patients are psychiatrically disturbed. This is untrue. There are a few patients with deliberate voluntary dislocation who do have personality or other psychiatric disorders[18] but the majority of patients with habitual instability are normal. Nevertheless this does introduce the idea that in the classification of both voluntary and habitual instability there are those patients with psychiatric abnormalities and those who are psychiatrically normal.

Aetiology

In the classification of shoulder instability an important distinction is between traumatic and atraumatic. The reader might think that the differentiation into these two groups would be easy. Unfortunately that is not always the case. The individual who has a previously normal shoulder, goes into a tackle on the football field, sustains a major contact injury to the shoulder and ends up with an anterior dislocation of the shoulder clearly has a traumatic aetiology. The difficulty arises because patients frequently look in retrospect for a traumatic cause and then site some relatively minor injury. Some patients with relatively lax shoulders do sustain an injury, which initiates their subsequent recurrent episodes of instability, but the injury is of such a relatively minor nature that it would not have been expected to render a normal shoulder unstable. There is a spectrum ranging between the obviously traumatic and those with no injury; these latter should clearly be classified as atraumatic. It is important to try to categorize the patients into a broadly traumatic group as against a mainly atraumatic group. To achieve this requires a good history of the initiating episode. To be clearly traumatic the initial injury should be of sufficient severity that it would be reason-

able to have expected it to cause structural damage.

There are the difficult group of patients who gradually stretch out their shoulders as a result of repetitive overuse at the limits of normal physiological performance. These are the high-level throwing athletes. Whether they should be separately classified is debatable but what is certain is that their treatment needs to be specific. An appreciation of the aetiology is therefore important.

CLASSIFICATION

The terms TUBS (traumatic, unidirectional, Bankart, surgery) and AMBRI (atraumatic, multidirectional, bilateral, rehabilitation, inferior shift) were coined by Thomas and Matson[19] and have achieved a certain popularity. They are easy to remember and essentially classify instability into two major groups. Not only do the acronyms indicate aetiology, clinical presentation and pathology but also give guidance about treatment. Although this is a good starting point it is probably too simplistic for a comprehensive classification today.

The algorithmic approach proposed by Silliman & Hawkins[20] is, in the author's opinion, preferable. This includes all the clinical elements that have been discussed in the preceding paragraphs: volition, trauma, direction, chronology and degree. The algorithm illustrated in Figure 11.1 is a modification of that described by Silliman & Hawkins.

The first question to ask and answer is whether there is a voluntary component to the instability. A small group of patients will have a voluntary component. The question 'can you put the shoulder out yourself?' can be surprisingly revealing. If there is a voluntary component, then it is necessary to decide whether there is an associated emotional or psychiatric abnormality. Most are normal.

The great majority of patients with shoulder instability fall into the involuntary group. The next major division is between traumatic and

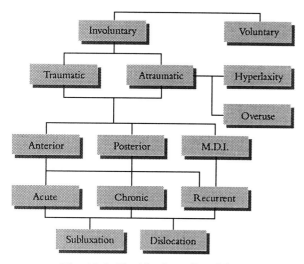

Fig. 11.1 Classification of instability.

atraumatic ensuring that the trauma associated with the initial episode of instability is sufficient to cause structural damage.

The next thing to determine is direction; this is usually possible after a good history and clinical examination but may require some ancillary tests such as examination under anaesthesia or arthroscopy. Then a question about chronology needs to be asked. Is the instability a single acute episode? If it is repeated acute episodes, then the instability is recurrent. If the shoulder subluxed or dislocated and has remained in that situation, then it is chronic; the usual example of this is the chronic missed posterior dislocation. Finally the degree or extent of the instability completes the classification. Is it subluxation or dislocation?

At the end of this exercise it should be possible to classify the instability and therefore move on to management (Figure 11.1).

MECHANISMS OF GLENOHUMERAL STABILITY

In order to understand and classify the various pathological lesions which may contribute to instability it is necessary first to consider those mechanisms that maintain the normal stability of the joint.

The glenohumeral joint is remarkable for its great range of movement. There is virtually no intrinsic bony stability. It must therefore depend on other mechanisms to retain the humeral head centred in the glenoid. These can be divided into static and dynamic restraints. In general terms the static stabilizers consist of the labrum, the capsule and ligaments whereas the dynamic component of stability is provided by the muscles. Although it is possible to categorize them in this fashion for the purposes of analysis, in reality each affects the other and, as will be seen from the ensuing discussion, their effects are interrelated.

Anatomical shape of the glenoid–labrum complex

Although the bony contour of the glenoid appears rather flat as seen on a plain radiograph, this is a misleading representation of the true situation as anyone who has looked into the shoulder with an arthroscope will know. First the articular cartilage on the glenoid is thicker at the margins than in the centre;[21] this in itself produces some degree of concavity with a radius of curvature similar to that of the humeral head. The labrum provides an extension of this concavity and it has been suggested that the labrum contributes as much as 50% to the total depth of the glenoid.[22] This leads on to the concept of concavity compression. If there is an axial loading force, then even a relatively small concavity becomes important for resisting translation forces. Matsen's group[16,23] have investigated this; they applied a compressive load perpendicular to the glenoid surface and then applied increasing tangential forces until the humeral head dislocated over the glenoid rim; because the shape of the glenoid fossa is not ovoid and the anatomy varies according to the position on the circumference, the forces were applied in eight different directions at 45° angles. Doubling the compressive force from 50 to 100 N increased the required translational force by about 75%. As one might expect, they found that the least translation force was required in the anterior and posterior directions and the greatest in the directly superior or inferior directions; this correlated with the greater depth of the concavity in the supero-inferior plane. In addition, resection of the labrum reduced the average effective depth of the concavity from 4.9 to 3.4 mm and the required translational force was reduced by 20%. It follows from these basic scientific experiments that anything that reduces the glenoid concavity would be expected to encourage instability. Hence glenoid rim fractures, a torn labrum or a flat glenoid would all be expected to contribute to instability, which is exactly what one finds in practice.

Capsuloligamentous restraints

In order to permit the great range of motion that is characteristic of the normal shoulder, the capsule must be relatively loose and mobile. It would be impossible for the shoulder to have strong isokinetic ligaments as exist, for example, in the knee and ankle. Nevertheless there are some condensations of the capsule which form the superior, middle and inferior glenohumeral ligaments (SGHL, MGHL, IGHL). Until the advent of shoulder arthroscopy, these were not properly appreciated as anatomical structures. Once identified considerable attention has been focused upon their function. Warner,[24] amongst others, using cadaveric specimens has looked at the role of these in maintaining glenohumeral stability. What has been shown is that the contribution of the ligaments varies according to the position of the arm. With the arm by the side the SGHL was the most important ligament for resisting inferior translation. At 45° of abduction all three ligaments were in their loosest position but with increasing amounts of abduction the IGHL became the more important restraint. In the abducted shoulder with neutral humeral rotation, the SGHL, MGHL and IGHL contributed equally in preventing anterior humeral translation. When the humeral head was externally rotated, the importance of the IGHL increased markedly and the restraining effect of the other two became insignificant. At 90° of abduction, internal and external rotation causes reciprocal tightening of the anterior and posterior parts of the IGHL.

Mechanically these ligaments can be regarded as check reins which tighten in different positions of the humerus. Another analogy is that of the hammock in which the two supporting ropes sag equally when the occupant lies in the middle. As he rolls to one side the rope on that side tightens and prevents spillage over the edge.

The other possible role of the glenohumeral ligaments is a biological one as the site of joint position receptors. This is an attractive concept because it would help to explain why even small disruptions of such relatively flimsy structures appear to have such a great effect on stability. Nerve endings characteristic of joint position receptors have been found histologically concentrated particularly in the IGHL but the physiological significance of this finding has yet to be established.

The state of the rotator interval seems also to be important when considering capsular restraints. Harryman et al[25] investigated this aspect in a cadaveric study. Resistance to anterior, posterior and inferior translation was tested with the capsule in the rotator interval in its normal state, after it had been divided and after it had been plicated. Division increased posterior and inferior instability to passive translational forces whereas placation decreased it. Once more this tallies with the clinical experience that the rotator interval is often deficient in those patients with unstable shoulders and some degree of capsular laxity. Operatively it is important to identify and correct this deficiency if it is present.

An extension of this type of capsular deficiency is the older patient who sustains a traumatic dislocation of the shoulder with an associated rotator cuff rupture. This has been well documented and can lead to instability. The rotator cuff tear in this situation is usually a long radial split extending along or just posterior to the rotator interval in the substance of the supraspinatus with an avulsion of the anterior attachment of the supraspinatus. The cuff posterior to the tear tends to fall backwards over the humeral head compromising both the static and dynamic contributions to stability. It is essential to identify and correct this lesion in order to restore stability, hence the importance of recognizing it in any pathological classification.

Negative intra-articular pressure

Two studies[26,27] have demonstrated that there is a contribution, at least in the experimental situation, to stability as a result of a negative intra-articular pressure gradient. Certainly such a negative pressure exists. When a needle or the arthroscope is inserted into the joint without predistension, there is an audible inrush of air. Venting the glenohumeral joint with a needle in cadaveric specimens reduces the amount of translational force required to displace the humeral head in relation to the glenoid. Habermeyer[27] also demonstrated that increasing traction caused a decrease in intra-articular pressure in stable shoulders but not in those with unstable shoulders and a Bankart lesion. This suggests that repairing the Bankart lesion not only restores the static capsuloligamentous restraints but may also be important in restoring the integrity of the 'suction cup' which allows the negative pressure to work. The reader can verify this himself with a simple experiment using any item such as a child's arrow which has a rubber sucker on its end. When the sucker is pushed down on to a smooth hard surface such as glass it sticks firmly. If one cuts even a small piece out of the circumference of the sucker it ceases to stick.

Dynamic restraints

Tension in the rotator cuff muscles is important in retaining the humeral head centred in the glenoid. Blasier et al[28] showed in a cadaveric model that tension in all of the rotator cuff muscles was important in resisting anterior dislocation of the humeral head on the glenoid. If one considers again the hypothesis of concavity compresssion, then the only mechanism whereby an axial force at 90° to the glenoid can be applied, when the shoulder is in neutral abduction, is by contraction of the rotator cuff muscles. In the situation where the humerus is abducted in relation to the scapula, it is possible for other muscles such as the deltoid to contribute to such a perpendicular force. In the ultimate situation where the scapula is fully rotated and the glenoid pointing directly upwards, it is theoretically possible for the humeral head to

remain balanced on the glenoid without any applied force. This is akin to the juggler who balances a ball on the end of a stick. Provided that the downward force through the centre of gravity of the ball passes directly down the stick it will stay there. A minor deviation to one side and it falls off. In reality this situation never exists in the shoulder because it is probable that the glenoid is never pointing exactly vertically upwards and, secondly, there are always muscle forces acting across the articulation. It does serve to introduce the concept of balance.

Balance (Figures 11.2 and 11.3)

This concept brings together all the factors that have been discussed in the preceding paragraphs. For the humeral head to remain stable in the glenoid in all positions, the resultant of all the forces (F) acting on the humeral head must pass somewhere through the glenoid arc (XY). The more centrally orientated this force the more stable is the articulation. Anything that serves to tip the glenoid in relation to the axis of the humerus decreases the stability. Hence scapula position in relation to the humerus is important for stability as is proper balanced action of the scapulothoracic muscles. Anything that shortens the arc of the glenoid reduces the stability in the direction of the deficiency because the resultant force more easily falls outside the glenoid arc. Hence rim fractures or labral deficiency reduce stability. The greater the depth of the concavity,

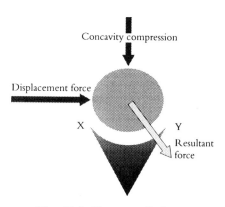

Fig. 11.2 Concept of balance.

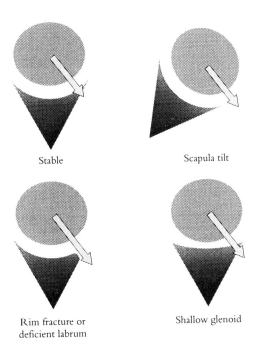

Fig. 11.3 Mechanisms of instability.

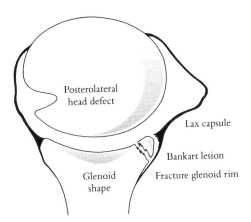

Fig. 11.4 Pathology of anterior instability.

the easier it is for the juggler to balance the ball on the pole and the greater is the arc through which the forces are still acting through the glenoid; a shallow glenoid for whatever reason reduces stability. Finally the muscles themselves must remain balanced in their action. If one component of the muscle couple is contracting inappropriately, then this in itself can cause instability. Even more dramatic is where both components of a muscle couple are out of phase so that what should be contracting is relaxed and vice versa. This is the mechanism of instability for both the habitual and the voluntary dislocator.

PATHOLOGICAL LESIONS

If one has understood the theory of the stabilizing mechanisms, it is a short step to understanding the pathological lesions. It also becomes clear why it is important to classify the instability both clinically and pathologically. It is only by so doing that it becomes possible to apply an appropriate treatment. The easiest way to describe the pathological

lesions is by a composite illustration showing the various possibilities (Figure 11.4).

Diagnosis

It has been agreed that it is necessary to identify the clinical type and the pathology of the instability in order to apply appropriate treatment. The question therefore arises as to how to achieve this end. It should be possible in 90% of instances of instability to arrive at the correct diagnosis after a careful history, a thorough clinical examination and possibly a few well-chosen plain radiographs. Ancillary sophisticated investigations such as magnetic resonance scans and arthroscopy should rarely be necessary.

The history is probably the most important tool. It is easy to arrive at the correct diagnosis when the patient presents with a clinically obvious anterior dislocation, a history of a significant injury to the shoulder on the sports field or in a fall and previous episodes of radiologically proven similar dislocations. No further evidence is required. However, not all patients with recurrent anterior instability present in this manner; some may even present with pain alone.

The patient with recurrent anterior subluxation may present with a history of injury in which the arm was forcibly abducted and extended as, for example, in going into a rugby football tackle. The shoulder may have been painful at the time and for a few days to a few weeks after the event.

There is no documented dislocation or even subluxation except that sometimes the patient will say 'I felt the shoulder pop-out'. Subsequently the patient reports that every time he goes into a tackle it is painful and 'gives way'. Similarly the patient who complains that the arm 'feels dead' when she serves at tennis is probably suffering from recurrent anterior instability.[11]

The exact history of the initial episode is essential. It must include the presence or absence of significant trauma and precisely what happened both during the event and subsequently. An accurate description of what movements or actions cause further symptoms can help to establish both the diagnosis of instability and its direction; in racquet sports, pain with overhead shots is more likely to indicate an anteroinferior direction whereas pain on a backhand is more indicative of a posterior instability. Questions such as 'are you very bendy' or 'can you ever put the shoulder out yourself' can be most revealing in the diagnosis of joint laxity or voluntary instability.

The age of the patient is in itself an important piece of information. In the older patient with a history of significant injury and subsequent instability a rotator cuff tear must be considered. Beware the patient under 40 years of age who presents with what appears to be an impingement syndrome. This may well be secondary to instability. The importance of recognizing this factor lies in the response to treatment. If the impingement alone is treated, then only about 10% good results will be achieved, whereas if the instability is addressed, 90% response can be expected. There is a spectrum ranging from pure instability to pure impingement and it is clearly important to recognize where in that spectrum any particular patient lies. The age of the patient is the most important factor in prognosis for recurrence after a first dislocation[6–8] as has already been discussed; this is clearly important when advising about treatment.

The history of previous treatment is important. In a young patient with impingement secondary to instability the usual good response to local steroid injections is often absent and should be another factor that alerts the clinician to the true diagnosis. Many patients will have had some form of physiotherapy treatment. It is not good enough to merely record the fact that physiotherapy has taken place. One wants to know exactly what modalities of treatment were used. If an exercise programme was prescribed, what was its nature. It is quite possible that inappropriate regimes have been applied because the exact nature of the problem had not been appreciated. In that situation it may be relevant to discuss with the therapist the possibility of further treatment of a different type. If an operation has been performed and symptoms persist or recur, then the history of the original problem becomes doubly important as does the response to the operation. It is important to remember that amongst the commoner causes of failure of surgical treatments for instability are incorrect diagnosis, incorrect classification, particularly with respect to direction of the instability, and failure to address the pathology, particularly a Bankart lesion. In the patient with a failed operation for instability a good history will usually direct the clinician to which of these causes is most likely.

Examination

The general approach to examination has already been covered in Chapter 1 and will not be repeated here. Some of the important aspects of the examination specifically related to instability will be highlighted.

The features of an acute anterior dislocation are well known with loss of the normal rounded contour of the shoulder which has become squared and the humeral head palpable anteroinferiorly. Acute and even chronic posterior dislocation is frequently missed. This should not happen if a careful examination is carried out. Inspection of the contour of the shoulder will reveal a prominence posteriorly which is the humeral head. Anteriorly the coracoid is more prominent and there is a dip where the humeral head would normally be felt anteriorly. The other feature of a posterior dislocation that should give a clue to the diagnosis is the fixed internal rotation.

Any features of generalized joint laxity should be recorded. When examining the range of movement it is worth noting that a high proportion of those with recurrent anterior instability have a greater than average range of external rotation. Whether this is caused by anterior capsular laxity or by altered humeral torsion is a moot point but from a practical point of view it is important to know about the range before contemplating any surgical repair. There is a wide range of 'normal' external rotation but those patients with limited external rotation cannot afford to lose any more whereas in those with, for example, 80° of external rotation a loss of even 30° will not be disastrous and may even be desirable.

The specific laxity tests (see Chapter 1), namely the sulcus sign, anterior and posterior drawer, should be evaluated. The apprehension tests both for anterior and posterior instability are essential. The anterior apprehension test is more valuable than is the posterior. It is important that the anterior test be carried out in various positions of elevation (90°, 120°, 150°) and the level at which it becomes positive recorded. A positive test is when the patient looks apprehensive, visibly resists the manoeuvre by contracting the pectoralis major and says that he is experiencing his feeling of instability. This is often expressed in terms such as 'that feels as if my shoulder is going to come out'. The relocation test of Jobe can be useful in distinguishing instability from impingement but is a difficult test to perform and interpret; however, a clear positive can be extremely useful. This test must be performed with the patient lying down and a positive test is when the pain or apprehension produced by the anterior apprehension test is abolished by repeating the manoeuvre but with posterior pressure on the humeral shaft as opposed to an anterior pull.

Radiographs

An AP and axillary view are the basic projections which should always be obtained. Sometimes in the acute situation an axillary view is not possible. Nevertheless a lateral view of some description must be obtained. If this rule is never broken, then posterior dislocations will not be missed radiologically. A tangential scapula lateral view is a very acceptable alternative. It is more difficult to interpret than an axillary view but is preferable to a transthoracic lateral view which is of virtually no value. To obtain a tangential scapula lateral the X-ray beam is directed along the plane of the scapula perpendicular to the glenoid. Further information can be obtained about posterior displacement of the humeral head from a Stripp view in which the X-ray beam is directed from above downwards with the patient leaning backwards and the X-ray plate placed flat on the table.

A West point view is designed to visualize the anterior glenoid and can be useful in delineating lip fractures.

For recurrent instability the best view to determine the presence of a posterolateral head defect is the Stryker notch view. This is taken by asking the patient to place the hand on the head with the elbow pointing forwards and then taking an AP projection of the shoulder. Small defects can be difficult to interpret and comparison with the same view of the other shoulder is often useful.

Investigations

As already stated it should be possible to diagnose and classify the majority of patients with instability after a careful history and physical examination. If doubt still exists about either the diagnosis or type of instability then possible investigations include arthrography, computed tomography (CT), CT arthrography, magnetic resonance imaging (MRI), examination under anaesthesia and arthroscopy. Each modality has its advantages and disadvantages. Plain arthrography is nowadays of little value for investigating problems relating to instability. CT is good for showing bony defects and glenoid orientation. It is non-invasive but, without the addition of contrast injection into the joint, little information is obtained about the capsule or labrum. CT arthrography is probably the best imaging modality for visualizing labral tears and evaluating the degree of capsular laxity. MRI has its advocates and is undoubtedly the best method for imaging the rotator cuff with published accuracies of between 90 and 100% for sensitivity and specificity. However it is less reliable for labral pathology and most published series quote accuracies of between 80 and 90% for equivalent sensitivities and specificities. Probably the best and most accurate method for evaluating instability is arthroscopy. Although it is invasive, it gives the opportunity to examine the shoulder under anaesthesia (regional or general) and to directly visualize the pathology. In the patient in whom the direction of the instability is uncertain, the arthroscope should provide the diagnosis; even a small posterolateral chondral humeral head defect and some damage to the anteroinferior labrum confirms the direction as being anterior, whereas no posterolateral humeral head damage and scuffing of the posteroinferior labrum makes the posterior direction certain. If there is no arthroscopic abnormality, then the diagnosis of voluntary or habitual instability should be reconsidered.

Furthermore arthroscopy allows an opportunity to decide whether treatment should be surgical and, if so, whether arthroscopic or open operation is preferable in the individual case. These subjects are covered in detail in Chapters 13 and 14.

Examination under anaesthesia

This is fully covered in Chapter 6 and the reader is referred to the excellent papers by Cofield and co-workers[29,30] on this subject, which are essential reading.

TREATMENT

Treatment of the various types of instability is not really the subject of this chapter and is covered in detail in other chapters. It will not be described in any depth here. Nevertheless it seems appropriate for completeness to give a brief outline of treatment strategies for the various types of instability.

Acute traumatic anterior dislocation

This requires immediate closed reduction by a suitable method of manipulation. Although there is currently some interest in carrying out an immediate arthroscopic stabilization in the high-class athlete after one dislocation, this cannot be justified at the present time in the average indivi-

dual. Hovelius has shown that even in the younger age groups the percentage requiring surgical stabilization over a 10-year period is no more than 75%. Hence immediate operation would result in 25% unnecessary procedures.

Recurrent traumatic anterior dislocation or subluxation

Once two or certainly three episodes of instability have occurred the chances of achieving stability without operation are small. Burkhead and Rockwood[13] showed that less than 20% of patients with recurrent traumatic subluxation responded well to an exercise regime. The patient may choose to modify their lifestyle in order to avoid operation and the appropriate decision needs to be made for each individual. The choice of operation depends on the exact nature of the pathology and the demands of the patient. There are several open procedures for dealing with recurrent traumatic anterior instability; all are between 90 and 95% successful in terms of achieving stability but some (e.g. Putti–Platt) limit external rotation more than others, whereas others (e.g. Bristow) have a slightly greater rate of complication. If there is a large Bankart lesion, it is important to repair it, and, if there is an element of capsular laxity, it is necessary to deal with it in order to avoid failure. The aim of a good operation for instability is to restore stability without losing range of motion. The best approach is to identify the pathology and address it directly.

There is increasing interest in arthroscopic stabilization. At present the overall published results for this method are not as good as for an open procedure. If, however, patients are carefully selected with appropriate pathology, then excellent results can be achieved. The ideal patient is one with several episodes of recurrent traumatic anterior dislocation or subluxation, a labral detachment, good-quality soft tissues and no significant capsular laxity.

Recurrent traumatic posterior instability

This is much rarer and more difficult to diagnose and treat than its anterior equivalent.[31,32]

Reported failure rates for operative treatment range from 12 to 50%. Most agree that first-line treatment should be conservative in the form of an exercise regime. This should be specifically directed at the rotator cuff muscles, in particular the infraspinatus and teres minor. Only if conservative measures fail should operative treatment be considered. There are a number of available operative options: reattachment of a detached posteroinferior labrum (reversed Bankart), reversed Putti–Platt, posterior capsular shift, posterior bone block, Scott glenoplasty, a rotational humeral osteotomy or a combination.

Ideally the chosen procedure should address the pathology, have a high rate of success and low incidence of complications. It is unusual to find a true detached posterior labrum, but if this is present it should be reattached. The usual pathology is posterior capsular redundancy which makes the posterior capsular shift an attractive option. It is logical to add an iliac crest bone graft if there is glenoid deficiency. If the glenoid is retroverted, then the Scott glenoplasty can be used but it should be noted that this is technically difficult and associated with a high rate of complication.

Atraumatic instability

Burkhead and Rockwood[13] have shown that as many as 80% of patients in this category will respond to a conservative treatment programme. This should be given a proper trial and operative treatment reserved for those in whom it fails. There is nearly always an element of capsular redundancy in this group of patients and any operative procedure needs to address this. Therefore some form of capsulorrhaphy will need to be included in the chosen operation. The extent of the capsular tightening and whether it is performed from the anterior or posterior side will depend on an accurate classification of the direction and degree of the instability.

Voluntary and habitual instability

There is virtually no place for operative treatment in this group of patients.[33] In those who are truly voluntary and dislocate the shoulder at will it is necessary to persuade them to stop the voluntary act. In the majority, particularly adolescents, the pattern has usually become established in the subconscious and is no longer voluntary but is involuntary and habitual. The strategy of treatment is to identify the abnormal muscle couple and teach the patient to relearn the normal pattern of muscle action. A standard strengthening regime is of no value; the muscles are not weak but acting in the wrong phase. Biofeedback has been used but the author and a specifically interested physiotherapist have been successful with a protocol which involves the three elements of explanation, analysis and retraining. In a group of 26 patients a normal pattern of muscle action has been established within an average of 2 days. A small proportion of these patients have psychiatric or emotional disturbance. Although it is rare it is important to identify and treat this problem if it is present.

Chronic dislocation

It is more common to be presented with an unreduced posterior rather than anterior dislocation. If this is more than a few days old it is likely that open reduction will be required to reduce it. With a posterior dislocation it may be worth trying a gentle closed manipulation with good image intensifier control up to 3 weeks after the event but great care is required. If reduction is achieved then the shoulder will need to be held in a spica with the shoulder in about 20° of abduction and 10° of external rotation for about 3 weeks.

If, as is more usual, the shoulder has been dislocated too long to even consider manipulation, the first decision to make with either direction is whether the disability is sufficient to warrant any intervention. The elderly patient with a chronic anterior dislocation and relatively little pain may well be best left alone and the loss of motion accepted. In most patients particularly with posterior dislocations the functional gain from relocating the joint makes it worth while. These operations are technically difficult and should be performed by someone who is experienced in shoulder surgery. An anterior approach is best for the chronic dislocation in either direction. Once the head has been relocated it is necessary to decide whether it can be preserved and what else is required to achieve stability. For posterior dislocations the head can be preserved if the head defect involves less than about 35% of the head and the version has not been altered by a fracture. If the head is preserved, the subscapularis will need to be sutured or otherwise fixed into the anterior head defect. If the head cannot be salvaged then a hemiarthroplasty is required. In either instance a spica should be used for 3 weeks in the position described in the preceding paragraph. For anterior dislocations it is necessary to identify and deal with the pathology to restore stability; a large anterior glenoid defect must be reconstructed, a rotator cuff tear in the older patient must be repaired, and a large posterolateral head defect may merit an anterior bone block. The surgeon must have the experience to execute all the available options.

REFERENCES

1. Kazar, B. & Relovszky, E. (1969) Prognosis of primary dislocation of the shoulder. *Acta Orthop. Scand.* **40:** 216.
2. Kroner, K., Lind, T. & Jensen, J. (1989) The epidemiology of shoulder dislocations. *Arch. Orthop. Trauma Surg.* **108:** 288–290.
3. Hovelius, L. (1982) Incidence of shoulder dislocation in Sweden. *Clin. Orthop.* **166:** 127–131.
4. Nordqvist, A. & Petersson, C.J. (1995) Incidence and causes of shoulder girdle injuries in an urban population. *J. Shoulder Elbow Surg.* **4:** 107–112.
5. Gerber, C. & Ganz, R. (1984) Clinical assessment of instability of the shoulder with special reference to anterior and posterior drawer tests. *J. Bone Joint Surg.* **66B:** 551–556.
6. Hovelius, L., Eriksson, K., Fredin, H., Hagberg, G., Hussenius, A., Lind, B., Thorling, J. & Weckstrom, J. (1983) Recurrences after initial dislocation of the shoulder. Results of a prospective study of treatment. *J. Bone Joint Surg.* **65A:** 343–349.
7. Hovelius, L. (1983) Anterior dislocation of the shoulder in teenagers and young adults. Five year prognosis. *J. Bone Joint Surg.* **65A:** 343–349.
8. Hovelius, L. (1995) Primary anterior dislocation of the shoulder in the young: treatment and prognostic aspects. In M. Vastamaki & P. Jalovaara (eds) *Surgery of the Shoulder.* Amsterdam: Elsevier Science B.V.
9. Rowe, C.R. (1956) Prognosis in dislocations of the shoulder. *J. Bone Joint Surg.* **38A:** 957–977.
10. Blazina, M.E. & Saltzman, J.S. (1969) Recurrent anterior subluxation of the shoulder in athletes – a distinct entity. *J. Bone Joint Surg.* **51A:** 1037–1038.
11. Rowe, C.R. & Zarins, B. (1981) Recurrent transient anterior subluxation of the shoulder. *J. Bone Joint Surg.* **63A:** 863–872.
12. Rowe, C.R. (1987) Recurrent transient anterior subluxation of the shoulder. The 'dead arm syndrome'. *Clin. Orthop.* **223:** 11–19.
13. Burkhead, W.Z. & Rockwood, C.A. (1992) Treatment of instability of the shoulder with an exercise program. *J. Bone Joint Surg.* **74A:** 890–896.
14. Rockwood, C.A. & Matsen, F.S. (eds) (1990) *The Shoulder.* Philadelphia: W.B. Saunders.
15. Neer, II C.S. & Foster, C.R. (1980) Inferior capsular shift for involuntary inferior and multidirectional instability of the shoulder. A preliminary report. *J. Bone Joint Surg.* **62A:** 897–908.
16. Matsen, F.A., Lippitt, S.B., Sidles, J.A. & Harryman, D.T. (1994) *Practical Evaluation and Management of the Shoulder.* Philadelphia: W.B. Saunders.
17. Emery, R.J.H. & Mullaji, A.B. (1991) Glenohumeral joint instability in normal adolescents. Incidence and significance. *J. Bone Joint Surg.* **73B:** 406–408.
18. Rowe, C.R., Pierce, D.S. & Clark, J.G. (1973) Voluntary dislocation of the shoulder. A preliminary report on a clinical, electromyographic and psychiatric study of twenty-six patients. *J. Bone Joint Surg.* **55A:** 445–460.
19. Thomas, S.C. & Matsen, F.A. (1989) An approach to the repair of avulsion of the glenohumeral ligaments in the management of traumatic anterior glenohumeral instability. *J. Bone Joint Surg.* **71A:** 506–513.
20. Silliman, J.F. & Hawkins, R.J. (1993) Classification and physical diagnosis of instability of the shoulder. *Clin. Orthop.* **291:** 7–19.
21. Flatow, E.L., Soslowsky, L.J., Ateshian, G.A., Ark, J.W., Pawluk, R.J., Bigliani, L.U. & Mow, V.C. (1991) Shoulder joint anatomy and the effect of subluxation and size mismatch on patterns of glenohumeral contact. *Orthop. Trans.* **15:** 803.
22. Howell, S.M., & Galinat, B.J. (1991) The glenoid-labral socket. A constrained articular surface. *Clin. Orthop.* **261:** 128.
23. Lippitt, S. & Matsen, F. (1993) Mechanisms of glenohumeral joint stability. *Clin. Orthop.* **293:** 20–28.
24. Warner, J.J., Deng, X., Warren, R.F. & Torzilli, P.A. (1992) Static capsuloligamentous restraints to superior–inferior translation of the glenohumeral joint. *Am. J. Sports Med.* **20:** 675–685.
25. Harryman, D.T., Sidles, J.A., Harris, S.L. & Matsen, F.A. (1992) The role of the rotator interval capsule in passive motion and stability of the shoulder. *J. Bone Joint Surg.* **74A:** 53–66.
26. Gibb, T.D., Sidles, J.A., Harryman, D.T., McQuade, K.J. & Matsen, F.A. (1991) The effect of capsular

venting on glenohumeral laxity. *Clin. Orthop.* **268:** 120–127.

27. Habermeyer, P., Schuller, U. & Wiedemann, E. (1992) The intra-articular pressure of the shoulder: an experimental study on the role of the glenoid labrum in stabilising the joint. *Arthroscopy* **8:** 166–172.

28. Blasier, R.B., Guldberg, R.E. & Rothman, E.D. (1992) Anterior shoulder stability: contributions of rotator cuff forces and the capsular ligaments in a cadavar model. *J. Shoulder Elbow Surg.* **1:** 140–150.

29. Cofield, R.H. & Irving, J.F. (1987) Evaluation and classification of shoulder instability with special reference to examination under anesthesia. *Clin. Orthop.* **223:** 32–43.

30. Cofield, R.H., Nessler, J.P. & Weinstabl, R. (1993) Diagnosis of shoulder instability by examination under anesthesia. *Clin. Orthop.* **291:** 45–53.

31. Pollock, R.G. & Bigliani, L.U. (1993) Recurrent posterior shoulder instability. Diagnosis and treatment. *Clin. Orthop.* **291:** 85–96.

32. Tibone, J.E. & Bradley, J.P. (1993) The treatment of posterior subluxation in athletes. *Clin. Orthop.* **291:** 124–137.

33. Huber, Gerber, C. (1994) Voluntary subluxation of the shoulder in children. A long-term follow-up study of 36 shoulders. *J. Bone Joint Surg.* **76A:** 118–122.

12

Anatomy of Portals for Arthroscopy of the Shoulder

C Kelly

INTRODUCTION

Arthroscopy of the knee has been conquered, so the next challenge is the shoulder. However several factors combine to make 'routine' shoulder arthroscopy potentially more hazardous than the knee.

1. The shoulder is covered by layers of muscle with their vascular and nerve supply. This compares with the knee which is a subcutaneous joint especially in relation to portal placement.
2. The bony anatomy of the knee is readily palpable. This may not be the case in an obese or muscular shoulder.
3. Routine diagnostic and instrument portals in the shoulder lie close to important nerves and vessels.[1] In the knee most of the 'clockwork' is posterior and is relatively easily avoided during portal placement.

Good knowledge of anatomy allows proper placement of arthroscopic portals and helps avoid complications. Inappropriate portal placement risks injury to these structures and makes the procedure technically more difficult. There are many good textbooks on basic arthroscopy and some have well–illustrated step-by-step accounts of safe portal placement.[2] As with any new surgery, a period of time spent training with a shoulder arthroscopist will increase the surgeon's skill and confidence and thus improve surgical outcome.

Possible complications of shoulder arthroscopy are many and varied. In a study of staple capsulor-rhaphy in 1986, Small[3] reported a 5.3% incidence of complications that excluded re-dislocation. A prolonged procedure combined with awkward positioning of the patient can increase the risk to the brachial plexus.[4] Lee et al[5] reported three cases of pneumomediastinum after subacromial decompression.

CONSIDERING PORTAL PLACEMENT

The position of the patient will depend on the planned surgical procedure. The lateral decubitus position can be used for subacromial decompression and the beach chair position for diagnostic and instability arthroscopy. The surface anatomy of the important structures will change according to the amount of forward flexion and abduction of the arm. For instance, when the patient is in the lateral position the axillary nerve and posterior humeral circumflex vessel lie closer to the inferior glenohumeral joint than when a beach chair position is used. Therefore the anterior portals must be kept high.[6]

When the lateral decubitus position is used, the effect of traction and positioning must be considered in order to avoid injury to the brachial plexus. There is no real agreement on the safest position except that some forward flexion and some abduction is favoured. When subacromial decompressions are performed in the lateral decubitus position, an average 10 lbs traction weight is used with 45° of abduction and 20° of forward flexion (Figure 12.1). In this position the gleno-

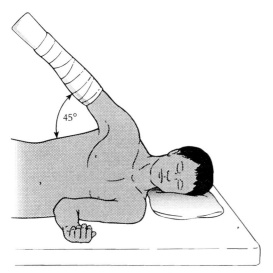

Fig. 12.1 The lateral decubitus position.

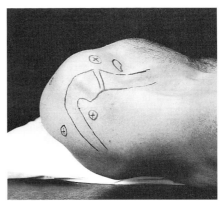

Fig. 12.2 Marking the skin over the bony surface anatomy aids in correct localization of the portals.

humeral joint can be inspected and the subacromial bursa entered using lateral and anterior portals. The acromioclavicular joint is also amenable to surgery in this position.

By avoiding traction and using the beach chair position, brachial neuropraxia can be avoided. This position is useful especially in assessment of instability. The shoulder laxity can be tested while the intra-articular structures of the joint are inspected. However, it is not completely without risk, and a safe head position should be used. Rotation and lateral flexion especially to the same side should be avoided.[4] Hypoglossal nerve palsy has been reported and was due to compression of the contralateral nerve by a head support.[7] The safest position is with the head in a neutral position facing forward with no extension.

INCISIONS AROUND THE SHOULDER

Minimally invasive surgery of the shoulder claims good cosmetic results. This assumes the incisions in the skin are kept small and heal with no ugly scar. Basic principles tell us that incisions along the Langer's lines of stress heal best. A longitudinal incision is used for most anterior and posterior

portals and a transverse incision for the lateral portal. The lines of tension can be seen by gentle side-to-side compression of the skin over the proposed portal site.

Marking the bony landmarks before incising the skin is standard practice especially during the learning of shoulder arthroscopy. The acromion, coracoid process and acromioclavicular joint are marked (Figure 12.2). Continuous infusion of fluid will inevitably cause some tissue swelling, which can make location of the bony anatomy difficult if the skin is not marked.

Closure of portals with a suture or 'steristrip' may not be necessary; a simple dressing only may be used. This allows escape of haematoma or fluid in the early post-operative phase. When the swelling settles, scarring is minimal and patient satisfaction with cosmesis is high.

CHOOSING THE PORTALS

The posterior portal is used for inspecting the joint and bursa. It can be used alone for diagnostic arthroscopy but other portals are needed if probing is required. This portal must be mastered before proceeding to therapeutic shoulder arthroscopy. Subacromial decompression is usually performed with two or three portals: a posterior portal for the arthroscope, a lateral or posterolateral portal for the shavers and possibly a third anterior portal for drainage of the bursa. Arthroscopic stabilization of the glenohumeral joint requires anterior instrument portals. Access to the anteroinferior labrum and capsule can be difficult and portals may need to be sited low and medial. Portal placement in this situation requires particular care.

The posterior portal

The posterior portal is the most commonly used portal for visualization of the joint and subacromial bursa. For many trainees it will be the first and only portal used in diagnostic shoulder arthroscopy. The surgeon must be comfortable in the knowledge of the anatomy and placement of this portal before proceeding to the more hazardous anterior portals.

The exact location of this portal varies in description. The objective is to enter the glenohumeral joint in its upper half through the interval between the teres minor and infraspinatus. The location of the portal has been described by palpation of the 'soft spot'.[8] The important bony landmark is the posterolateral corner of the acromion. The portal is located 2–3 cm inferior and 1 cm medial to this point. The skin only is incised in a longitudinal direction along Langers line. A pointed number 11 blade is used to try to keep the size of the portal smaller than the size of the 4 mm arthroscope used. This gives a snug fit to the scope and reduces extravasation of blood and irrigation fluid. The blunt trocar and cannula is inserted through the skin and with the opposite hand the index finger locates the tip of the coracoid process. The cannula is then directed towards the coracoid process. It traverses subcutaneous fat, the posterior fibres of deltoid and the interval between infraspinatus and teres minor. The cannula then pierces the thin upper half of the posterior capsule entering the glenohumeral joint. With the 30° angled arthroscope, the anterior glenoid and long head of biceps origin should be immediately identifiable. In elderly patients with osteoporosis, damage to the posterior humeral head can be caused by too forceful an entry. Anatomy at risk using this portal include the following.

The axillary (circumflex humeral) nerve[9]

The axillary nerve arises from the posterior cord. Its fibres are derived from the fifth and sixth cervical ventral rami. It begins lateral to the radial nerve then posterior to the axillary artery and anterior to the subscapularis, at the lower border of which it curves back inferior to the glenohumeral capsule and with the posterior circumflex humeral vessels it transverses to the quadrangular space. The nerve divides into anterior and posterior branches. The anterior branch with the posterior circumflex humeral vessel curves around the humeral neck deep to the deltoid to its anterior border, supplying it and giving a few small cutaneous branches which pierce the muscle to ramify into the skin over its lower part. The posterior branch supplies the teres minor and the posterior part of the deltoid; on the branch to teres minor an enlargement or pseudo-ganglion usually exists. The posterior branch pierces the deep fascia low on the posterior border of the deltoid continuing as the upper lateral cutaneous nerve of the arm and supplying the skin over the lower part of the deltoid and the upper part of the long head of triceps. The axillary trunk supplies branches of the shoulder joint below the subscapularis. The nerve is located approximately 5 cm inferior to the tip of the acromion with the arm at the side. It is therefore the limiting factor in locating accessory posterior portals inferior to the standard portal.

The suprascapular nerve[9]

This nerve is a large branch of the superior trunk; it runs laterally deep to the trapezius and omohyoid entering the supraspinous fossa through the suprascapular notch inferior to the superior transverse scapular ligament. It runs deep to the supraspinatus and curves around the lateral border of the scapular spine along with the suprascapular artery to reach the infraspinous fossa where it gives two branches to the supraspinatus and articular rami to the shoulder and the acromioclavicular joints. The suprascapular nerve may have a cutaneous branch and, when present, it pierces the deltoid muscle close to the tip of the acromion. The posterior portal is 1 cm lateral to the main nerve. Portal misplacement or angulation of the cannula that is too medial is hazardous to the axillary nerve.

The anterior portals

The anterior portal can be located by an inside-out technique or by direct puncture of the anterior skin of the shoulder. Direct portal placement may be more hazardous. Using the inside-out technique the interval between the biceps tendon and the upper tendinous border of the subscapularis is identified. This interval contains no important vascular or neural structures and can be penetrated with safety. Several anterior portals have been described in this interval. An anterior portal that passes medial to the coracoid has been described.[10]

The arthroscope is directed into the superolateral interval tissues, and is then replaced with the sharp trocar. The trocar is then pushed through the rotator interval producing a prominence on the skin of the anterior shoulder. It should be confirmed that the exit point is above and lateral to the coracoid process. A small incision is made in the skin and the sharp trocar pushed through. A plastic cannula can then be inserted over the trocar and 'rail-roaded' back into the glenohumeral joint. Alternatively a Wissinger rod can be used in a similar manner.

The following anatomy must be considered when making the anterior portals.

The brachial plexus[9]

The brachial plexus is a union of the lower four cervical ventral rami and the greater part of the first thoracic ventral ramus. Contributions from C4 and T2 vary. The fifth and sixth rami form the upper trunk, the eighth and T1 rami form the lower trunk and the seventh cervical ramus forms the middle trunk. These trunks incline laterally and behind the clavicle and divide into anterior and posterior divisions. The divisions then join to form three cords, the lateral, medial and posterior cords. In the neck the plexus is in the posterior triangle. It emerges between the scalenus anterior and medius and its proximal part is superior to the

third part of the subclavian artery with the lower trunk posterior to it. The plexus passes posterior to the medial two-thirds of the clavicle, the subclavius and the suprascapular vessels and lies on the first digitation of the serratus anterior and the subscapularis. In the axilla the lateral and anterior cords are lateral to the first part of the axillary artery, the medial cord being behind it. The cord surrounds the second part of the artery, and, in the lower axilla, it divides into the principal nerves of the upper limb. The brachial plexus lies approximately 5 cm medial and caudal to the coracoid process and therefore is usually well out of the way. Inexperience with incorrect angulation of the instruments can put the plexus at risk.

The musculocutaneous nerve

The musculocutanous nerve is probably most at risk as it is the most lateral structure in the plexus. It is derived from the lateral cord opposite the lower border of pectoralis minor and is derived from the fifth and seventh cervical ventral rami. It pierces the coracobrachialis and ascends laterally between the biceps and the brachialis to the lateral side of the arm. A line drawn from the lateral side of the third part of the axillary artery across the coracobrachialis and biceps to the lateral side of the biceps tendon is a surface projection for the nerve. Its point of entry into the coracobrachialis is variable and is approximately 5 cm from the coracoid. By staying medial to a longitudinal line from the coracoid process, injury to the nerve can be avoided. Increased abduction puts the nerve at greater risk.

The lateral portal

The lateral portal was popularized by Ellmann in his description of the subacromial decompression.[11] The patient is placed in the lateral decubitus position. A 20° posterior tilt brings the acromion horizontal and allows a more comfortable position for the surgeon. The portal is located 3–4 cm lateral and 1 cm posterior to the anterior border of the acromion. The skin incision should be transverse in the lines of skin tension and once again should be kept small to minimize extravasation of fluid. This portal is commonly used for the arthroscopic shaver and diathermy. The blunt trocarter is inserted through the skin and subcutaneous fat and passes obliquely through the muscle fibres of the deltoid entering the subacromial bursa in its subdeltoid portion. The obliquity of the portal means that the axillary nerve is rarely at risk. During prolonged procedures fluid will inevitably escape from the bursa into the intervening tissues. Swelling may appear alarming, but it does resolve rapidly as the fluid is absorbed over the next hour. Compartment syndrome in the arm has not been described secondary to shoulder arthroscopy.

The superior (supraclavicular fossa) portal

This portal can be used to gain access to the glenohumeral joint and was popularized by Neviaser.[12] It is commonly used for irrigation of the joint; however, the use of instruments is restricted by the surrounding bony anatomy.

The portal is located in the V-shaped 'soft spot' formed by the clavicle and acromioclavicular joint anteriorly and the spine of the scapula posteriorly. A needle will pass through the trapezius muscle and the supraspinatus muscle or tendon. It should be directed laterally to enter the glenohumeral joint at the posterosuperior glenoid sulcus. It can also provide access to the subacromial bursa. If the arm is abducted more then $45°$, the supraspinatus tendon may be penetrated and potentially damaged.[13] The suprascapular nerve and vessels pass through the muscle approximately 2 cm medial to this portal and can be injured if the cannula is directed too medially. The portal is used with greatest safety when the arm is at the side with no forward flexion and the cannula directed lateral. This portal is rarely required.

THE SUBACROMIAL SPACE

This space can be entered using anterior, posterior, superior and lateral portals. It is safe to use an outside-in technique. The bursa is normally a potential space and provides a smooth gliding surface between the coracoacromial arch and the rotator cuff muscles. It is probably misnamed in that, with the arm at the side, the bursa is located anteriorly, more underneath the coracoacromial ligament than the acromion. It extends for a variable degree underneath the deltoid muscle laterally. The bursa provides much grief for the trainee surgeon. Entry can be difficult and common mistakes include:

1. entry too medial into the fat pad underneath the acromioclavicular joint;
2. entry too posterior behind the posterior 'veil' of the bursa;
3. entry too inferior into the substance of the rotator cuff;
4. entry too anterior into the substance of the deltoid; this is easily recognized when red muscle fibres are seen as the 'bursa' is distended with fluid.

Errors number 1 and 2 are most common. If the peribursal tissues are infused with fluid in error, the second attempt at entering the bursa will be even more difficult.

When distended, the bursa appears as a synovial lined space occasionally divided by a 'plica'. When viewed from the posterior portal, the coracoacromial ligament can be seen anteriorly inserting into the undersurface of the acromion. The two bands of this ligament spread out in the shape of an inverted Y to their insertion on the coracoid process. On the medial side of the ligament the thoracoacromial artery branches. This area may cause troublesome bleeding if penetrated by instruments. Also this is the area that bleeds during subacromial decompression as the ligament is excised from the acromion. The medial fat pad is extrabursal and hides the acromioclavicular joint. The pathological impingement lesions on the undersurface of the acromion and on the bursal side of the rotator cuff can be easily seen. Partial and full-thickness tears of the cuff can be assessed.

The subacromial bursa is usually inspected after a routine glenohumeral joint survey. The arthroscope is withdrawn from the glenohumeral joint and replaced with the blunt trocar and cannula. The trocar is withdrawn to just underneath the skin and redirected into the subacromial bursa. By placing a finger on the anterolateral acromion, the surgeon can guide the trocar through the sub-cutanous fat, piercing the posterior deltoid and passing superficially to the rotator cuff tendons. The trocar pierces the posterior wall of the bursa to enter the space. By moving the trocar from side to side, the coracoacromial ligament can be palpated and the trocar can be seen to enter the lateral recess of the subacromial bursa. The arthro-scope is then inserted and the bursa distended with fluid. The normal bursa should demonstrate a smooth walled cavity indented by the coraco-acromial ligament anteriorly. Pathological bursae may be difficult to enter due to scarring. Some surgeons distend the bursa with fluid before insertion of the trocar. This can aid localization of the subacromial space provided that the fluid is actually injected into the bursa itself. If the fluid is injected into the peribursal tissues, this makes the procedure more difficult. In approximately one-third of cases, is necessary to debride the bursal tissue in order to identify the abnormal pathology. In subacromial decompression the lateral portal is used for diathermy and the shavers. Rarely an accessory anterior portal is necessary for drainage of the bursa in cases of excessive bleeding.

THE ACROMIOCLAVICULAR JOINT

Arthroscopic excision arthroplasty of this joint can be performed alone or in association with sub-acromial decompression. It is most useful to mark the surface anatomy, as extravasation of fluid makes portal placement difficult. Access for sha-vers is via the subacromial bursa or by separate anterior portal. A direct portal can be located 2 cm anteroinferior to the joint. The bursal approach is used for inferior osteophyte excision and a com-bination of both for excision arthroplasty. The variation in inclination of this joint means exci-sion can be difficult and more than two portals may be needed.

CONCLUSIONS

Safe placement of arthroscopic portals in the shoulder requires a knowledge of the anatomy of surrounding nerves and vessels. The suprascapular and axillary neurvascular bundles are most at risk in posterior portal placement. The brachial plexus and musculocutaneous nerve are in danger in anterior portal placement. The more complex arthroscopic procedures require more variation in portal placement and therefore should only be attempted by the experienced shoulder arthro-scopist.

REFERENCES

1. Nottage, W.M. (1993) Arthroscopic portals: anatomy at risk. *Orthop. Clin. North Am.* **24:** 19–26.
2. Bunker, T.D. & Wallace, W.A. (1991) *Shoulder Arthroscopy.* London: Martin Dunitz.
3. Small, N.C. (1986) Complications in arthroscopy: the knee and other joints. *Arthroscopy* **2:** 253–258.
4. Cooper, D.E., Jenkins, R.S., Bready, M.D. & Rock-wood, C.A. (1988) The prevention of injuries of the brachial plexus secondary to malposition of the patient during surgery. *Clin. Orthop.* **228:** 33–41.
5. Lee, H.C., Dewan, N. & Crosby, L. (1992) Subcuta-neous emphysema, pneumonediastinum and potentially life-threatening tension pneumothorax. Pulmonary complications from arthroscopic shoulder decompression. *Chest* **101:** 1265–1267.
6. Johnson, L.L. (1986) *Arthroscopic Surgery: Principles and Practice.* St. Louis: C.V. Mosby.
7. Mullins, R.C., Drez, D. & Cooper, J. (1992) Hypoglos-sal nerve palsy after arthroscopy of the shoulder and open operation with the patient in the beach-chair position. *J. Bone Joint Surg.* **74A:** 137–139.
8. Andrews, J.R., Carson, W.G. & Ortega, K. (1984) Arthroscopy of the shoulder: technique and normal anatomy. *Am. J. Sports Med.* **12:** 1–7.
9. Williams, P.L., Warwick, R., Dyson, M. & Bannister, L.H. (1989) *Gray's Anatomy,* 37th edn. Edinburgh: Churchill-Livingstone.
10. Wolf, E.M. (1989) Anterior portals in shoulder arthroscopy. *Arthroscopy* **5:** 201–208.
11. Ellmann, H. (1987) Arthroscopic subacromial decom-pression: analysis of one to three year results. *Arthroscopy* **3:** 173–181.
12. Neviaser, T.J. (1987) Arthroscopy of the shoulder. *Orthop. Clin. North Am.* **3:** 361–372.
13. Souryal, T.O. & Baker, C.L. (1990) Anatomy of the supraclavicular fossa portal in shoulder arthroscopy. *Arthroscopy* **6:** 297–300.

13

Arthroscopic Evaluation of the Unstable Shoulder

G Declercq

INTRODUCTION

Before undertaking shoulder arthroscopy one should carefully go through the patient history, complete the physical examination and finally study the radiographic evaluation. This should be sufficient to establish the diagnosis of shoulder instability. A knowledge of anatomy and the possible normal variations is important. They have been well documented but subtle differences between normal variations and real pathology can make life difficult for the arthroscopist. Examination under anaesthesia of both shoulders should be performed before the arthroscopy is started. Translation and load and shift tests are performed in all directions, and this should confirm the clinical diagnosis.

Arthroscopy can be performed with the patient in the beach chair or the lateral decubitus position. In my department, we prefer the lateral decubitus position with a double traction for instability work. Anterior and posterior kidney rests are used to stabilize the patient and the arm is placed in skin traction, with 2–4 kg traction to keep the arm slightly abducted and flexed forward. A second sling is applied at the upper arm which pulls at an angle of 90° to the chest of the patient, with 3–6 kg traction. Easier evaluation is possible when distraction force is applied to the glenohumeral joint.

Landmarks are outlined on the acromion, the clavicle and coracoid process. We routinely use normal saline for inflow. For diagnostic purposes elevation of the inflow bags is sufficient, but it is our experience that an inflow pump is mandatory

when performing a stabilization procedure. Routine knee arthroscopy instruments can be used, and an interchangeable cannula system is very helpful. Classic shoulder arthroscopy portals can be used for diagnostic examination.

It is necessary to evaluate the shoulder from both the posterior and anterior view to complete the examination. A double-anterior portal is used for a stabilization procedure. This will be explained in detail in Chapter 20.

NORMAL VARIATIONS IN ANATOMY OF THE LABRUM AND GLENOHUMERAL LIGAMENTS

The labrum is a wedge-shaped structure that is circumferentially attached to the glenoid. Sometimes it is very thin and firmly attached to the glenoid; the transition zone between glenoid and labrum can only be felt with a probe. Detrisac & Johnson[1] have also described a more meniscus-appearing wedge with a free central margin that overlaps the articular surface cartilage.

The labrum has one attachment point directly to the glenoid zone via a fibrocartilaginous transition zone, and one to the periosteum of the scapular neck. The labrum should be considered as part of the capsular ligaments of the shoulder.

The superior, middle and inferior glenohumeral ligaments are thickened bands of the anterior capsule and are characterized by their attachment to the humeral head rather than their scapular attachement. The superior glenohumeral ligament (SGHL) is attached near the top of the lesser tuberosity and inserts at the superior glenoid tubercle near the base of the coracoid, running almost parallel to the biceps tendon. The middle glenohumeral ligament (MGHL) is attached on the lesser tuberosity and runs obliquely across the subscapular tendon and inserts at the superior portion of the labrum. Possible variations will be discussed. The inferior glenohumeral ligament (IGHL) is attached low on the humeral neck, passes beneath the humeral head and inserts at the anterior inferior portion of the glenoid. There is often a firm thickening of the anterior portion (anterior band). The axillary pouch forms a sling of capsule, and a thickening of the posterior portion of the axillary pouch (posterior band) may complete the picture of a hammock-like IGHL complex.

There is one very consistent bursal recess in the anterior compartment of the shoulder, the subscapularis recess. It is located between the SGHL and MGHL. It is possible to look down into this recess from the anterior portal and this gives an excellent view of the superior tendinous portion of the subscapularis muscle.

Considerable variability exists in the pattern of the different ligaments and associated recesses and this has been well documented in the literature by De Palma,[2] Moseley & Overgard,[3] Detrisac & Johnson[1] and Morgan.[4] Exact understanding and precise recognition of these normal variants are essential when considering arthroscopic evaluation of a normal or possibly unstable shoulder.

The classic pattern (Morgan's series, 66%; De Palma's series, 30%)

Three ligaments and one recess. SGHL, MGHL and IGHL are distinct structures as described above and the subscapularis recess is situated between the SGHL and MGHL (Figures 13.1–13.3).

Sublabral hole (Figures 13.4 and 13.5)

A large number of patients have a large foramen extending from the midglenoid notch almost up to the biceps insertion. In this area the labrum is detached from the glenoid margin and through

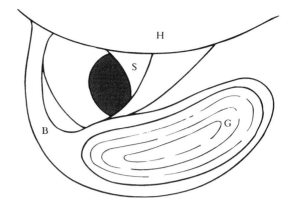

Fig. 13.1 The classic pattern. H, humeral head; G, glenoid; B, biceps tendon; S, subscapularis.

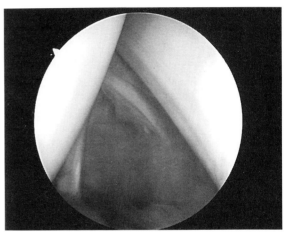

Fig. 13.2 Normal left shoulder. View from classic posterior portal. Top left humeral head and top right biceps tendon. The SGHL runs almost parallel to the biceps tendon.

the hole there is communication with the subscapularis bursa. Otherwise the ligament pattern is essentially classic. Stabilizing this 'loose' labrum will result in uniformly good results because the shoulder was probably not unstable from the beginning.

Cord-like MGHL (Figures 13.6 and 13.7)

The three ligaments are easily visualized and beside the classic subscapularis recess, there is an extra bursal recess between the MGHL and IGHL

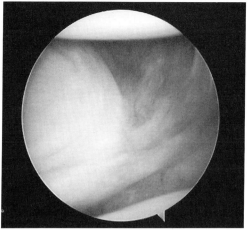

Fig. 13.3 Normal left shoulder. View from anterior portal. The humeral head is superior and the glenoid is left. Normal attachment of the IGHL with well-developed superior band.

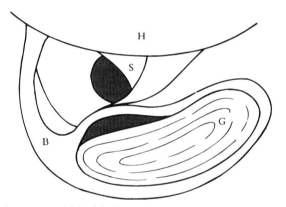

Fig. 13.4 Sublabral hole. H, humeral head; G, glenoid; B, biceps tendon; S, subscapularis.

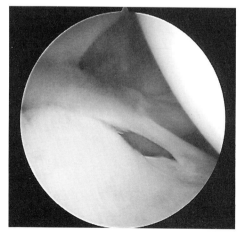

Fig. 13.5 Normal right shoulder with a sublabral hole, posterior view.

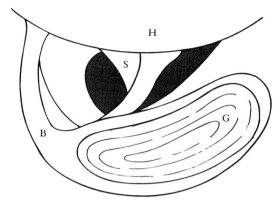

Fig. 13.6 Cord-like MGHL. H, humeral head; G, glenoid; B, biceps tendon; S, subscapularis.

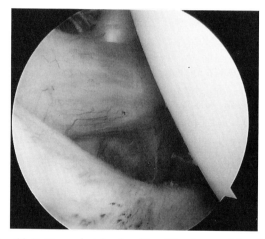

Fig. 13.7 Normal right shoulder. The humeral head is located on the right. The cord-like MGHL crosses the subscapularis tendon.

(De Palma's series 47% and Morgan's series 19%). The MGHL is strongly developed and appears like a cord attaching just beneath the biceps insertion.

Confluent MGHL and IGHL (De Palma's series, 9% and Morgan's series, 7%)

The MGHL and IGHL are blended together and a large subscapularis recess is located below the SGHL (Figures 13.8 and 13.9).

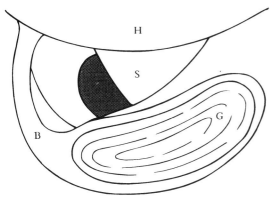

Fig. 13.8 Confluent MGHL and IGHL. H, humeral head; G, glenoid; B, biceps tendon; S, subscapularis.

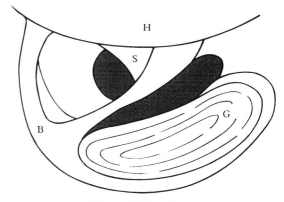

Fig. 13.10 A cord-like MGHL with a very large inferior recess: the Buford complex. H, humeral head; G, glenoid; B, biceps tendon; S, subscapularis.

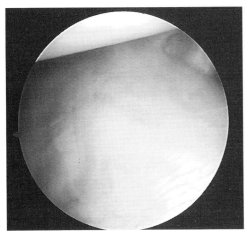

Fig. 13.9 Normal left shoulder. From a posterior portal we see the humeral head superiorly. The MGHL and IGHL are blended together. The subscapularis tendon is just visible at the top right of the picture.

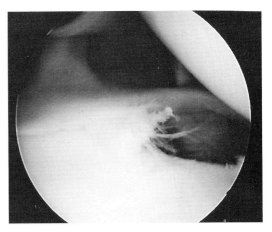

Fig. 13.11 Right shoulder with a cord-like MGHL and a huge recess. The humeral head is superior and the glenoid below. This can easily be mistaken for a Bankart lesion.

Absent ligament pattern (De Palma's series, 11% and Morgan's series, 8%)

There are no distinguishable thickenings in the anterior capsule. According to some authors this pattern may predispose to anterior shoulder instability.

Others

Sometimes a cord-like MGHL is associated with a large inferior recess, which can be easily mistaken for a Bankart lesion. However, careful palpation of the IGHL will show a normal ligament attachment from the mid-glenoid notch downwards.

This pattern has been called the 'Buford complex'[5]. (Figures 13.10 and 13.11).

Other minor variants are possible, but the key factor in normal ligament anatomy is the firm attachment of the IGHL up to the mid-glenoid notch.

ARTHROSCOPIC FINDINGS IN PRIMARY SHOULDER DISLOCATIONS

Several authors have described the lesions found at arthroscopy in acute initial shoulder dislocations.

Baker et al[6] in 1990 described three groups according to the stability examination under anaesthesia (EUA).

The first group was felt to be stable at EUA, and haemorrhaging was seen in the subscapularis tendon and the capsule between the MGHL and IGHL. The attachment of the glenoid labrum was normal and no glenoid fractures or Hill–Sachs lesions were identified.

Group 2 included shoulders that could be subluxed at EUA. Mild haemarthrosis was found at arthroscopy. The glenoid labrum was not completely separated but incomplete separation was palpable extending superiorly up to the biceps tendon insertion. A Hill–Sachs lesion or chondral fracture was present.

Group 3 included shoulders with gross instability at EUA and moderate haemarthrosis. Complete separation of the glenoid labrum or disruption of the ligaments with fragmentation of the labrum was the key feature. An identation at the posterolateral aspect of the humeral head with loose chondral fragments and a bleeding surface bed was a very consistent finding, indicating an acute Hill–Sachs defect. This group may include glenoid rim fractures and full-thickness rotator cuff defects.

Wheeler et al[7] reported in 1989 on nine patients. All patients showed complete disruption of the labrum, without appreciable interstitial damage to the glenohumeral ligaments. A large number (five), however, showed a glenoid rim fracture, but a chondral fracture or an osteochondral defect posterolaterally was invariably present.

In our department, we have retrospectively analysed the files of 28 patients who underwent arthroscopy after an initial acute traumatic anterior dislocation of the dominant shoulder. They were less than 25 years of age and were involved in contact or throwing sports. In the majority of patients (72%) a frank disruption of the labrum from the anteroinferior glenoid was present. Small flake avulsions from the glenoid rim were present in 25% of the patients in this group. One patient sustained a major fracture dislocation with a large glenoid fragment knocked off by the humeral head. All the other patients showed more or less damage to the ligaments without disruption or

fragmentation of the labrum. One patient showed a major tear of the whole MGHL and IGHL complex close to the humeral attachment, exposing the belly of the subscapularis muscle. All patients in this selected group of patients after a traumatic anterior dislocation showed chondral or osteochondral damage to the posterolateral aspect of the humeral head.

ARTHROSCOPIC FINDINGS IN RECURRENT ANTERIOR SHOULDER DISLOCATIONS

When the humeral head translates over the glenoid rim in an anterior–inferior direction, the glenohumeral ligament complex will fail. Failure can occur at different levels. Wolf[8] classified the pathology in recurrent anterior dislocation according to the location of the pathology.

Type 1: failure at the glenoid (73% of total)

This lesion occurs at the junction of the fibrocollagenous labrum and the cartilaginous glenoid surface, with an associated rupture of the anterior scapular periosteum. Most people would call this the classic Bankart lesion (Figures 13.12 and 13.13).

There are some potential subgroups or variations of this lesion.

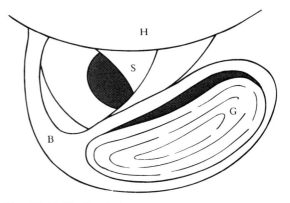

Fig. 13.12 Bankart lesion. Disruption of the IGHL from the anterior glenoid rim.

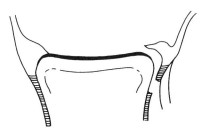

Fig. 13.13 Bankart lesion. Both the labrum and the periosteum are torn and separated from the glenoid.

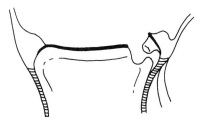

Fig. 13.15 Bony Bankart. Flake avulsion, pulled off the anterior–inferior scapular neck by the capsulolabral complex.

1. Perthes' lesion: when the failure occurs at the level of the scapular neck with stripping of the periosteum. In this case we find no complete separation of the labrum from the glenoid margin (Figure 13.14).
2. Bony Bankart: a fracture of the glenoid rim may occur by avulsion at the time of the initial dislocation, or may occur during recurrent episodes of shoulder dislocation. It appears that small flake avulsions, pulled off the anterior–inferior scapular neck by the capsulolabral complex, are far more frequent than previously thought. During arthroscopic evaluation of recurrent instability, larger bony fragments can be readily detected, but small flakes are easily overlooked unless the avulsed capsulolabral complex is debrided and carefully probed (Figure 13.15).
3. Anterior labral ligamentous periosteal sleeve avulsion (ALPSA), as described by Neviaser. This lesion is very similar to a classic Bankart lesion and consists of a stripping of the labrum and periosteum from the scapular neck. The whole complex drops down inferiorly and medially on the scapular neck, where it may

heal and eventually become covered with fibrous tissue and synovium. During arthroscopy this lession can easily be missed. One should look for the absence of the normal anterior–inferior capsulolabral buttress, and, with a probe, the labrum should be identified in a more inferior and medial position on the scapular neck (Figure 13.16).

Type 2: intrasubstance tears, or laxity of the glenohumeral ligaments (17% of total)

It has been shown *in vitro* that the IGHL stretches from 10 to 60% before tearing occurs either at the glenoid, intrasubstance or humeral attachment site. How much of this elongation is elastic is not really known, but some plastic deformation of the IGHL may be sufficient to cause anterior instability. We have no objective means of measuring laxity during arthroscopy, so this type of laxity is often diagnosed by exclusion. It can occur after chronic microtrauma with subsequent stretching or acute tearing with fibrous repair and elongation. The diagnosis of this type of capsular redundancy together with an intact labrum is usually

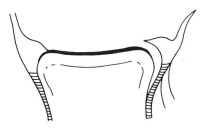

Fig. 13.14 In the Perthes' lesion there is stripping of the periosteum from the scapular neck, but no complete separation of the labrum.

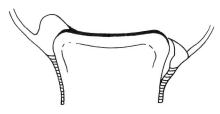

Fig. 13.16 ALPSA lesion. The labrum and periosteum are separated from the glenoid. They both slip down the scapular neck and heal down in a more inferior and medial position.

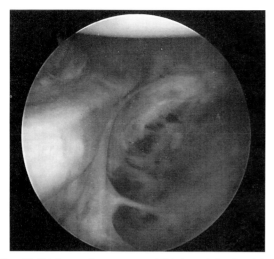

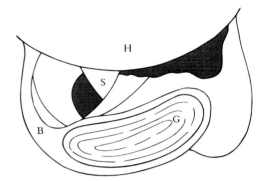

Fig. 13.18 HAGL lesion.

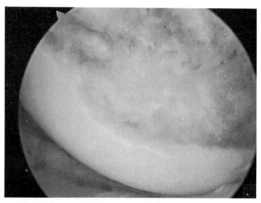

Fig. 13.17 Intrasubstance tear. This is a right shoulder, with a view on the anterior compartment through an anterior portal. The humeral head is above and the glenoid with the labrum still attached is on the left side. Centrally there is a rupture of the ligaments and through the rent the muscle fibres of the subscapularis muscle are visible.

Fig. 13.19 Large Hill–Sachs defect in a recurrent dislocating right shoulder.

made when anterior instability has been documented radiologically and/or by EUA.

Occasionally an intrasubstance tear is clearly visible with intact attachment sites at both the glenoid and humeral ends. Through the rent in the capsule the muscle of the subscapularis muscle can be identified (Figure 13.17).

Type 3: humeral avulsion of glenohumeral ligaments (HAGL) (9% of total)

This relatively rare lesion was first described by Nicola[9] in 1942. The importance of this lesion should not be underestimated and it should be looked for in all unstable shoulders, whether an open or arthroscopic method of stabilization is proposed. Again, subscapularis muscle fibres may be clearly visible through the defect in the capsule (Figure 13.18).

All these types of instability lesions can commonly occur with a posterolateral humeral head defect. This may be chondral or osteochondral. The so-called Hill–Sachs lesion (Figure 13.19) is caused by abutment of the anterior glenoid rim

against the posterior aspect of the humeral head when the head rotates and translates over the rim in an anterior–inferior direction. This manoeuvre can sometimes be reproduced arthroscopically by bringing the arm in abduction and external rotation. Additional anterior force on the humeral head will often dislocate the joint completely. We have to be aware of the fact that the Hill–Sachs lesion can be very superficial, purely chondral, and it should not be confused with the normal 'bare' area. This is the normal transition zone between the insertion of the rotator cuff and the cartilage of the humeral head. Furthermore, because of fragmentation of the bone and cartilage, small pieces of debris may float freely inside the joint and become loose bodies. As the result of gravity, they usually fall down into the axillary pouch, but they may become hidden in the

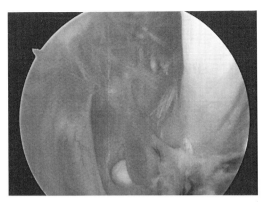

Fig. 13.20 Loose body hidden in the subscapularis recess. This is a left shoulder. Through the anterior portal we can look down into the subscapularis recess. The superior tendinous portion of the subscapularis is seen on the right.

subscapularis recess. Careful examination through the anterior portal should reveal the loose fragments (Figure 13.20).

ARTHROSCOPIC FINDINGS IN ATRAUMATIC SHOULDER INSTABILITY

Atraumatic instability can be defined as instability that is insidious or spontaneous in onset without a history of significant trauma inducing the first episode of instability. This instability is often referred to as multidirectional instability.

In this condition arthroscopy reveals glenohumeral ligaments that are attenuated or grossly lax. In fact, in most cases the thickening in the capsule that normally represents the ligaments is flattened or may not be visible at all. The capsule itself appears somewhat stretched out and voluminous, especially inferiorly. The labrum has a normal or somewhat hypoplastic appearance. In the typical case, a Bankart lesion is not found, nor a Hill–Sachs defect. During arthroscopic evaluation, the humeral head can usually be displaced anteriorly, posteriorly or inferiorly without exerting too much force.

A patient with atraumatic instability may also experience an episode of trauma, which might produce traumatic changes. In this instance a Bankart lesion and Hill–Sachs defect may be present in combination with obvious capsular laxity. When considering a stabilization procedure it might be necessary to correct both.

ARTHROSCOPIC FINDINGS IN POSTERIOR INSTABILITY

In normal stable shoulders the posterior capsular structures seem less well defined or developed. There is no characteristic thickening in the capsule, except for the posterior band. This band runs in a posterior–inferior direction, and, together with the axillary pouch and the anterior band, a hammock-like sling is formed.

As far as arthroscopic evaluation is concerned, the posterior labrum can be nicely evaluated from a posterior portal. However, complete examination of the posterior capsule should be carried out from an anterior portal.

In traumatic posterior instability one should look for a mirror image of the patterns seen in anterior dislocation. Detachment of the posterior labrum, especially in the posterior–inferior area, together with a reverse Hill–Sachs lesion is somewhat pathognomonic for posterior instability. The reverse Hill–Sachs lesion is an indentation at the anterosuperior aspect of the humeral head, because of impaction of the posterior glenoid rim during posterior dislocation. Again, this area is best visualized through the anterior portal.

We have no exact data on the incidence of complete disruption of the capsulolabral complex at the glenoid attachment site, but it seems that capsular laxity due to tearing or stretching of the capsule itself is far more frequent than in anterior instability. So, EUA and careful evaluation of the posterior capsule and anterosuperior aspect of the humeral head are the key features in posterior instability (Figure 13.21).

LABRAL LESION

The glenoid labrum provides some contribution to stability of the shoulder. It deepens the socket

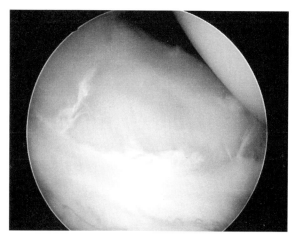

Fig. 13.21 Recurrent posterior instability in a right shoulder. Through the posterior portal, the disruption of the posterior–inferior labrum can be seen. The glenoid is below, the humeral head above.

and may play a role as a 'chock block' in controlling glenohumeral translation. Consequently, the presence of a labral lesion, without any visible or palpable capsular lesion or stretching, should alert the arthroscopist for possible instability.

Snyder and Karzel[5] introduced the concept of superior labrum from anterior to posterior (SLAP) lesions. The superior portion of the labrum serves as a site of attachment for the superior and middle insertions of the glenohumeral ligaments and posterosuperior capsule (Figure 13.22). The true

contribution of this lesion to glenohumeral instability is still controversial. Recent work by Pagnani et al[10] showed that *in vitro* creation of a complete disruption of the superior portion of the labrum (SLAP type 2) resulted in significant increases in anteroposterior and superoinferior glenohumeral translations.

In my department, we have retrospectively analysed 45 patients with labral lesions, diagnosed by arthroscopy, in order to analyse the relationship between labral lesions and instability. All patients were participating in different types of sport and were examined by arthroscopy because of inability to continue their sport despite conservative therapy, or a palpable click was found during stability testing. Only full-thickness defects (bucket-handle tears or well-defined flap tears) or

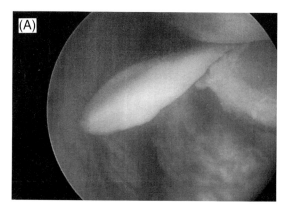

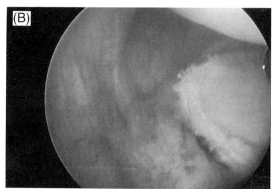

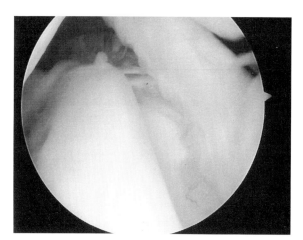

Fig. 13.22 SLAP lesion type III. Bucket-handle tear of the superior labrum. The biceps anchor remains firmly attached.

Fig. 13.23 (A) Well-defined flap tear of the anterior inferior labrum. View through an anterior portal in a right shoulder. (B) After debridement of the flap the attachment and integrity of the IGHL can be appreciated.

capsulolabral disruptions were included, with the exception of Bankart lesions.

Substantial evidence of instability (by stability testing of both shoulders) was found in all anterior and posterior–inferior lesions. Instability was suspected in 50% of the superior (SLAP) and posterior–superior lesions. We concluded that in the presence of labral pathology, instability should be ruled out (Figure 13.23).

REFERENCES

1. Detrisac, D.A. & Johnson, L.L. (1986) *Arthroscopic Shoulder Anatomy: Pathologic and Surgical Implications*, pp. 69–89. Thorofare, NJ: Slack.
2. De Palma, A.F. (1983) *Surgery of the Shoulder*. Philadelphia: Lippincott.
3. Moseley, N.F. & Overgard, B. (1962) The anterior capsular mechanism and major dislocation of the shoulder. *J. Bone Joint Surg.* **44B:** 313–327.
4. Morgan, C.D. (1992) Arthroscopic shoulder anatomy and pathology of anterior instability. Arthroscopic Association of North America Book of Abstracts, 11th Annual Meeting, April 23–26.
5. Synder, S. & Karzel, R.O. (1990) SLAP lesions of the shoulder (lesions of the superior labrum both anterior and posterior). *Arthroscopy* **14:** 274–279.
6. Baker, C.L., Uribe, J.W. & Whitman, C. (1990) Arthroscopic evaluation of acute initial anterior shoulder dislocations. *Am. J. Sports Med.* **18:** 25–28.
7. Wheeler, J.H., Ryan, J.B. & Anciero, R.A. (1989) Arthroscopic versus non operative treatment of acute shoulder dislocations in young athletes. *Arthroscopy* **5:** 213–217.
8. Wolf, E.M. (1992) Arthroscopic capsulo-labral reconstruction using suture anchors. AANA Book of Abstracts, Instructional Courses and Symposia, November 19–22, 1992.
9. Nicola, T. (1949) Acute anterior dislocation of the shoulder. *J. Bone Joint Surg.* **31A:** 153–159.
10. Pagnani, M.J. et al (1995) Effect of lesions of the superior portion of the glenoid labrum on glenohumeral translation. *J. Bone Joint Surg.* **77A:** 1003–1010.

FURTHER READING

Bankart, A.S.B. (1938) The pathology and treatment of recurrent dislocation of the shoulder joint. *Br. J. Surg.* **26:** 23–29.

Declercq, G. (1994) *Proceedings 8th Congress of the European Society for Surgery of the Shoulder and Elbow,* Barcelona 16–18 June, 1994.

Johnson, L.L. (1986) *Arthroscopic Surgery. Principles and Practices.* St Louis: C.V. Mosby.

Rogerson, J.S. (1993) Shoulder arthroscopy: normal anatomy versus pathology in the glenohumeral joint. AANA Book of Abstracts and Instructional Courses. 12th Annual Meeting, April 1–4, 1993.

Rowe, C.R. & Zarins, B. (1981) Recurrent transient subluxation of the shoulder. *J. Bone Joint Surg.* **63A:** 863–871.

Turkel, S.J., Panio, M.W., Marshall, J.L. & Girgis, F.G. (1981) Stabilising mechanisms preventing anterior dislocation of the glenohumeral joint. *J. Bone Joint Surg.* **63:** 1208.

14

Arthroscopy of the Shoulder

SA Copeland

Arthroscopy of the shoulder is a procedure that the modern orthopaedic surgeon has to master. The basic skills of triangulation and use of the endoscopic instruments will almost certainly have been learnt on the knee which is the most commonly endoscoped major joint and the same and familiar arthroscopic equipment may be used. There are, however, some important differences particularly relating to the variability of the normal anatomy that may be found.[1] The basic techniques of portal placement and joint entry may be learnt adequately on plastic models, but the variation of normal anatomy can only be appreciated with time and experience of many diagnostic arthroscopic procedures. This can be done by working with an experienced shoulder surgeon as an observer with the video monitor before 'going solo'.

INDICATIONS FOR SHOULDER ARTHROSCOPY

There is no substitute for taking a good history and detailed clinical examination which will give the diagnosis in the vast majority of shoulder disorders. The arthroscope may be used to confirm the diagnosis, or in the minority of cases where the diagnosis remains unclear. As experience increases, then the frequency of arthroscopy alone decreases and the need for arthroscopic surgery increases. One of the major indications is assessment of the unstable shoulder. This is an excellent opportunity to learn the basics of diagnostic arthroscopy before performing an open

stabilization. Familiarity with the joint may be gained along with the exact pathology of the unstable shoulder which can then be used to tailor the surgery to the problem. Later, as experience is gained, arthroscopic stabilization may be considered. Assessment of the arthritic shoulder may be aided by arthroscopy so that the detailed plan of treatment may be worked out for the patient. Assessment of the rotator cuff is a common indication for arthroscopy. Impingement may be confirmed and both the articular and bursal side of the cuff inspected. If a rotator cuff tear is present the size may be determined, and the repairability and quality of the remaining muscle may be assessed. Problems arising from the intra-articular portion of the long head of biceps and glenoid labrum may be seen and possibly treated using the arthroscope. It must be stressed that the intra-articular structures only may be seen and hence any changes must be taken in conjunction with the clinical findings.

EQUIPMENT

The standard knee arthroscope may be used. This is commonly the 30° fore-oblique 4 mm scope. Small diameter and short arthroscopes are available but have not been found to be necessary or useful as the shoulder is a very large volume joint and light through a small scope may be inadequate. The length of the scope is also important as sometimes in the fat or very well muscled patient the joint may be deeply placed. A compact camera system in conjunction with a television monitor is highly desirable. Diagnostic arthroscopy alone may be carried out with inflow and outflow fluid through the scope alone, intra–articular pressure being varied by raising or lowering the saline-fluid inflow bag. Obviously a tourniquet cannot be used on the shoulder and sometimes bleeding may have to be controlled. If bleeding is a problem this can be controlled in several ways. The intra-articular pressure may be increased above arterial pressure and through-flow increased by a second puncture drain. This may be done using a knee arthroscopy draining needle attached to cannula drainage tubing, or a large-bore outflow cannula. A 5 mm disposable plastic cannula with a rubber diaphragm is very useful as this allows instrumentation probing to gain more information. During the early stages triangulation skills may be improved by the use of a probe. For basic diagnostic arthroscopy an arthroscopic pump is not required but it may be very useful if arthroscopic surgery is indicated.

POSITIONING THE PATIENT

Lateral decubitus position (Figure 14.1)

This is perhaps the easiest position to start learning arthroscopy as no assistant is required, the arm being held in balanced traction. The patient lies in the mid-lateral position with the affected side uppermost. If the patient is rolled 30° backwards, this brings the plane of the glenohumeral joint horizontal. The trunk is stabilized by a pelvic support posteriorly and a chest support anteriorly. General anaesthesia is most commonly used although it is possible to do this under scalene block anaesthesia alone. Traction is applied using a paediatric skin traction set with a weight and pulley system. Some excellent shoulder holders are available which allow more accurate positioning of the arm both in abduction, adduction and flexion extension, but for most uses an adequate system can be made by

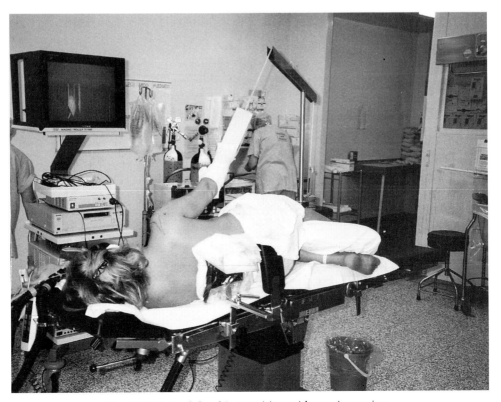

Fig. 14.1 Lateral decubitus position with arm in traction.

taking the top of a drip stand and attaching it to the foot of the table in front of the patient to act as a fulcrum for traction. This allows approximately 15° of forward flexion of the shoulder and 30° of abduction. The sponge-rubber type of paediatric skin traction set is preferred to those using skin adhesives because skin avulsion has been described in the rheumatoid patient. The rubber type is also reusable, keeping the cost of the procedure down. For the average patient, approximately 10 lb traction weight is used. This is reduced in the lighter patient and increased in the heavy, muscular male.

Beach chair position

The type of position used is entirely surgeon preference and how the surgeon feels most comfortable. I personally use the lateral decubitus position for assessment of the rotator cuff and impingement problems, but use the beach chair position for assessment of instability. If the patient is in this position and the decision is made to proceed to open surgery, no repositioning or redraping of the patient is required. The patient is placed supine on the operating table with the head on a neurosurgical headpiece and then flexed at the hips giving a relaxed reclining position like sitting in a beach chair. Traction is helpful and may be applied using an assistant to pull down on a limb towards the hip or by using balanced traction through a bivalved elbow shell. This position has been described by Resch & Betk.[2]

TECHNIQUE

It is useful at this stage to infiltrate the portal sites with bupivacaine 0.5% and adrenaline to reduce bleeding and postoperative pain (Figure 14.2). In the average patient 20 ml are used and after infiltration of the portal sites the remaining 10 ml are used to inflate the glenohumeral joint. If local anaesthetic has been used for a scalene block, then these volumes must be reduced accordingly. When first learning the technique of shoulder

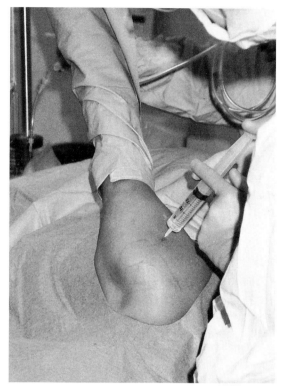

Fig. 14.2 Portal track and joint injected with bupivacaine with adrenaline.

arthroscopy it may be an advantage to inflate the joint before insertion of the scope. As the shoulder is a deeply placed structure, entry may not be as easy as the knee. Hence, when the joint is entered the back flow of fluid confirms entry into the joint. As experience is gained, however, the joint may be entered dry.

POSTERIOR PORTAL

This is the common utility portal and most structures can be viewed through this portal alone. It is situated one thumb's breadth inferior and 1.5 cm medial to the angle of the acromion. A skin puncture wound 5 mm long is made parallel to the skin tension lines. In this position the incision should be vertical. At this site there is a 'soft spot' which can be palpated with the thumb. With the middle finger on the coracoid and the thumb on the soft spot the arthroscope sheath

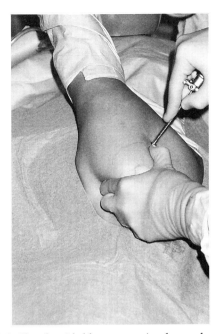

Fig. 14.3 Sheath with blunt trocar is advanced towards the coracoid.

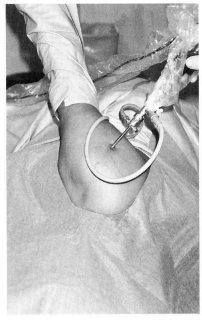

Fig. 14.4 Inspection of joint with light source, fluid inflow and camera connected.

with blunt cannula is pushed through the skin and subcutaneous tissue towards the coracoid marked by the middle finger. This gives the approximate line of the glenohumeral joint. There are two structures which need to be avoided when using the posterior portal: medially lies the suprascapular nerve as it winds around the base of the acromion, inferolaterally lies the axillary nerve. The blunt obturator is used to enter the joint. It is better to err on the supralateral side and pass through the muscle layer and palpate the bulge of the humeral head through the joint capsule with the tip of the obturator. The scope is then 'walked' inferomedially until the posterior edge of the glenoid is palpated and with a firm push the joint entered (Figure 14.3). A sensation of 'give' is felt and once the blunt obturator is removed an outflow of fluid should confirm the position of the sheath. The fluid inflow is connected to the side arm of the cannula and the scope inserted and television camera connected (Figure 14.4). If the view is not immediately clear it may be obscured by some joint fluid or blood staining. It may be enough at this stage to remove the scope and allow free inflow and outflow of fluid to wash the joint out.

The scope is reconnected and the view should be clear. If the joint cannot be adequately visualized because of bleeding, then adequate through-flow must be established. If inspection alone is adequate rather than probing, then a second portal wide bore needle is connected to the drainage tubing to allow adequate flow of fluid. More usually, however, much more information may be obtained by manipulating the intra-articular structure with a probe and this may be done with a second formal portal anteriorly.

ANTERIOR PORTAL

The anterior portal is located superiorly and laterally to the coracoid process but the exact site is located from within the joint. It is easiest to establish this second portal from within out. The joint is inspected and the telescope driven into the triangular area bordered by the long head of biceps, the anterior border of the glenoid and the superior border of subscapularis. The light may be seen transilluminating the skin anteriorly. The

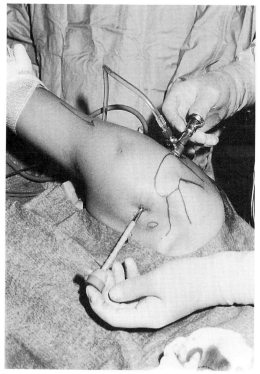

Fig. 14.5 The cannula is 'railroaded' into the joint from the anterior portal.

telescope is removed leaving the sheath in place. The sharp obturator is then inserted through the sheath and through the soft tissues anteriorly until this is just underneath the skin. A second puncture wound is made anteriorly and then the trocar passed through and through the skin anteriorly (Figure 14.5). In the large patient the sharp obturator may not be long enough and a Wissinger rod is used instead to railroad the second portal. The 5 mm cannula is then mated with either the sharp obturator or the Wissinger rod and railroaded back into the joint. This method ensures that the cannula enters the joint at exactly the correct point. A through and through irrigation system is then set up so that the inflow goes in via the side portal of the scope and the outflow through the side portal on the accessory anterior cannula. Gravity drainage alone is all that is required; suction is not needed. The anterior portal may now be used for passage of the probe for the palpation of intra-articular structures.

INSPECTION OF THE JOINT

A standard routine of inspection must be developed so that all positive and negative findings may be recorded. Everybody develops their own routine, but as long as it is the same routine each time then no structures will be missed. The long head of biceps is a good starting point for orientation as this is the most obvious intra-articular structure, its origin being found at the apex of the glenoid. The tendon is inspected from its origin to its disappearance in the biceps groove on the anterolateral aspect of the humerus. By positioning the arm, the scope may be passed some way down the long head of biceps canal. The scope is then passed back along the long head of biceps to the supraglenoid recess and the posterior structures are then inspected. Sweeping the scope down the posterior glenoid recess leads into the infraglenoid recess and the inferior capsule is inspected. The scope is then passed over the posterior humeral head to inspect the bare area and posterior rotator cuff insertion and posterior humeral head articular cartilage. The undersurface of the rotator cuff is inspected by rotating the 30° scope to look superiorly.

The scope is then passed across the face of the glenoid to inspect the anterior structures. Assessment of the anterior structures may be greatly helped by using the probe from the anterior portal. The upper border of the subscapularis may be seen and appears as an intra-articular structure. This is because the intra-articular pressure of fluid pushes the capsule out through the rotator interval, making the superior aspect of the subscapularis much more prominent. The glenoid labrum is a ring of dense fibrous connective tissue connected to the osseous glenoid rim. A thin transitional zone of fibrocartilage may be demonstrated at the point of osseous attachment. The labrum is an extremely variable structure. It is triangular in cross-section with the free edge directed towards the centre of the glenoid. It may be very loosely attached anteriorly above the equator of the glenoid but in the normal shoulder should always be firmly attached below the equator of the glenoid. This loose upper attachment superiorly can be mistaken by the inexperienced to be a Bankart lesion, but is in fact a normal variant and is only pathological if detached below the equator. The anterior band of the inferior glenohumeral ligament arises from the anteroinferior half of the labrum and blends with the labrum as it extends superiorly. The biceps tendon and superior glenohumeral ligament also merge with the labrum at its superior aspect. The superior recess may now be visualized as a common variant which communicates freely with the subscapular bursa. The middle glenohumeral ligament is a constant finding which may be very variable in structure. It is seen to arise on the superoanterior aspect of the glenoid and sweep inferolaterally obliquely across the subscapularis. Isolated pathological detachment of the superior labrum is rarely seen. Pathological detachment of the superior labrum frequently develops as an extension of a pre-existing inferior labral detachment caused by traumatic anterior dislocation. An anterosuperior labral detachment in association with a posterosuperior labral detachment (SLAP lesion) is rarely seen and is abnormal.[3] Glenohumeral ligaments are extremely variable. The inferior glenohumeral ligament and its anterior band normally attaches to the inferior half of the anterior labrum and sends its superior band upwards as it blends with the labrum. The anteroinferior labrum may be quite obvious and well developed, but in other instances it may be impossible to identify as a separate distinct structure. Flap tears, scuffing and fraying may be observed as a consequence of shoulder subluxation or recurrent dislocation. In the recurrent anterior dislocating shoulder all these anterior structures may be detached, scarred and stretched. Sometimes a bony Bankart can be seen involving a small flaky fracture of the anterior lip of the glenoid. Posterior labral injuries are commonly seen in athletes involved in throwing sports.[4] The hyperlax individual who is very easy to examine by arthroscopy with multidirectional instability may show few labral abnormalities. The joint is so capacious that scuffing does not occur.

The glenoid articular surface is inspected for fibrillation and thinning of articular cartilage, areas of chondromalacia and pitting. In older individuals there may be a normal central 'blue' spot. This does not indicate early osteoarthritis but is simply a normal variant.

The humeral head articular cartilage is examined next. If the arthroscopy has been indicated for assessment of anterior instability, then a detailed inspection should be made of the posterior humeral head for a Hill–Sachs lesion. This should not be confused with the intracapsular portion of the humeral neck or 'bare area'. The humeral head is rotated in front of the scope and a Hill–Sachs lesion may be encountered medial to the bare area. This may be variable such that there may be only cartilaginous damage or a large deep impacted fracture.

Returning to the anterior structures, the subscapular recess should be inspected in detail. The recess lies between the intra-articular surface of the subscapularis and the neck of the glenoid. Reactive changes of synovitis are commonly seen here and intra-articular loose bodies may be found in this region. If a loose body is being chased, palpation by a finger placed anteriorly may be used to coax it out of this recess.

If the arthroscopy is being carried out in order to assess instability, at this stage the arm may be unhooked from the traction and with the scope still in place, translational forces applied to the humeral head. If the arm is taken into abduction external rotation, then the edge of the Hill–Sachs lesion may be seen to engage with the anterior glenoid lip. Posterior and inferior instability is assessed by stressing the joint in these positions.

Tendons of the supraspinatus, infraspinatus and teres minor insert into the superior and posterior aspects of the greater tuberosity. The articular capsule is adherent to the undersurface of these tendons and the individual tendons cannot be identified arthroscopically as they merge into one sheath. However, it may be taken that the supraspinatus extends from the rotator interval delineated by the long head of biceps anteriorly to the upper portion of the bare area on the head. The infraspinatus extends roughly over the circumference of the bare area. Increasing abduction and external rotation facilitate inspection. Partial tears involving the articular surface of the cuff may be seen at this stage, noted and recorded.

ANTERIOR INSPECTION

At this stage of a complete and thorough intra-articular inspection it will have been noted that the anterior aspect of the humeral head has not been seen and the anterior neck of the glenoid may not have been clearly inspected. These structures may be viewed by swapping the scope from the posterior to the anterior portal. This manoeuvre may be achieved by removing the scope from the posterior portal leaving the sheath in place. The blunt obturator is inserted and locked in place so that the inflow may be maintained. The unsheathed scope may then be passed to the anterior portal to inspect the anterior neck of the glenoid and the anterior humeral head.

SUBACROMIAL BURSOSCOPY

No arthroscopic inspection of a shoulder joint is complete without a thorough subacromial bursoscopy.[5] After a standard glenohumeral arthroscopy, the telescope is removed, the blunt obturator inserted into the cannula and withdrawn into the subcutaneous tissues posteriorly. The same posterior skin portal is used. A finger is then placed over the anterior bony margin of the acromion and the obturator and cannula are advanced to this point. While pushing the obturator forward, a slight 'give' is felt and the bursa entered. This position can be checked by swishing the obturator laterally and medially flicking under the coracoacromial ligament. Sometimes a sensation of give is not felt and there is some doubt as to whether the bursa has been entered. Sweeping the obturator laterally from this point usually ensures entry into the bursa. The scope is then inserted and inflow fluid switched on. If 'cobwebs' are only seen, then the bursa has probably not been entered. The fluid is quickly switched off and a further attempt made.

Occasionally despite a few attempts the bursa cannot be entered. In this case a limited bursectomy with a power shaver may be necessary to allow adequate inspection of the bursal structures. Bleeding may be a problem after entry into the bursa and increased flow pressure may be required. Lack of bony landmarks makes orientation within this space more difficult, but feeling the bony tip of the acromion with the scope is a useful manoeuvre. Needle insertion on either side of the coracoacromial ligament may be helpful for orientation. The whole of the bursa is inspected into the lateral recess and under the surface of the coracoacromial ligament. The acromion is assessed for inflammatory change and wear. The bursal surface of the rotator cuff is inspected for inflammatory change and evidence of partial or full-thickness tearing and calcification. The arm is removed from traction and rotated in front of the scope to view the whole of the the intrabursal surface of the cuff. A useful technical point at this stage is that, if on entering the bursa there is fluid flow-back, this indicates that there is a full-thickness tear of the rotator cuff and any fluid that has entered the glenohumeral joint has passed through the rotator cuff tear and into the bursa. This is the technique used in arthrography to determine the presence or absence of a rotator cuff tear. Therefore, if there is fluid flow back on entering the bursa, then every effort must be made to find the communication between the bursa and the main glenohumeral joint (Figure 14.6). When examination is complete, the bursa is flushed out and the skin puncture sites left unsutured to prevent formation of localized haematoma and outflow of remaining fluid.[6]

POSTOPERATIVE MANAGEMENT AND PATIENT INSTRUCTIONS

If only diagnostic arthroscopy is performed, the patient is told to mobilize the joint as freely as possible within the limits of discomfort, and discomfort will resolve over a few days only. Simple analgesics only are required.

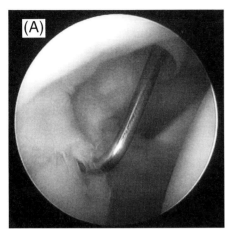
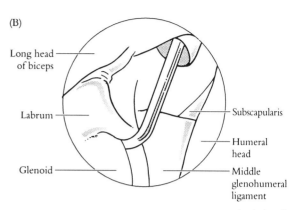

Fig. 14.6 (A) The glenohumeral joint is viewed from the posterior portal. The probe is seen entering the joint from a cannula in the anterior portal. (B) Line drawing of (A).

REFERENCES

1. Detrisac, D.A. & Johnson, L.L. (1986) *Arthroscopic Shoulder Anatomy: Pathological and Surgical Implications,* pp. 69–89. Thorofare, NJ: Slack.
2. Resch, H. & Betk, E. (1992) *Arthroscopy of the Shoulder.* New York: Springer Verlag.
3. Snyder, S.J., Karzel, R.P., Del Pizzo, W., Ferkel, R.D. & Fiedman, M.J. (1990) S.L.A.P. lesions of the shoulder. *Arthroscopy* **6:** 274–279.
4. Andrews, J.R., Kupferman, S.P. & Dillman, C.J. (1991) Labral tears in throwing and raquet sports. *Clin. Sports Med.* **10:** 901.
5. Matthew, L.S. & Fadale, P.D. (1989) Subacromial anatomy for the arthroscopist. *Arthroscopy* **5:** 36–40.
6. Copeland, S.A. & Williamson, D. (1988) Suturing of arthroscopy wounds. *J. Bone Joint Surg.* **18:** 145.

15

Throwing Injuries

R Hackney and WA Wallace

INTRODUCTION

Throwing is an action familiar to everyone. The overhead throw has a similar movement whether it is used in throwing a cricket ball, serving in tennis or throwing a javelin in an athletics stadium. In the United Kingdom the most popular sports involve kicking rather than throwing, in contrast with the United States of America where baseball is a passion. Indeed, it is from America that the great volume of research into throwing and its related injuries has originated.[1,2] The incentive for such interest derives from the fact that baseball pitchers are among the world's most highly paid sportsmen. The injuries suffered by such athletes are as a consequence of the extremes of speed, range of movement, force and power that are involved in throwing.

In the last decade there have been great advances in the understanding of how throwing injuries arise and their subsequent management. An aim of rehabilitation must also be to reduce the chances of recurrence. Of necessity this must involve correction of any errors in throwing technique.

A major difference between caring for sportsmen and women and the normal population is that the athlete's treatment is not completed until a return to full sport and competition has been achieved. As a general rule in sports medicine, an athlete will respond much better if the practitioner has an understanding of the sport concerned. In order to understand the cause of throwing injuries and to provide a logical approach to their management, it is a fundamental principle that the mechanisms and biomechanics of throwing are understood. Failure of synchrony of the movement from whatever cause predisposes to injury. Fatigue from excess throwing, training errors, minor injury, extremes of effort, all lead to errors in throwing technique and increased risk of injury. A knowledge of training methods is required, as injuries occur in training as well as competition.

Local muscle endurance is important and so the thrower uses high repetition, light resistance work and repetitive drills. Strength training with heavier weights does form some part of the training programme. Free weights, as opposed to apparatus, improve three-dimensional control and hence proprioception. The complex lifts used with free weights require good technique to avoid injury. For example, some weight-training exercises put the shoulder in the classical position of the apprehension test. The initial injury may occur in the weight-training room but is manifested in the stadium. Throwing athletes use only very little aerobic training such as running, but may use cross-training with swimming and cycling

MECHANISMS OF THROWING

It is important to emphasize that the whole body participates in the throwing action. The shoulder is part of a chain running from feet to hand. The shoulder acts as a funnel for forces developed against the ground by the legs and trunk. The kinetic energy is then transferred on to the elbow and wrist. Using the shoulder alone, only 30% of maximum throwing velocity can be produced. For a tennis serve, the forces produced by the shoulder are just 21% of the total. The lower extremity develops 51% of kinetic energy in the tennis serve, the shoulder only 13%, the difference required to constrain the shoulder.

The majority of sports medicine literature related to throwing technique deals with baseball pitching. Analyses have been performed using high-speed multiple-camera cinematography with video digitization, electromyographic analysis and various muscle-testing devices.

Baseball pitching

The baseball pitch has been divided into five different phases. The pitcher stands upon a 10 inch high mound and throws off one step only. The first step off the mound involves quite a significant drop. The pitcher is effectively throwing down at the batsman.

Wind up

Wind up phase runs from the start of the movement until the ball is transferred from the non-throwing (gloved) hand. The wind up establishes the rhythm of the movement and begins the forwards motion of the body as the opposite foot strides forward. Balance is crucial, though imbalance is more likely in sports such as American football where the thrower (quarterback) is running and has the added risk of being tackled by a 350 pound opponent! The pitcher begins standing sideways to the direction of delivery. When body weight is shifted from stride foot on to the support foot, the wind up is initiated. The body rotates backwards 90° with the stride leg externally rotated. The trunk remains rotated in a position of extension and rotation as the stride is taken. This phase takes 1500 ms.

Arm cocking

As the stride is taken, the trunk remains externally rotated. The sequence that follows involves hip rotation, trunk rotation following the hip, and the upper trunk follows the lower. The arm flexes at

the elbow and is brought up to 90° abduction at the shoulder, which externally rotates to up to 180°. The arm has not yet been brought forward whilst the legs, hips, pelvis and trunk have already been accelerated. The arm is left behind as long as possible. This phase takes an average of 60 ms. There is a force of 380 N stressing the anterior structures.

Arm acceleration

This phase is very explosive. As the arm follows the trunk, the humerus begins internal rotation and horizontal flexion about the shoulder. There is a slight delay between this and the beginning of elbow extension. Elbow extension during the acceleration phase reduces the inertia that must be generated at the shoulder allowing the torque produced to provide greater angular velocity. When the ball is released the trunk flexes, continuing the rotation. This phase ends with ball release. In baseball the average time from foot contact of the stride leg until ball release is 145 ms while the ball is accelerated from 4 to up to 95 miles per hour. The acceleration phase itself takes 50 ms. The peak angular velocities of internal rotation achieved have been measured at up to 9100° per second. Pappas et al[3] measured shoulder internal rotation from 122 to 48° during the 10 ms prior to ball release. Peak accelerations approaching 600 000 degrees per se per sec were found.

Arm deceleration

After ball release, the elbow continues to extend and internally rotate at the elbow. Deceleration reduces the angular velocity to zero, with deceleration values of 500 000 degrees per second. The baseball pitcher aims to confuse the batsman with a variety of differing velocities and spins of the ball. The forearm pronates to a degree which is dependent upon the nature of the throw. After ball release, 440 N of posterior force, 1090 N of compressive force and 97 N m of horizontal abduction torque are generated.

Follow-through

Follow-through ends with the stride leg extended and flexed at the hip to prevent further forward motion. The shoulder adducts, the elbow flexes and the forearm supinates from varying amounts of pronation. The body catches up with the arm as it adducts across the chest.

Individual pitchers are very consistent in their speeds and range of motion through the pitch. There is a much greater inter-pitcher variation. The entire excursion of the arm is 225° with respect to the horizontal plane. Throwing is a composite movement of glenohumeral, scapulothoracic and trunk extension, flexion and rotation. The proportion of the velocity derived from the step and trunk has been estimated at about 47%.

Throwing in track and field athletics

Javelin (Figure 15.1)

Of the throwing disciplines in athletics only the javelin involves an overhead technique. The principles of overhead throwing as described for baseball pitching apply to the javelin throw, but with some obvious differences. The javelin weighs 800 g and is shaped like a spear. The aim is to hold the binding quite firmly either side of the ledge on the grip. This prevents slipping and allows spin to be imparted to the javelin on release. Javelin differs from baseball in that a run up is used to increase the speed at which it is thrown. The throw has to take place along the line of the length of the spear. The shoulder comes into play when the wind up phase is reached. The javelin is left behind the thrower as he/she runs forward in a position of extension, external rotation and 45° of abduction. The javelin is held in the line of the throw, with the palm facing the sky with the tip of the javelin held just above the eyeline. The pelvis and chest are perpendicular to the direction of the run (in external rotation), but the eyes are facing forward. The runner accelerates until the cross-over stride. The left foot lands (for a right handed thrower), to provide the athlete with a solid base. The right knee, then pelvis and trunk are thrust forward in a rotational movement as in the baseball pitch. The

left arm is pulled across the body (Figure 15.2). Throughout this part of the throw, the throwing arm remains as far behind the body as possible, for as long as possible. The shoulder is brought around on the trunk as the arm is whipped forwards. The elbow should be above shoulder height as the shoulder reaches neutral flexion, i.e. the shoulder should be abducted more than 90°. The trunk may well be leaning to the left in this phase, giving a false impression of the amount of abduction at the shoulder. This is important to observe in the prevention and management of injuries to the shoulder and elbow. The throw imparts a spin to the javelin, as it is launched at an angle of around 40–45° from horizontal to obtain ideal length of throw. The follow-through continues the supination of the forearm used to impart the spin, of note in the causation of medial elbow pain. Javelin throwers tend to be the lightest of the track and field throwers, technique and speed of movement being of greater importance than strength.

Hammer throw

The hammer is an event of Celtic origin, deriving from country fairs where sledge hammers were thrown. The event progressed to the use of a ball on a wooden shaft and then on to the chain used in the modern event. The hammer event is held inside a cage on a 7-foot concrete circle. The hammer is swung through three rotations at a 45° angle to the ground. The thrower rotates on his heels leaning backwards to counterbalance the weight of the hammer (Figure 15.3). Hammer throwers tend to be bigger than javelin throwers, the implement being that much heavier. However, the hallmark of the event is controlled rotational speed and power pivoting upon the hindfoot. There is a much greater proportion of upper body and trunk strength used in the throw as the ground contact surface is very small for such forces.

Discus

The discus dates back to ancient Greek times. The implement is a flat circular 2 kg piece of wood

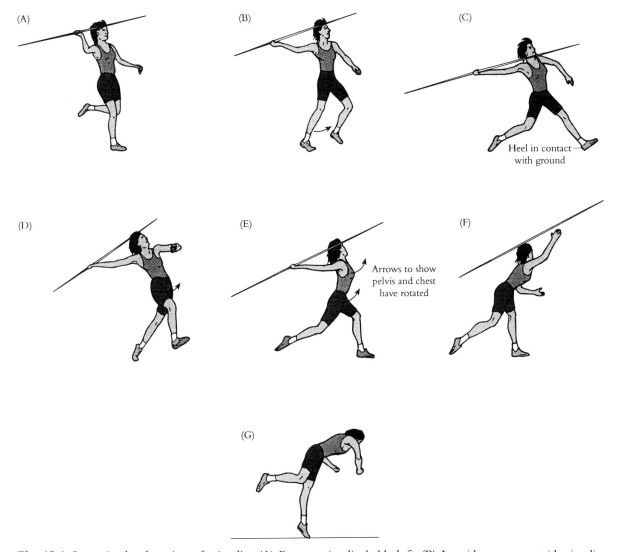

Fig. 15.1 Stages in the throwing of a javelin. (A) Run up, javelin held aloft; (B) In mid cross-over stride, javelin withdrawn, right leg crossing but pelvis and trunk still perpendicular to line of throw; (C) Leg has crossed, pelvis has not moved but javelin still held back; (D) Wide stance from stride, front (left) leg braces the body, pelvis about to be thrust round; (E) Pelvis trunk rotated, javelin still held back, the spine is extended; (F) Release of javelin, final rotation and flexion of spine; (G) Follow-through and will land on right leg.

with a metal rim. The arm is held straight throughout the throw. The body is rotated, twisting one and a half turns on the circle leaving the arm behind, with the shoulder in an extended and abducted position. The left foot (for a right handed thrower) is planted to block further rotation on the left, but the right side continues to move against the left. The shoulder pulls the discus around projecting it forwards with flexion of the shoulder girdle in the 90° abducted position (Figure 15.4).

Shot put

The shot put involves projecting a metal ball from a position with the shot tucked into the neck. The arm action is flexion and abduction of the shoulder with extension of the elbow. The

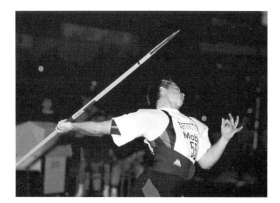

Fig. 15.2 Throwing a javelin. Courtesy of Mark Sheaman.

shoulder is not particularly susceptible to injuries during the discus, hammer and shot putt events, but the weight training required is heavy, involving sets of lifts with 150 kg weights for top throwers. Shoulder injuries are more likely to be caused by the weight training used to prepare for these events.

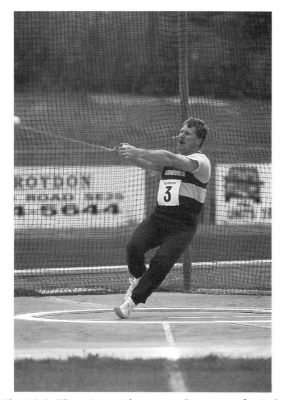

Fig. 15.3 Throwing a hammer. Courtesy of Mark Sheaman.

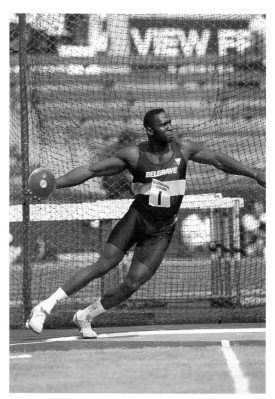

Fig. 15.4 Throwing a discus. Courtesy of Mark Sheaman.

ELECTROMYOGRAPHIC (EMG) ANALYSIS

EMG analysis of the shoulder girdle muscles during a baseball pitch have helped towards the understanding of mechanisms of injury and the rehabilitation necessary for overhead throwing activities.[2]

In the throwing athlete, the supraspinatus acts to produce humeral abduction but its peak activity occurs in *late cocking* when the arm is already abducted and is most susceptible to subluxation. The supraspinatus contributes to stability by pulling the humeral head into the glenoid. Amateur throwers use the supraspinatus more than professional athletes. Fatigue of this muscle will occur more readily in amateurs than properly conditioned professionals.

The infraspinatus and teres minor are responsible for external rotation and stabilization by drawing the humeral head into the glenoid. Activities are similar for both muscles with peak activity during late cocking, deceleration and follow-through. In contrast with the excess external rotation found in throwing athletes, there is usually a reduction in internal rotation to 75° or less. The reason for the loss of internal rotation is poorly understood, with loss of flexibility of both the musculature and the posterior capsule.

The subscapularis has its peak activity in late cocking when it contracts eccentrically to protect the anterior joint capsule which is under extreme tension. It then functions as an internal rotator to help carry the arm across the chest during acceleration and follow-through.

Professional athletes demonstrate selective use of the individual cuff muscles, and are able to use the subscapularis exclusively during the acceleration phase. Amateurs tend to use all the cuff muscles and biceps. Proper co-ordination of the trunk renders the supraspinatus, infraspinatus, teres minor and biceps unnecessary for acceleration.

The biceps brachii muscle fires in a similar pattern to the brachialis suggesting that the biceps is acting mostly at the elbow. The long head of biceps contributes to anterior stability by increasing the torsional rigidity in the shoulder and thereby resisting the excessive external rotational forces occurring in the cocking position. Pitchers with instability have increased firing of the biceps. The pectoralis major and latissimus dorsi function together as internal rotators and eccentrically contract to protect the joint along with the subscapularis during late cocking. They contract in acceleration providing internal rotation and arm depression to power the throw. The serratus anterior controls the scapula and provides a stable glenoid. Serratus anterior activity is important for scapular protraction during late cocking. The scapula is then able to keep pace with the humerus as it flexes horizontally and externally rotates. The trapezius is relatively inactive during cocking, but provides some scapular stabilization in acceleration. In follow-through the trapezius decelerates scapular protraction.

CLASSIFICATION OF INJURIES

There are important differences in both the nature of the injuries of the shoulder in throwing (Table 15.1) and the mechanisms of injury. There are specific injuries that are attributed to the throwing action. The biomechanics of throwing detailed in the previous section give some insight into the tremendous forces involved in throwing a javelin the length of a football pitch. The extreme range of movement required and the speed at which that movement takes place is repeated many times both in competition and training. The part of the throw in which symptoms are experienced is relevant to the diagnosis, as different injuries are related to the stages of throwing. The nature of the difficulty is that frequently the athlete presents with secondary complaints.

IMPINGEMENT INSTABILITY AND ROTATOR CUFF LESIONS

Pathophysiology

The 180° of external rotation of the shoulder at 90° of abduction during a throw is beyond what is considered a normal range of movement, but is an integral part of the throwing technique. The arm is left behind the rest of the body to give as great a

Table 15.1. Injuries in throwing athletes

Impingement, internal and subacromial
Rotator cuff lesions, tendinitis, tears partial and full-
   thickness
Anterior instability, including subluxation and dislocation
SLAP lesions
Posterior instability
Dead arm syndrome
Acromioclavicular joint pathology
Stress fractures
Nerve lesions, thoracic outlet syndrome, quadrilateral space
   syndrome, suprascapular nerves
Long thoracic nerve injury
Avascular necrosis of the humeral head
Referred pain from the neck, pleura

SLAP, superior labral anterior to posterior.

slingshot effect as possible. The anterior stabilizing structures, in particular the inferior glenohumeral ligament, must be able to stretch to achieve this. When the shoulder is in the cocked position, the static stabilizer holding the shoulder in joint is the inferior glenohumeral ligament. This ligament is at risk of attenuation with time. The athlete is thus treading a fine line between a powerful throw derived from a wide range of movement on the one side and developing a loose shoulder with subluxation of the glenohumeral joint on the other.

Recurrent episodes of injury alter the musculotendinous structure of the rotator cuff resulting in decreased tensile strength and elasticity. Healed tendon has decreased tensile strength and elasticity heals as sclerotic tissue. When athletes have been throwing and weight training since they were 9–10 years of age, the build-up of recurrent injury leads to increased incidence with age.

With repeated stresses upon the stabilizing structures, injury occurs to both the dynamic and static elements. The competitive athlete throws close to his limits, where poor technique is more likely to occur. Fatigue of the rotator cuff, the dynamic stabilizers, with repeated throwing leads to increased anterior and superior translation of the humeral head. Posterior capsular tightness contributes towards increased migration of the humeral head. The normal translation allows up to 4 mm of movement. When translation exceeds 6 mm, the humeral head rides up over the glenoid labrum causing fraying or even tearing. Abrasion of the labrum together with attenuation of the inferior glenohumeral ligament leads to anterior instability.

This description of a mechanism of causation of anterior instability is only part of the picture. Superior translation of the humeral head as a consequence of poor rotator cuff control has been thought to lead to subacromial impingement.[4–6] The deceleration phase of the throw forces the posterior rotator cuff musculature to work eccentrically. The distraction forces in deceleration reach 90% of body weight. Repeated trauma has been thought to lead to primary tensile failure,[7] usually of the infraspinatus, which is manifested as damage to the humeral side of the

rotator cuff. This theory has been challenged by Chris Jobe.[8] The measured EMG activity of the rotator cuff in the deceleration phase is low, as the cuff muscles are not working particularly hard to withstand a distraction force. Jobe reports an impingement of the undersurface of the rotator cuff against the posterosuperior labrum in throwers with anterior instability. This phenomenon can be observed arthroscopically; the humeral head can be seen to hinge upon the posterior superior labrum. This accounts for both the fraying of the undersurface of the rotator cuff and the damage to the labrum frequently seen in elite baseball pitchers. It explains why the injury to the rotator cuff is on the undersurface and not the subacromial side. This 'internal impingement' occurs in the late-cocking phase and is aggravated by posterior tightness. Throwing athletes frequently complain of posterior pain which can be attributed to this mechanism. Subacromial impingement in conventional terms is quite rare. At the Kerlan–Jobe clinic, a number of cases have been seen where impingement against the medial coracoacromial ligament has produced scarring of the bursa in baseball pitchers. This probably occurs in the follow-through phase. Arthroscopic cleaning of the adhesions produces symptomatic relief.

The scapula is also implicated in the mechanism of the instability complex.[9] Repeated throwing movements may cause fatigue of the muscles controlling scapular motion. This results in altered movement of the scapula which adversely affects the control and rhythm of the throwing action aggravating any instability present.

Diagnosis

The time of onset of pain during the throwing action is helpful in determining the cause. Pain at late cocking is most probably due to instability, and pain that is increased after activity is associated with rotator cuff tendinitis. Rotator cuff tears give night pain. Pain associated with the shoulder in the at-risk position of abduction and external rotation when weight training may be diagnostic of instability. A shooting pain and reduced use of the arm immediately after a throw is called dead arm syndrome.[10] This indicates underlying anterior instability. The athlete may be unaware of any subluxation during the throw. It is therefore vital that a throwing athlete with a history of pain be thoroughly assessed for instability.

Examination for rotator cuff lesions and instability in the throwing athlete is carried out as for the normal population. In the throwing arm, however, there is likely to be a loss of internal rotation and excessive external rotation compared with the opposite side. An altered glenohumeral rhythm with winging of the scapula may be seen in the shoulder of an athlete with instability. Muscle strength must be assessed, although these athletes are powerful individuals and the examiner must place himself in a position of biomechanical advantage. Assessing muscle strength by an iso-kinetic device such as the Cybex system will be useful for both diagnosis and as a baseline for rehabilitation purposes.[11]

Stability tests are particularly important. The signs of instability may be very subtle. The classic apprehension test may give equivocal results because the athlete experiences pain from tendinitis and impingement in this position. Of much more value are the Jobe relocation test and examination under anaesthesia (EUA). Jobe believes that the pain produced in the position of abduction and external rotation is caused by internal impingement of the rotator cuff against the posterior superior labrum. The pain on release of the humeral head is caused by the humeral head hinging upon the posterior superior labrum.

Investigations

Standard radiographs are of limited use in this situation. Magnetic resonance imaging (MRI) scans are of value in assessing labral damage and tendinitis but may be oversensitive and the report must be measured against the clinical situation. Miniaci et al[12] scanned the shoulders of 30 young asymptomatic volunteers. The results are summarized in Table 15.2. They concluded that non-enhanced MRI may be of limited value in defining rotator cuff tears in a patient with shoulder pain.

Shoulder arthroscopy after EUA and probing

Table 15.2. Classification of MRI results from 30 asymptomatic volunteers

Grade	MRI signal	Percentage
0	Normal	0
1	Focal lesion, intermediate signal	100
2	High signal less than grade 3	23
3	High signal throughout	0

of the labrum and glenohumeral ligaments is an important part of the diagnostic work-up. EUA is performed with the arm at varying degrees of abduction and external rotation, and comparison with the normal side is made. Stability in all directions is assessed. The drive-through sign is positive when the arthroscope can be pushed across the glenohumeral joint from the posterior portal to the anteroinferior glenoid. This indicates capsular laxity.

Classification

Jobe & Kvitne[5] proposed a classification of athletes with impingement and instability. This classification precedes the concept of internal impingement, which is now believed to be the predominant cause of pain in the throwing athlete. True subacromial impingement is less common in the patient population.

Group one: pure impingement no instability

This group includes older throwers aged 35 years or more who will have positive impingement but negative apprehension and relocation tests. Severe impingement will give rise to pain on apprehension testing but no pain relief on testing with the relocation test.

Neer's stages of impingement are detailed elsewhere. Jobe has modified this to include a fourth category. The classification is open to misinterpretation in that the stages should not necessarily be regarded as being a path along which an individual can pass. The classification is for athletes. Stage 1 is early changes of oedema and mild haemorrhage commonly caused by overuse from overhead activity in young athletes under 25 years of age. This responds well to reduced activity and conservative measures. Stage 2 is observed in throwers suffering recurrent episodes of impingement. The supraspinatus tendon is inflamed. This stage usually responds to adequate rest and conservative measures, and is found in older athletes (25–40 years of age). Stage 3 is usually seen in older sportsmen who give a previous history of multiple episodes of pain and impingement. A small (<1 cm) rotator cuff tear is present and is associated with a bony osteophyte of the acromion and clavicle inferolaterally. Conservative treatment at this stage may fail but should be attempted. Stage 4 consists of rotator cuff tears greater than 1 cm. Surgical management may be necessary, although Wilk et al[13] amongst others report acceptable results using conservative treatment in professional pitchers with full-thickness tears.

Group two: primary instability due to chronic labral micro-trauma with secondary impingement

This group consists of throwing athletes who have developed a chronically unstable shoulder as a result of their throwing activity. Examination reveals impingement and pain but not apprehension until the relocation test is performed. EUA may not detect instability as the findings can be subtle. There may be increased anterior movement of the humeral head. Arthroscopic findings are undersurface cuff tears, anterior labral damage and attenuation of the inferior glenohumeral ligament. There may be minor posterior labral damage and posterior humeral head chondromalacia, the so-called kissing lesion, associated with internal impingement.[18] The kissing lesion is caused by impingement in the cocking and early acceleration phases of throwing.

Skilled throwers with isolated anterior glenohumeral instability have altered patterns of activity on EMG testing. The differences fail to compensate for the instability. The supraspinatus is generally more active whereas the infraspinatus fires more in early cocking but not late cocking. There is mildly increased biceps activity during late cocking and accelerating may represent a compensatory mechanism to provide increased anterior stability. The pectoralis major, subscapularis and latissimus dorsi all have markedly decreased activity during the throw in patients with instability. Inhibition of the synergistic activity of these muscles may predispose to anterior instability. The serratus anterior also shows decreased activity and hence develops reduced horizontal protraction of the scapula which adds to the stress upon the anterior restraints. Poor scapular stability is reflected in winging.

Group three: instability due to generalized increased ligamentous hyperelasticity with subsequent impingement

The findings on clinical examination are the same as for group two except that there is evidence of generalized laxity. Scapular winging is common. These shoulders are unstable on EUA, frequently bilaterally. Arthroscopically they may have fraying of the rotator cuff. The inferior glenohumeral ligament is loose on probing and it does not tighten on external rotation. The humeral head can be seen to be pushed over the edge of the glenoid labrum which is small but intact. The arthroscope can be passed easily between the humeral head and the anteroinferior glenoid.

Group four: pure instability without impingement

These patients will usually have had a major traumatic episode with anterior subluxation or dislocation. There is a negative impingement test but pain with apprehension testing and relief of pain with the relocation test. EUA reveals anterior instability. Arthroscopy shows anterior labral damage due to subluxation, with corresponding humeral head defects and capsular injury. The rotator cuff is normal.

Treatment

Treatment depends upon the category into which an individual falls. The correct diagnosis is essential. The athletes in group two do require a high index of suspicion of instability to make the diagnosis of secondary impingement.

The majority of athletes will respond to conservative measures. The steps in returning to competitive throwing are based on a recognition and correction of the pathophysiology of the injury. An understanding of the specific adaptation to imposed demands (SAID) principle is essential. The aim is to return the athlete to function in as short a time as possible.

PRINCIPLES OF REHABILITATION IN THE THROWING ATHLETE

1. Rest from aggravating activity, throwing or upper body training that induces symptoms. N.B. The athlete should be encouraged to exercise the non-injured parts and maintain cardiovascular fitness.
2. Settle acute inflammation and pain with non-steroid anti-inflammatory drugs (NSAID), use up to three injections of corticosteroid and cryotherapy.
3. Range of motion, stretching, strengthening for power and endurance, in the scapular plane using exercises with rubberized cord, e.g. cliniband or theraband. Proprioceptive feedback techniques.
4. Progression to free weights, scapular stabilization, Cybex testing and strengthening isokinetics.
5. Functional sports-orientated work, including plyometrics and specific drills with coaches to correct faulty technique. The five 'S's of sport are regained: speed, strength, suppleness, skill, stamina.

Rehabilitation must also address the technical errors found in throwing athletes with injuries; liaison with the coach is essential.

Range of motion exercises

Range of motion exercises include stretching of internal rotation to counter the commonly observed restriction of internal rotation in throwing athletes. Passive and active stretching of a tight posterior capsule will reduce anterior translation and relieve symptoms. Overstretching the ante-

rior capsule will aggravate any instability. Many overhead athletes use anterior stretches as part of their programme to achieve a greater external rotation. They should only be performed in the rehabilitation programme when subluxation and instability have been excluded. The exercises include: pendular; pulley; active assisted; stretching posterior muscles, internal rotation and scapular protraction.

Strengthening programme

The principles of the strengthening programme are to provide a graduated progression along a series of steps on a ladder of return to competition. Attempting to climb too fast or miss steps may lead to a slide back down the ladder.

The strengthening programme begins when the athlete is pain free. Rubberized cord is available in various thicknesses to provide a gradation of effort. The cord can be used for concentric and eccentric exercises. Initially short lever arms are used, with the elbow bent with gravity eliminated. Movements are slow, comfortable and controlled within the pain-free range. Re-establishing the synchrony of movement is extremely important. As the athlete improves, gravity is introduced, the elbow is extended to provide a longer lever arm and increased resistance from the cord. Isolated movements are used to strengthen a particularly weak muscle, whereas a combined movement pattern re-establishes and enhances a functional movement or activity.

Key muscle groups are identified to focus the rehabilitation:

1. protectors: the four rotator cuff muscles;
2. pivoters: the 17 muscles controlling scapular movement;
3. positioners: the deltoid;
4. propellors: the muscles providing the force to the arm, e.g. pectoralis major, latissimus dorsi, biceps.

The first muscle groups to be focused upon are the rotator cuff muscles, the protectors whose function is to hold the humeral head in the glenoid and reduce the stresses upon the capsular structures. A relatively new concept in shoulder rehabilitation, particularly in overhead athletes, is the importance of the scapula. The scapula provides a stable platform for the glenohumeral joint. The humeral head on the glenoid can be compared with a golf ball on a tee. If the tee is unstable, then the ball will fall off. Normal scapula biomechanics are essential to prevent winging, impingement and instability. Strengthening the scapular pivoters is undertaken first in association with the rotator cuff exercises. The rotator cuff muscles are exercised in the functional scapular plane, and not in direct abduction. The scapular plane is 30° of forward flexion from abduction in the neutral plane.

The powerful propellor muscles are worked upon last as they are related to throwing performance. If these muscles are strengthened too early they overpower the compromised rotator cuff control and lead to further impingement.

Rotator cuff 'protectors'

Isometric exercises are begun, progressing to dynamic contraction. A progression is made from short to long lever arms and from rubberized cord (cliniband) on to free weights. Isometric contraction of the infraspinatus is in varying positions of external rotation and of the supraspinatus in the scapular plane. Internal and external rotational strengthening exercises are performed at the side and up to 90° abduction to optimize rotator cuff strengthening. The teres minor is not active with the arm at the side, but is important in the control of the throwing action and requires active consideration in the rehabilitation programme. As improvement occurs, resisted dynamic external rotation and scapular plane movement rotation are introduced. These exercises should be both concentric and eccentric, with care to avoid any positions exacerbating anterior instability. The athlete must always be made aware of the position of the scapula when exercising the rotator cuff to avoid winging.

Scapular 'pivoters'

A variety of exercises may be used to enhance scapular control. Once again there should be a step-like progression in difficulty of action. Shoulder shrugs work the trapezius, levator scapulae and the rhomboids. The shoulder is rotated in a posterior direction emphasizing correct posture. Shoulder retraction and seated rowing strengthen the rhomboids. Push ups or press ups can be performed with a progression. Initially the athlete may stand against a wall and push away from it, concentrating on scapular retraction and protraction, preventing winging. This can also be performed as an eccentric exercise. The athlete then adds gravity by lying in the standard position for a press-up but not allowing the trunk to fall below elbow level to avoid overstressing the anterior capsule. The initial position of the arms is close together. As function improves, the grip or hand position is widened adding further stress to the stabilizers. The final exercises for the scapula add movement in a further plane and add a degree of proprioceptive control, for example, walking on hands and knees or feet, then adding sideways movements. As exercises in scapular control they are very tiring and should be tried by the surgeon and therapist! The endurance element of scapular exercises is important, so many repetitions are performed against relatively light resistance.

Shoulder 'positioners'

These muscles should only be worked when the protectors and pivoters are strong and synchronous. The deltoid is strengthened by performing flexion in the sagittal plane, again progressing from short weight arm to long weight arm. Abduction in the scapular plane and extension is prone to the horizontal.

Shoulder 'propellors'

These primary movers of the shoulder are trained last. The latissimus dorsi has a significant role in deceleration, and may be exercised with pull downs, introducing internal rotation as the arm is brought down from the horizontal. Biceps curls are included in recognition of the importance of these muscles in the control of the humeral head. The pectoralis major work is performed in protraction and internal rotation.

Open and closed chain exercises and proprioception

The concept of open and closed kinetic chain exercises should be understood. A closed kinetic chain is one where the distal segment is fixed relative to an immovable object. An example of this is the press up exercise where the hands are resting upon the floor. Closed kinetic chain exercises are useful in producing forces which promote glenohumeral joint compression by ensuring both agonist and antagonist contraction, the so-called co-contraction concept. This enhances dynamic joint stability. Proprioceptive work is increasingly recognized as important in rehabilitation. All closed kinetic work will help develop proprioception. In open chain exercises the patient has to replace his/her arm in the same position in space with the eyes closed, to enhance proprioception. The use of mirrors in the gymnasium helps the athlete. A wobble board, piece of foam or a physio ball require a great deal of strength and proprioceptive control and are excellent pieces of apparatus for shoulder rehabilitation. Proprioception is very important, and training is most beneficial when the shoulder is fatigued.

Proprioceptive neuromuscular facilitation

The therapist can use a technique called proprioceptive neuromuscular facilitation (PNF). This involves stretching a muscle group which the athlete then contracts against resistance provided by the therapist. A longer stretch can then be achieved with little effort. An advantage of this technique is that it works muscles at extremes of their range – an intrinsic requirement of sport. PNF techniques are used to strengthen specific functional movement patterns.

RETURN TO THROWING

After completing the programme outlined above, the athlete is ready to commence rehabilitation related to throwing. The cocking phase in throwing involves prestretching the flexors/internal rotators which facilitates the rapid acceleration phase. This stretch shortening cycle is common to many sporting activities and can be enhanced by a technique termed plyometric training. The intention is to train the elastic and reactive component of muscle to increase muscle recruitment over minimal amount of time, creating a rapid onset of maximum force. Gentle throwing against an inclined surface and catching the return provides excellent rehabilitation for endurance.

Wilk et al[13] use 'movement awareness drills' to enhance neuromuscular control of the shoulder. Their advanced drills place the shoulder in a position that maximally challenges the dynamic stabilizers. They use a 9 lb medicine ball in the position of apprehension requiring the patient to control the movement. Examples include the following: throwing exercises; two-handed overhead soccer throw in; two-handed chest pass; one-handed stop and pass; two-handed side throw; wall ball catching; exercise tubing for external and internal rotation in 90° of abduction with and without elbow flexion; plyometrics (jumping) off a 6 inch box.

When the athlete is ready to return to throwing, he/she will have improved power and control of his/her shoulder, and will have performed many drills which simulate the throwing action. At this stage, coaching input is essential to prevent a return to errors in throwing technique or tennis serve. The effort the athlete puts into the throw should gradually increase from a slow controlled movement up to full speed over a period of time. The coach will ensure that the correct run up or preparation for the throw is regained; a full-effort throw cannot be performed off balance. Errors in throwing technique will be assessed. The commonest error is allowing the elbow to drop below shoulder height. This exerts extra tension upon the anterior stabilizers of the shoulder and the medial ligament of the elbow.

The legs and trunk contribute over 50% of the kinetic energy of a throw. The rehabilitation programme must include suitable training of the trunk, back and abdomen in particular.

PRESEASON CONDITIONING

Many of these exercise should be part of the preseason conditioning of the overhead athlete. Indeed, there is evidence that not only is the risk of injury reduced, but performance is improved. As has been stated, amateur pitchers have markedly greater use of the supraspinatus hence the need for preseason conditioning for all, as fatigue from overuse predisposes to shoulder injuries. The dominant arm in tennis players is stronger, but in internal rotation and not in external rotation. Strengthening internal over external rotation occurs as an adaptive mechanism. This may create muscle imbalances across the shoulder which predispose to injury to the external rotators as they attempt to stabilize the humeral head in the deceleration phase of the throwing or serving action. Certainly in tennis players, Mont et al[11] have shown that a training programme increased serve velocity by 11%. In baseball no statistical difference between dominant and non-dominant arms in terms of internal and external rotation has been shown, but there is a trend. Other authors have shown an increase in strength of internal rotation and a reduction in strength of external rotation in the dominant arm.

FAILURE OF CONSERVATIVE TREATMENT

The vast majority of athletes, some 95%, can be expected to respond to rehabilitation. Some do not settle with conservative measures. In this situation the diagnosis must be re-examined. The commonest error is that underlying instability has been missed, but other causes of pain should be excluded.

Breakdown during the rehabilitation phase may also be due to attempts to progress too fast along the training ladder or poor exercise technique. The usual error introduced is the use of exercises that are standard in weight training, moving the shoulder into a position of impingement or potential instability. If the athlete has not received correct coaching input and returns to the same throwing technique, then he/she is quite likely to suffer recurrence.

SURGERY FOR IMPINGEMENT AND ROTATOR CUFF PATHOLOGY

The history of development of the surgical management of throwing injuries is one of improved recognition of the true underlying pathology. The published series of results of surgery for throwing athletes are not well known and numbers are small. Tibone[14] in 1986 reported that of 18 throwing athletes treated by open decompression, only four returned to their previous level, despite satisfactory pain relief. In a later paper from the same centre for athletes treated by acromioplasty and rotator cuff repair, the results improved to 41% success for throwers, although only 32% for professionals.[6] However, the rotator cuff pathology had no influence on the ultimate result. Partial and total-thickness tears were repaired at the same open operation. These papers preceded the wide recognition that instability is frequently the primary cause of impingement and it is likely that the poor results were due to unrecognized instability.

Arthroscopic subacromial decompression in the athlete has the advantage of being a less traumatic procedure with reduced damage to the deltoid origin, and earlier rehabilitation is possible. In addition, associated pathologies can be identified within the glenohumeral joint which would be missed with the open procedure. Glousman[4] made a comparison in results at the Kerlan–Jobe clinic from a further review of results. In this later series, symptoms had been present for 14 months and those with full-thickness rotator cuff tears were excluded; 77% returned to sport, but only 25% of those with capsular laxity or labral pathology were able to return to the same level of activity. No pitchers or swimmers were able to return to their previous level. The conclusion was that the results of subacromial decompression alone were unpredictable. Certainly those with primary instability and secondary impingement do not respond well to subacromial decompression because the underlying instability is not treated. With time the pain recurs.

Damage to the rotator cuff caused by internal impingement/tensile failure on the humeral surface is visible at arthroscopy. Andrews et al[15] reported a group treated with debridement followed by a rehabilitation programme. They obtained excellent results in 85% of patients including 64% baseball players. The results are, as perhaps what might be expected from a rehabilitation programme. These authors considered that complete tears should be repaired. Baker and Lui[16] recommend arthroscopically assisted repair of the rotator cuff, citing satisfactory results with reduced morbidity and earlier return to function.

It is imperative not to miss underlying instability which is the primary cause of internal and subacromial impingement and associated rotator cuff pathology. The instability is best treated by stabilization if rehabilitation fails. Frank Jobe no longer repairs small cuff tears associated with internal impingement.

SURGERY FOR INSTABILITY

Surgery on the glenoid labrum

In the throwing athlete, it is recommended that arthroscopic examination of the shoulder precedes the stabilization procedure. Arthroscopic findings include rotator cuff tears, fraying and tearing of the glenoid labrum, SLAP lesions and damage to the humeral head. Loose bodies can be removed.[17]

Pappas[18] put forward the concept of functional glenohumeral instability due to flap tears of the glenoid labrum successfully treated by open excision in 1983. Since that time other authors have not been so successful. Altchek and co-workers[19] reported a series of patients all of whom were active in shoulder-involved sports. Before surgery 38 of 40 had a positive impingement test which settled. The relocation test was published after the patients were treated, but using EUA and drawer signs, 24 of 40 had laxity. Although initial results were satisfactory, after 3 years, 72% noted dete-

rioration with time, 7% had mild pain, 70% had moderate pain and 23% severe pain. Similarly, others have reported a deterioration with time. Occult instability was found in 70% of patients with SLAP lesions, all others had instability on EUA. At 1 year, 78% of patients with superior lesions had excellent relief and 30% with anteroinferior lesions, but at 2 years the success rates had fallen to 63% and 25% respectively. Only 45% and 25% had returned to the previous level of sport. Four required reoperation, two each for instability and impingement.

Terry et al[20] reported that results of arthroscopic labral debridement depended upon associated damage to the glenohumeral ligaments. Follow-up averaged 3.2 years. The results were 14% excellent, 71% satisfactory, 15% poor. The poor results were associated with grade 3 glenohumeral ligament tear in which only a partial excision of torn labrum was performed. Although 82% returned to their sport, only 48% thought that they were able to perform at their previous level. The paper suggests that minor tears with no significant ligament damage can be treated arthroscopically.

Martin[21] in 1995 also reported a long-term follow-up. Emphasizing the importance of rehabilitation after surgery, 62% of baseball pitchers were unimpaired after arthroscopic debridement without gross instability or a Bankart lesion. The average age of patients in this series was 19 years, which is before chronic attenuation of the glenohumeral ligaments associated with prolonged throwing occurs. This separates the patients in this series from others.

To summarize, arthroscopic debridement of the glenoid labrum may be of use in treating the young thrower with only mild damage to the glenohumeral ligaments and without instability. A rehabilitation programme is essential.

STABILIZATION PROCEDURES IN THROWING ATHLETES

Instability in the throwing athlete may present as popping or clicking with shoulder pain, secondary impingement, or the dead arm syndrome. The instability is due to capsular laxity (occasionally multidirectional), trauma to the glenoid labrum and is associated with failure of the dynamic stabilizers. The problem is of subluxation rather than frank instability. Surgery must be performed to correct these deficiencies.

Stabilization procedures for throwing athletes must treat glenoid labral lesions and reduce excess capsular laxity. It is axiomatic that procedures must not reduce external rotation, cause weakness or fail to correct instability, or throwing performance will be impaired.

Many operations have been described for stabilizing the shoulder. Loss of external rotation is a well-recognized effect of many of them. Historically, Dickson & Devas[22] reported a 20° loss of external rotation after the Bankart procedure in 1957. Carter Rowe[23] reported a series using the Bankart procedure which included 30 throwing athletes; only 10 of these returned to their previous level of competition. Lombardo[24] in 1976 concluded that throwers were not capable of returning to high-performance levels after the Bristow procedure. Few throwing athletes are included in the studies of surgery for shoulder instability. Careful reading of the results frequently demonstrates that the results for throwers are not as good as for other athletes.[25]

The rationale behind a superior shift of the inferior capsule in reducing loss of external rotation yet reducing glenohumeral instability was demonstrated by Speer and co-workers.[26]

Bigliani et al[27] published their experience with an anterior–inferior capsular shift in 1994 in 31 overhead throwing athletes. The operation included a capsular shift in addition to repair of a Bankart lesion when present. They justify the procedure by noting the need to address inferior capsular laxity together with the requirement to reattach the capsule to the glenoid labrum. Athletes with strictly anterior instability and those with posterior instability were not included in this study. Of 68 shoulders in 63 athletic patients, 31% had Bankart lesions that required repair, and in a further 43%, significant wear on the anteroinferior labrum was found. The subluxors had a much lower incidence of Bankart lesions than in the

frank dislocators (5% versus 43%). Of the throwers, half returned to the same level of competition, and the others were able to throw but at a reduced level. Loss of external rotation in the series averaged 7°, range 0–30°. Spreading of the rotator interval was common, and was repaired when present, a finding also noted by Rowe and Zarins.[10]

Jobe and coworkers[28] published a series of stabilization procedures in athletes in 1991 that used an anterior capsulolabral reconstruction. This was followed up with a series on the functional outcomes.[29] In the first paper, six of 12 pitchers returned to throwing at 1 year, although only three of eight were professionals. This included three who, although they had gained almost full range of motion, strength and speed, decided to retire for personal reasons. In the follow-up study, 81% returned to their previous level of sport, including 12 of 16 pitchers (75%), six of seven professionals. The average loss of range of motion was 1°. The importance of preservation of external rotation can be exemplified by one pitcher who lost just 5° of external rotation, yet was unable to regain his throwing velocity.

Jobe uses a subscapularis splitting approach which reduces the operative damage to the muscle. Persistent posterior shoulder pain is due to tightness of the posterior structures; this settles with stretching of the posterior capsule. In later work, the concept of posterior or internal impingement was introduced to account for the findings of a partial-thickness tear and posterosuperior labral damage. The subscapularis splitting approach permits very early active movement and external rotation. The shoulder is placed in an aeroplane splint at 90° of abduction and 45° of flexion. Partial-thickness tears of the rotator cuff are not repaired, as the underlying pathology has been corrected. They are allowed to recover with time. The rotator interval cannot be directly visualized with this technique. The importance of prolonged rehabilitation of a year to full throwing speed is emphasized.

There are many controversies related to the diagnosis and management of patients with anterior shoulder instability. The majority of information is based on a number of case series. There is little evidence of an experimental nature and therefore no proof to decide on one method of management over another.[30]

DEAD ARM SYNDROME

Dead arm syndrome is the name given to the situation where a throw is accompanied by a sudden sharp or paralysing pain. The athlete complains that the arm goes 'dead' and may hang useless by the side after a throw with maximum effort. The arm may ache afterwards. Performance deteriorates with time. The syndrome was described in athletes who complained of subluxation of the shoulder in 1969 by Blazina and Satzman.[31] Dead arm syndrome was first attributed to occult anterior instability of the shoulder in 1981 by Rowe and Zarins.[10] Thirty-two of their 60 athletes were unaware of the shoulder 'popping in and out' preceding the dead arm feeling.

Presumably the shooting pain is caused by traction upon the brachial plexus as the humerus is thrown out of joint at the end of the acceleration phase, and the decelerators fail to control the integrity of the joint.

BICEPS TENDON

The biceps works during a throw to resist humeral distraction, applying a compression force to the arm. The biceps is active not only in acceleration but also deceleration, with increased activity in the unstable shoulder where its action as a stabilizer of the glenohumeral joint is increased. Biceps pathology may be classified into four types.

1. Secondary biceps tendinitis, which accounts for 95% of biceps pathology. The biceps tendon pathology is secondary to impingement syndrome. Burkehead[32] states that both Charles Neer and Charles Rockwood stress that 95–98% of patients with the diagnosis of biceps tendinitis have in reality a primary diagnosis of impingement syndrome. They

have condemned biceps tenodesis. Treatment must address the underlying pathology.[33]
2. Primary biceps tendon tendinitis. This is now recognized to be extremely uncommon. Where it does occur it is usually secondary to an inflammatory aetiology or to an abnormality in the groove secondary to trauma. This excites a synovitis and may progress to rupture. Post[34] reported a 94% success with good to excellent results treating tendinitis with primary tenodesis in a selected group of young patients with impingement excluded. Where difficulties arise in separating those with or without impingement it is advisable to perform an arthroscopic subacromial decompression at the time of biceps tenodesis.[4]
3. Biceps tendon instability. This is infrequent but can be seen in younger patients who participate in throwing sports. The tendon may be palpated as it flicks out of the groove with rotation of the shoulder in abduction. In older patients the biceps tendon may dislocate after a tear occurs in the rotator cuff and coracohumeral ligament. O'Donaghue[35] treated subluxation of the biceps tendon with tenodesis and reported a 77% success in returning athletes to their previous sport and resuming throwing.
4. Biceps tendon rupture as an acute or chronic event. This is usually found in the older athlete and follows repeated bouts of subacromial impingement, with bicipital and rotator cuff tendinitis.

INSERTIONAL PATHOLOGY OF THE GLENOID LABRUM (SLAP LESIONS)

Andrews et al[15] were the first to report the incidence of tears of the glenoid labrum related to the long head of biceps in 1985. They reported tears of the glenoid labrum in 73 pitchers. They noted that in many cases the anterosuperior portion of the labrum had been pulled off by the biceps tendon. They observed tension of the biceps tendon and the superior glenoid together with compression of the humeral head into the glenoid as the biceps muscle was electrically stimulated. Snyder and co-workers[17] coined the term SLAP lesion in 1990. They classified tears of the insertion of the biceps tendon into the superior glenoid labrum into four categories.

type 1: fraying of the superior labrum with degeneration but no separation;
type 2: separation of the biceps tendon–superior labrum complex from the superior glenoid with or without fraying;
type 3: bucket-handle tears of the superior labrum;
type 4: bucket-handle tears extending into the substance of the biceps tendon.

Maffet et al[36] proposed a further three types to be added to this classification:

type 5: an anterior extension continuing to an anteroinferior Bankart lesion;
type 6: unstable flap tear of the labrum in addition to the type 2 separation;
type 7: anteroinferior extension extending beneath the middle glenohumeral ligament.

SLAP lesions are associated with instability, clicking or a vague shoulder pain which may give rise to diagnostic difficulties. About 75% of Maffet's patients had a pre-operative diagnosis of impingement syndrome. Detachment of the superior glenoid labrum is detrimental to anterior stability, as it decreases the shoulder's resistance to torsion and places a greater strain on the inferior glenohumeral ligament. In throwing athletes, SLAP lesions may be the result of a sudden pull on the long head of biceps in the deceleration phase. Posterior–superior labral lesions may be caused by internal impingement.

The diagnosis is made by arthroscopy of the shoulder. The biceps tension test may be useful although it can be far from diagnostic. A downward-directed force is applied to the shoulder in 90° of abduction with the elbow extended and the forearm supinated. This pulls the labrum from the torn glenoid rim, reproducing the patient's symptoms.

Treatment of SLAP lesions

The frayed labrum is debrided, but stabilization of the type 2 lesion or higher may be indicated. Arthroscopic stabilization is becoming increasingly popular.[36,37] Co-existing instability or impingement should be dealt with at the same time.

POSTERIOR INSTABILITY

The throwing athlete with posterior instability may present in a variety of ways. Athletes may complain of posterior shoulder pain and/or clicking, tendinitis secondary to instability, or posterior subluxation. Recurrent posterior subluxation is associated with the stresses on the posterior structures in the deceleration phase, and the follow-through phase when the shoulder is in a position of adduction, internal rotation and flexion where there is a posterior translational force on the humeral head. Frank posterior dislocation is very rare in the athlete.

The findings of posterior instability are frequently associated with voluntary subluxation and multidirectional instability which must not be missed. In contrast to this, it should be recalled that reduced internal rotation is a more common finding in throwers and that posterior shoulder pain may be caused by a tight posterior capsule aggravating internal impingment.

Examination

The posterior draw sign will be positive, and there is a posterior subluxation of the shoulder with the patient supine which can be reduced with a clunk. Voluntary subluxation must not be missed and the patient should be asked to reproduce the effect. Voluntary subluxation uses asynchronous movement of muscles. Shoulder elevation and the rhythm of movement should be observed, and spontaneous subluxation and relocation should be looked out for.

Posterior subluxation occurs most often in a position of 100° of abduction with the shoulder in mild internal rotation and in either neutral or slight adduction.

Investigations

EUA and arthroscopy are important in the confirmation of the diagnosis and assessment of the direction of the laxity. The posterior glenoid labrum is often frayed and may be avulsed. Radiography may reveal a Bennett's lesion, which is a hypertrophic area of bone at 8 o'clock on the posterior glenoid lip in throwers.

Treatment

Conservative

Posterior instability should be managed conservatively where possible with a scapular and rotator cuff strengthening programme. Psychological issues may be significant.

Surgical

Posterior fraying of the labrum may be treated by arthroscopic excision; the labrum may be reattached arthroscopically. Many open procedures have been described including osteotomies of glenoid and humerus subscapularis or biceps tendon transfers. Posterior capsular reconstructions have included posterior Bankart repairs, reverse Putti–Platt and other capsulorrhaphy procedures. Surgery has limited success with only 30% returning to sport in the study of Tibone and co-workers[39] on posterior staple capsulorrhaphy. Fronek et al[40] achieved a 70% return to sport but mostly at a diminished level or altered position.

Hurley[41] in a retrospective study compared conservative with surgical treatment. Voluntary subluxation was evident in 50% of their patients. They noted a low incidence of degenerative changes: 50% of those treated surgically and 68% treated conservatively found their shoulders were improved. The recurrence rates were 72% (surgical) and 96% (conservative), but the latter could often cope with their condition. Hawkins & Cash[42] have abandoned glenoid osteotomy because of the unacceptable risks of degenerative

changes in the mid-term. Results of surgery are variable. Tibone has concluded that his posterior staple capsulorrhaphy is not an acceptable procedure and does not allow athletes to return to throwing.[39] He noted the incidence of associated anterior instability and stated that an operation should only be performed in certain patients who have pain or decreased function when performing the activities of daily living.

NERVE LESIONS IN THROWING SPORTS

Long thoracic nerve

This usually presents as a result of direct trauma, but has been described as a consequence of throwing. Patients complain of weakness of the shoulder girdle, a dull burning ache, and winging of the scapula. Pressing on a wall with the arms outstretched reveals the winging. The scapula fails to protract with shoulder elevation, and failure of synchrony movement leads to secondary impingement from poor elevation of the acromion. The treatment is expectant with anticipation that recovery will occur. Muscle transfers have been described but will not permit return to competitive throwing.

Suprascapular nerve

The suprascapular nerve can be injured in sport (in throwing and weight training) as well as in a fall and as a complication of surgery. There is a similar presentation to rotator cuff injury, occasionally with secondary impingement. Sensation remains intact but weakness and atrophy of the infraspinatus and supraspinatus are evident.

Suprascapular nerve entrapment may occur in the suprascapular notch or around the base of the acromion where it supplies the infraspinatus. Examination reveals wasting of the infraspinatus with the supraspinatus, depending upon the position of the entrapment. Diagnosis is by EMG studies with plain X-ray to observe the notch for any bony pathology. A cyst or ganglion arising from the sublabral region may cause direct compression of the nerve.

Treatment

Rest from aggravating activity, NSAIDs, electrical stimulation and corticosteroids are the main forms of treatment. The finding of a cyst or ganglion should lead to prompt drainage, which can be performed arthroscopically. Traction injuries usually recover in a few months. If no recovery is seen at 6 months, then surgical release of the nerve and removal of space-occupying lesions is indicated. Surgery is not very useful for the entrapment around the base of the acromion but aggressive rehabilitation of the infraspinatus may produce alleviation of symptoms and permit return to sport.

Musculocutaneous nerve

This is vulnerable where it lies under subscapularis. Injury occurs after strenuous activity and has also been described after throwing. It frequently recovers but if it does not, then surgical release should be attempted at 3 months.

Quadrilateral space syndrome

This very rare syndrome is caused by compression of the posterior circumflex artery and axillary nerve in the quadrilateral space. The symptoms are insidious with poorly localized intermittent onset of pain and paraesthesia in the upper arm. The pain is exacerbated by flexion abduction and external rotation. Throwers are susceptible. Palpation over the quadrilateral space with the shoulder held in the position that it adopts during the acceleration phase causes the symptoms after a few minutes. The diagnosis is confirmed by arteriography of the subclavian artery. With the arm dependent, the posterior circumflex humeral artery is visible. With the arm abducted and in external rotation the occlusion is demonstrated. If rest fails to settle the pain then surgical release is indicated.

Differential diagnosis of shoulder pain

Referred pain from C5, C6 is characterized by a deep burning pain in the rhomboid area associated with paraesthesia radiating down the forearm to the fingers. The patient may be more comfortable with the arm elevated, and the forearm resting on the head.

THE ACROMIOCLAVICULAR JOINT IN THROWERS

Acromioclavicular joint pathology is usually the result of direct trauma to the shoulder or via a fall. The acromioclavicular joint is very close to the supraspinatus tendon. The joint may be affected by the inflammatory process of impingement. Degeneration of the acromioclavicular joint produces osteophytic lipping which may affect the rotator cuff. Acromioclavicular joint pain is exacerbated by adduction, extremes of abduction and direct palpation. Local anaesthetic into the joint may be diagnostic by removing the pain from these movements, and local steroid may be therapeutic.

Atraumatic clavicular osteolysis is found most commonly in weight lifters. Throwers are also susceptible. In an epidemiological study of 25 weight lifters, with age-matched controls, 28% had radiological changes and 16% had symptoms but no radiological changes.[43] The more they lifted for longer, the more changes were visible. Treatment is by excision of the distal end of the clavicle leaving the coracoacromial ligament, which gives good relief of pain.

SCAPULOTHORACIC BURSITIS

Sisto & Jobe[44] reported on the operative treatment of scapulothoracic bursitis in professional baseball players. Pain is localized to the inferomedial angle of the scapula and is caused by high speed repetitive throwing and friction between the anterior scapula, the underlying muscles and the rib cage. The shoulder is characteristically painful in cocking and acceleration. Pain is relieved by the follow-through. There is often a mass palpable at the inferomedial border when the scapula is elevated by 60° of abduction and 30° of flexion. Symptoms may be associated with impingement or instability.

STRESS FRACTURES

Branch[45] published a series of 12 cases of spontaneous fracture of the shaft of the humerus during pitching. These fractures were in pitchers returning to pitching after a long lay-off of an average of 14 years. They were experienced pitchers who had been pitching for 11 years before their first retirement. The average age was 36. About 75% had symptoms before the fracture, mostly (75%) spiral fractures. Stress fractures of the coracoid have been reported whilst pitching in a game after a 3-week history of pain. Treatment is expectant.

SUMMARY

The challenge of managing an athlete with a throwing injury is an exacting one. The practitioner must be aware of the biomechanics of the throwing technique used in a given sport and the relevant basic scientific research. The advances in knowledge of the pathophysiology of throwing injuries, in examination and surgical techniques, have made this area one for the specialist. Equally, rehabilitation is the cornerstone of treatment which must be understood if good results are to be achieved.

REFERENCES

1. Fleisig, G.S., Andrews, J.R., Dillman, C.J. & Escamilla, R.F. (1995) Kinetics of baseball pitching with implications about injury mechanism. *Am. J. Sports Med.* **23:** 233–239.
2. Glousman, R.E. (1993) Electromyographic analysis and its role in the athletic shoulder. *CORR* **288:** 27–34.
3. Pappas, A.M., Zawacki, R.M. & Sullivan, T.J. (1985) Biomechanics of baseball pitching. *Am. J. Sports Med.* **13:** 216–222.
4. Glousman, R.E. (1993) Instability versus impingement syndrome in the throwing athlete. *Orthop. Clin. North Am.* Shoulder arthroscopy and related surgery. **1:** 89–99.
5. Jobe, F.W. & Kvitne, R.S. (1989) Shoulder pain in the overhand or throwing athlete. The relationship of anterior instability and rotator cuff impingement. *Orthop. Rev.* **18:** 963–975.
6. Tibone, J.E., Jobe, F.W. & Kerlan, R.K. (1988) Shoulder impingement syndrome in athletes treated by an anterior acromioplasty. *Clin. Orthop.* **198:** 134–140.
7. Kupferman, S.P. (1994) Tensile failure of the rotator cuff. In Andrews, J.R. and Wilk, K.E. (eds) *The Athlete's Shoulder*, pp. 113–120. New York: Churchill Livingstone.
8. Jobe, C.M. (1993) Evidence for superior glenoid impingement upon the rotator cuff. *J. Shoulder Elbow Surg.* **2:** 51–54.
9. Litchfield, R., Hawkins, R., Dillman, C.J., Atkins, J. & Hagerman, G.B. (1993) Rehabilitation for the overhead athlete. *J. Orthop. Sports Phy. Ther.* **18:** 433–441.
10. Rowe, C.R. & Zarins, B. (1981) Recurrent transient subluxation of the shoulder. *J. Bone Joint Surg.* **60A:** 863–872.
11. Mont, M.A., Cohen, D.B., Campbell, K.R., Gravare, K. & Mathur, S.K. (1994) Isokinetic concentric versus eccentric training of shoulder rotators with functional evaluation of performance enhancement in elite tennis players. *Am. J. Sports Med.* **22:** 513–517.
12. Miniaci, A., Dowdy, P.A., Willits, K.R. & Vellet, A.D. (1995) Magnetic resonance imaging evaluation of the rotator cuff tendons in the asymptomatic shoulder. *Am. J. Sports Med.* **23:** 142–145.
13. Wilk, K.E., Andrews, J.R., Arrigo, C.A., Keirns, M.A. & Erber, D.J. (1993) The strength characteristics of internal and external rotator muscles in professional baseball pitchers. *Am. J. Sports Med.* **21:** 61–66.
14. Tibone, J.E., Elrod Jobe, F.W., Kerlan, R.K. et al (1986) Surgical treatment of the rotator cuff in athletes. *J. Bone Joint Surg.* **68A:** 887–891.
15. Andrews, J.R., Broussard, T.S. & Carson, W.G. (1985) Arthroscopy of the shoulder in the management of partial tears of the rotator cuff: a preliminary report. *Arthroscopy* **1:** 117–122.
16. Baker, C.L. & Lui, S.H. (1995) Comparison of open and arthroscopically assisted rotator cuff repairs. *Am. J. Sports Med.* **23:** 99–104.
17. Snyder, S.J., Karzel, R.P. & Del Pizzo, W. (1990) SLAP lesions of the shoulder. *Arthroscopy* **6:** 274–279.
18. Pappas, A.M., Goss, T.P. & Kleinman, P.K. (1983) Symptomatic shoulder instability due to lesions of the glenoid labrum. *Am. J. Sports Med.* **11:** 279–288.
19. Altchek, D.E., Warren, R.F., Wickiewicz, T.L. & Ortiz, G. (1992) Arthroscopic labral debridement: a three year follow up study. *Am. J. Sports Med.* **20:** 702–706.

20. Terry, G., Friedman, S.J. & Uhl, T.L. (1994) Arthroscopically treated tears of the glenoid labrum: factors affecting outcome. *Am. J. Sports Med.* **22:** 504–512.

21. Martin, D.R. & Garth, W.P. (1995) Results of arthroscopic debridement of glenoid labral tears. *Am. J. Sports Med.* **23:** 447–451.

22. Dickson, J.W. & Devas, M.B. (1957) Bankart's operation for recurrent dislocation of the shoulder. *J. Bone Joint Surg.* **39B:** 114–119.

23. Rowe, C.R., Patel, D. & Southmayd, W.W. (1978) The Bankart procedure: a long term end result study. *J. Bone Joint Surg.* **60A:** 1–16.

24. Lombardo, S.J., Kerlan, R.K. & Jobe, F.W. (1976) The modified Bristow procedure for recurrent dislocation of the shoulder. *J. Bone Joint Surg.* **58A:** 256–261.

25. Altchek, D.W., Warren, R.F. & Skyhar, M.J. (1991) T-plasty modification of the Bankart procedure for multidirectional instability of the anterior and inferior types. *J. Bone Joint Surg.* **73A:** 105–112.

26. Speer, K.P., Deng, X., Torzilli, P.A., Altchek, D.A. & Warren, R.F. (1995) Strategies for an anterior capsular shift of the shoulder. *Am. J. Sports Med.* **23:** 264–269.

27. Bigliani, L.U., Kurzweil, P.R., Schwartzbach, C.C., Wolfe, I.N. & Flatow, E.L. (1994) Inferior capsular shift procedure for anterior–inferior shoulder instability in athletes. *Am. J. Sports Med.* **22:** 578–584.

28. Jobe, F.W., Giangarra, C.E., Kvitne, R.S. & Glousman, R.E. (1991) Anterior capsulolabral reconstruction of the shoulder in athletes in overhand sport. *Am. J. Sports Med.* **19:** 428–434.

29. Montgomery, W.H. & Jobe, F.W. (1994) Functional outcomes in athletes after modified anterior capsulolabral reconstruction. *Am. J. Sports Med.* **22:** 352–357.

30. Hawkins, R.H. & Mohtadi, N.G.H. (1991) Controversy in anterior shoulder instability. *CORR* **272:** 152–161.

31. Blazina, M.E. & Satzman, J.S. (1969) Recurrent anterior subluxation of the shoulder in athletes – a distinct entity. *J. Bone Joint Surg.* **51A:** 1037–1038.

32. Burkehead, W.Z. (1990) The biceps tendon. In Rockwood, C.A. Jr & Master, F.A. III (eds) *The Shoulder*, p. 791. Philadelphia: W.B. Saunders.

33. Curtis, A.S. & Snyder, S.J. (1996) Evaluation and treatment of biceps tendon pathology. *Orthop. Clin. North Am*. Shoulder arthroscopy and related surgery **24:** 33–43.

34. Post, M. (1989) Primary tendinitis of the long head of biceps. *Clin. Orthop.* **246:** 117.

35. O'Donaghue, D. (1982) Subluxating biceps tendon in the athlete. *Clin. Orthop.* **164:** 26.

36. Maffet, M.W., Gartsman, G.M. & Moseley, B. (1995) Superior labrum–biceps tendon complex lesions of the shoulder. *Am. J. Sports Med.* **23:** 93–98.

37. Field, L.D. & Savoie, F.H. (1993) Arthroscopic suture repair of superior labral detachment lesions of the shoulder. *Am. J. Sports Med.* **21:** 783–790.

38. Scarpinato, D.F. & Andrews, J.R. (1994) Posterior instability of the shoulder. In Andrews, J.R. & Wilk, K.E. (eds) *The Athlete's Shoulder*, pp. 205–214. New York: Churchill Livingstone.

39. Tibone, J.E., Prietto, C., Jobe, F.W., Kerlan, R.W., Carter, V.S., Shields, C.L., Lombardo, S.J., Collins, H.R. & Yocum, L.A. (1981) Staple capsulorrhaphy for recurrent posterior shoulder dislocation. *Am. J. Sports Med.* **9:** 135–139.

40. Fronek, J., Warren, R.F. & Bowen, M. (1989) Posterior subluxation of the glenohumeral ligament. *J. Bone Joint Surg.* **71A:** 205–216.

41. Hurley, J.A., Anderson, T.E., Dear, W., Andrish, J.T., Bergfeld, J.A. & Weiker, G.G. (1992) Posterior shoulder instability: surgical versus conservative results with evaluation of glenoid version. *Am. J. Sports Med.* **20:** 396–405.

42. Hawkins, R.H. & Cash, J.D. (1993) Complications of posterior instability repairs. In L.U. Bigliani (ed.), *Complications of Shoulder Surgery*, pp. 117–127. Baltimore: Williams and Watkins.

43. Scavenius, M. & Iverson, B.F. (1992) Nontraumatic clavicular osteolysis in weight lifters. *Am. J. Sports Med.* **20:** 463–465.

44. Sisto, D.J. & Jobe, F.W. (1986) The operative treatment of scapulothoracic bursitis in professional baseball players. *Am. J. Sports Med.* **14:** 192–195.

45. Branch, T., Partin, C., Chamberland, P., Emeterio, E. & Sabetelle, M. (1992) Spontaneous fracture of the humerus during pitching; a series of 12 cases. *Am. J. Sports Med.* **20:** 468–470.

16

Multidirectional Instability

PM Connor and LU Bigliani

INTRODUCTION

Multidirectional instability of the shoulder is more common than previously realized.[1–3] These patients have symptomatic glenohumeral instability in more than one direction: anterior, inferior and/or posterior. Standard unidirectional procedures may fail in the treatment of multidirectional instability because they do not correct all the directions of instability (e.g. a Bankart repair failure because of residual inferior or posterior instability), or conversely because excessive tightness created on one side of the hypermobile joint may cause a fixed subluxation in the opposite direction.[4–12] This may lead to glenohumeral arthritis, often at a very young age.[13]

There is a common misconception that multidirectional instability is limited to young sedentary patients with generalized ligamentous laxity who often present with bilateral symptoms and signs. Furthermore, the instability is classically thought of as acquired in an atraumatic fashion. While there does exist such a group of patients, shoulders with multidirectional instability are often found in athletic patients, many of whom have had a significant traumatic injury.[1,18] Repetitive micro-trauma, seen for example in butterfly swimming or gymnastics, can also lead to multidirectional instability by selectively 'stretching out' the capsule and ligaments of the glenohumeral joint in the absence of generalized ligamentous laxity.[4]

In addition, shoulders with multidirectional instability may have Bankart lesions[12] and humeral head impression defects,[1] although less commonly than unidirectional cases resulting from significant trauma. A previously normal shoulder without significant capsular laxity can acquire both inferior and anterior instability from trauma. Recent work in our laboratory on the material properties of the inferior glenohumeral ligament (IGHL), the principal static restraint against anterior glenohumeral instability, disclosed two predominant modes of failure: at the glenoid insertion (analogous to a Bankart avulsion) and in midsubstance (analogous to capsular stretching and laxity).[15] However, there was significant midsubstance ligament strain before failure even in the specimens that ultimately failed at the glenoid insertion. These findings are consistent with a recent biomechanical study, in a cadaver model, which demonstrated that a Bankart lesion alone did not increase instability enough to allow anterior dislocation.[16] This suggests that reconstructive procedures must correct capsular laxity in addition to repairing avulsions of the glenohumeral ligaments from the glenoid, and may explain some of the poor initial success of arthroscopic procedures aimed only at the Bankart lesions[2,17] (C. Jobe, unpublished work (1990), L. Johnson, unpublished work (1989)). Open procedures which only repair the Bankart lesion may rely for success, in part, on anterior capsular scarring from the open approach.

In our experience, patients with shoulder instability cannot always be easily separated into clear categories (unidirectional versus multidirectional). This is especially true of athletes, often lax to begin with, who subject their shoulders to repetitive micro-trauma on a daily basis, but may also suffer a superimposed injury. Therefore, if an athlete has recurrent traumatic dislocations, it is important to examine the patient for excessive capsular laxity so that this may also be corrected with the surgical repair. We have found patients with anterior instability to constitute a spectrum from unidirectional anterior instability to frank multidirectional instability with pronounced inferior capsular laxity, rather than simple discrete groups.[18] For this reason we have used the inferior capsular shift approach as described by Neer and Foster[19] in all cases, modifying the repair so that only as much capsule is shifted as is necessary to reduce the degree of laxity found in each instance. The primary pathology in shoulders with multidirectional instability is capsular laxity and redundancy, with instability in anterior, inferior and/or posterior directions. The inferior capsular shift is designed to reduce capsular volume on all sides, by both thickening and overlapping the capsule on the side of greatest instability, and tensioning the capsule on the inferior and opposite sides. Thus the soft tissues are balanced in a systematic way to meet the specific pathology present.

CLINICAL PRESENTATION

Patients with multidirectional instability may present in a variety of ways. The patient is often athletic, and swimmers, weight lifters and gymnasts may be particularly predisposed. The instability, either dislocation or subluxation, may have occurred without significant injury and spontaneously reduced. Extremely hypermobile shoulders can become symptomatic without unusual trauma and possibly even from activities of daily living; these patients are more apt to have a sedentary lifestyle. A common presentation appears to be an individual with a relatively loose shoulder who stresses it repetitively in athletic activities or work-related events.

Symptoms may suggest the directions of instability involved. Inferior instability may present with the patient's description of pain associated with carrying heavy suitcases or shopping bags. Occasionally these symptoms are accompanied by traction paraesthesias. Pain associated with pushing open heavy doors, revolving doors or use of the arm in a forward flexed and internally rotated position usually suggests a component of posterior instability, while discomfort in the overhead, abducted and externally rotated position might generally suggest anterior instability. However, an individual patient's symptoms may be vague and complex, thus precluding a diagnosis based on history alone.

The physical exam may demonstrate evidence of generalized ligamentous laxity such as hyperextension at the elbows, the ability to approximate the thumbs to the forearms, hyperextension of the metacarpophalangeal joints or patellofemoral subluxation. It is important to examine the acromioclavicular and sternoclavicular joints for tenderness as they may also be hypermobile and sources of symptoms. Inferior humeral subluxation with stress on the arm in adduction (the sulcus sign) or abduction suggests inferior laxity. In addition, close inspection of the scapulothoracic articulation should be performed, as concomitant scapulothoracic instability may occasionally be present.[1,20] There may be multiple positive findings using the following manoeuvres: anterior and posterior load and shift tests, anterior and posterior apprehension tests, the fulcrum test, relocation test, Fukuda test, and the push-pull or supine stress test.[1,20,30] The aim is to produce humeral translations anteriorly, posteriorly or inferiorly (relative to the glenoid), and to demonstrate that these translations are reliably accompanied by the patient's report of the usual pain and discomfort.

It can, at times, be difficult to determine the primary direction of instability on physical exam. Determining whether the shoulder is moving from a dislocated to a reduced position or from a reduced to a dislocated position can be challenging. Maintaining the fingers of one hand on the coracoid anteriorly and the posterolateral acromion can aid in this determination. For this reason multiple physical examinations, although difficult to achieve, are helpful in assessing these patients.

It is important that symptoms be reproduced with such manoeuvres, as laxity in and of itself is not an indication for surgical stabilization procedures. Asymptomatic shoulders may show substantial translation on clinical testing.[19,21,22] In addition, joint laxity may be remarkable enough to distract the examiner from the primary source of pain, such as a painful acromioclavicular joint or a cervical radiculopathy. Conversely, laxity may be hard to demonstrate, even in a shoulder with multidirectional instability, if pain, muscle spasm, and guarding prevent subluxation. It is helpful to examine the contralateral asymptomatic shoulder for laxity. If it is extremely loose, it may be a clue to the multidirectional nature of the affected side.

Plain radiographs are generally normal but should be evaluated for the presence of humeral head defects and/or glenoid lesions such as osseous Bankart fragments, reactive bone or wear. Double-contrast CT arthrograms may demonstrate an increased capsular volume and, less commonly, labral detachments. The MRI is less satisfactory in demonstrating the redundant capsule due to the lack of joint distension. However, labral lesions can be detected if present. Stress radiographs can demonstrate laxity, especially inferior subluxation, but are not generally needed. Cine MRI is currently investigational, but has the potential to demonstrate dynamically capsular and labral defects, in varying positions.[23]

INDICATIONS FOR SURGERY

Once the diagnosis of multidirectional instability has been established, a course of rehabilitation is instituted with emphasis on strengthening the deltoid and rotator cuff muscles with the arm below the shoulder. The scapulothoracic-stabilizing muscles are strengthened as well.[24] Patients with multidirectional instability may occasionally develop a secondary impingement syndrome. At times a subacromial injection of a xylocaine and steroid preparation will provide relief sufficient for the patient to resume his or her exercise regimen.

If the patient has prolonged symptoms which have not responded to conservative treatment, including an exercise regimen as well as the occasional use of anti-inflammatory agents, then surgery is recommended. Surgery may be considered sooner if additional factors such as a documented glenohumeral ligament avulsion via double-contrast CT arthrogram or MRI is noted. During the rehabilitation programme, the patient's motivation should be carefully assessed, both to be sure that he or she is mature enough to co-operate in the rehabilitation effort required after surgery, as well as to screen out those manipulating their disease for secondary gain.[25]

Patients with acquired instability may have developed the ability to dislocate the shoulder at will or on command. This is especially true if certain positions will reliably result in a dislocation (e.g. the humeral head falls out posteriorly whenever the arm is raised in the forward plane). Such 'positional dislocators' may demonstrate this for the examiner, if requested, but otherwise do their best to avoid such positions. Often these individuals have had an episode of trauma before which they could not voluntarily dislocate their shoulder. Although 'positional dislocators' can demonstrate instability on command, they do not necessarily have accompanying psychiatric disorders and are amenable to surgical correction.[26]

These patients must be differentiated, however, from true voluntary dislocators who have underlying psychiatric problems, and often use asymmetric muscle pull to dislocate their shoulder, or even to hold it out, to great dramatic effect. To complicate things further, there is a small group of patients who have developed a habitual initiation of improper muscle-firing patterns which also produce dislocations by asymmetric muscle pull. These patients can be unaware of this pattern and may be without psychiatric disturbance. Nevertheless, both groups of 'muscular dislocators' are poor candidates for stabilization procedures. Those with psychiatric disturbances need counselling, and the shoulder should be treated with skilful neglect. The group with habitually improper muscle use may be successfully treated with muscle retraining and biofeedback.[27]

OPERATIVE TECHNIQUE

As mentioned, the primary pathology in multi-directional instability is the presence of a loose redundant capsule. This pathological capsular laxity is directly addressed by the inferior capsular shift procedure, which reduces the volume of the glenohumeral joint anteriorly, inferiorly and posteriorly. The goal is to equalize tension on all sides and balance the humeral head. This can usually be performed from one surgical approach, anterior or posterior. The capsulorrhaphy is reinforced on the side of the direction of greatest instability which is also the side chosen for the approach.[1,28] Sometimes it is difficult to decide on the best side for the approach; a useful method for this determination is outlined in Table 16.1. Essentially, the side that dislocates takes precedence over lesser degrees of instability. Shoulders that dislocate both anteriorly and posteriorly should be approached from the anterior side as it is easier to stabilize the posterior structures from the anterior side than vice versa. These patients require special considerations with postoperative management, which will be discussed below.

We prefer interscalene regional block as the anaesthesia of choice when performing the anterior approach. Some infiltration of the skin and subcutaneous tissues of the axilla aids comfort, because of overlap with thoracic segmental nerves. The patient is placed in the beach chair position, and all bony prominences are carefully padded to avoid skin and neurovascular compromise. Head and neck positioning is greatly simplified in an awake patient under regional

Table 16.1. Indications for approach (anterior vs posterior)

Anterior approach

Anterior: subluxation + Posterior: stable or subluxation

Anterior: dislocation + Posterior: stable or subluxation or dislocation

Posterior approach

Posterior: subluxation or dislocation + Anterior: stable

Posterior: dislocation + Anterior: subluxation

---

anaesthetic. However, if the patient is asleep, hyperextension and/or hyperflexion of the cervical spine is avoided by securing the head and neck in a stable position. General anaesthesia, however, is required for the posterior approach and the patient is positioned in a lateral position to allow access to the posterior aspect of the shoulder.

Recent biomechanical studies have contributed to the fund of knowledge on the static stabilizers of the glenohumeral joint and this has helped in the performance of the examination under anaesthesia.[17,22,29] Because different portions of the capsule and ligament system are brought into play in different arm positions, the glenohumeral joint is stressed anteriorly, posteriorly and inferiorly in adduction, 45° of abduction, 90° of abduction and internal and external rotation. Usually, the direction of greatest instability has been determined before surgery after the assessment of the history, multiple repeat examinations, plain radiographs and any additional imaging. It is rare to change the intraoperative approach on the basis of the examination under anaesthesia. The upper extremity is then prepped and draped from the sternum, base of neck and medial border of the scapula with the upper extremity free. Prophylactic antibiotics are administered intravenously.

ANTERIOR APPROACH

An axillary skin incision is within the axillary crease skin folds beginning at a point midway between the tip of the coracoid and the inferior border of the pectoralis major and extending to the inferior border of the pectoralis major (Figure 16.1).[30] The incision is taken down through the subcutaneous tissues to the level of the deltopectoral interval. Haemostasis is carefully obtained by the use of needle tip electrocautery. The subcutaneous tissues are mobilized superiorly to the inferior aspect of the clavicle and anteroinferior acromion. The cephalic vein is mobilized with the deltoid laterally and retractors are placed beneath the pectoralis major for medial retraction and beneath the deltoid for lateral retraction. The

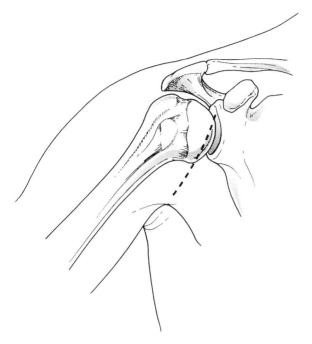

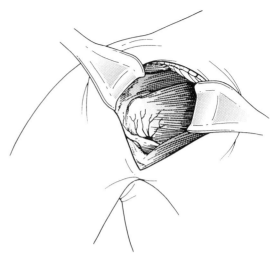

Fig. 16.2 Subscapularis tendon identification begins superiorly at the level of the rotator interval and inferiorly in the region of the anterior humeral circumflex vessels. The incision begins 1 cm medial to the lesser tuberosity.

Fig. 16.1 The skin incision begins at a point midway between the tip of the coracoid and the inferior border of the pectoralis major and extends to the inferior border of the pectoralis major, concealed within the anterior axillary skin crease.

superior third of the pectoralis major insertion may be taken down if needed and tagged for later repair, but this is not usually necessary. The long head of the biceps tendon is carefully protected during this manoeuvre.

The clavipectoral fascia is then incised lateral to the conjoined tendons, which are gently retracted medially. Osteotomizing the coracoid or incising these strap muscles may place the musculocutaneous nerve at risk, and is not necessary for exposure. The arm is then placed in a slight degree of external rotation to facilitate identification of the superior and inferior borders of the subscapularis. After excision of any overlying subdeltoid bursa, the lesser tuberosity is identified. The subscapularis tendon is then incised approximately 1 cm medial to its insertion on the lesser tuberosity. The incision is oriented from superior to inferior, perpendicular to the tendon fibres, and extends from the rotator interval superiorly to the lower border of the subscapularis inferiorly (Figure 16.2). The anterior humeral circumflex

vessels are cauterized to prevent bleeding and allow further release of the muscular portion of the subscapularis. A recent anatomical study has demonstrated that 40% of the subscapularis muscle insertion into the proximal humerus is inferior to the anterior humeral circumflex vessels.[31] Failure to adequately release the inferior subscapularis can limit visualization and mobilization necessary for proper superior shift of the inferior capsule. Compromise of humeral head blood supply is a theoretical consideration, but has not been seen clinically and one recent study has shown no significant reduction after circumflex vessel ligation.[32]

The entire subscapularis tendon and muscle belly is carefully elevated from the underlying capsule. Stay sutures are placed in the subscapularis tendon, which is retracted medially. The remaining lateral insertion of the subscapularis is elevated (undercut) from the underlying capsule. This facilitates differentiation of the capsular and subscapularis flaps, so that they may be later individually repaired. One must be cognizant of the position of the axillary nerve, as it courses quite close to the inferior portion of the capsule. This can usually be carefully palpated inferiorly at the border of the subscapularis muscle. The 'tug test' can be helpful in locating the anterior position of the axillary nerve if it cannot be easily located, such as in revision procedures.[33]

A stay suture is placed in the rotator interval for later repair. The capsule is then incised 5 mm medial to its humeral insertion. As the capsule is shaped like a funnel, wider laterally, we prefer to perform the vertical limb of the 'T' incision along the humeral neck. The capsule can be most effectively shifted to reduce capsular volume where the capsular circumference is largest. Also, the axillary nerve is usually close to the capsule more medially, and is more at risk with medial capsular incisions. The capsular incision is made close to the humerus, leaving a lateral remnant of tissue available for later repair. The incision is carried out inferiorly, and as the inferior aspect of the capsule is approached, the arm is maintained in external rotation to avoid injury to the axillary nerve (Figure 16.3). Stay sutures are placed in the capsule as it is mobilized. As the humerus is externally rotated and flexed, the capsule is incised around the neck of the humerus, extending as far posteriorly as necessary depending on the degree of instability (Figure 16.4). A finger may be placed in the inferior pouch to assess its size and how much redundant capsule needs to be released from the humerus before repair. In a shoulder with classic multidirectional instability, the capsule is taken down all the way to the posterior capsule,

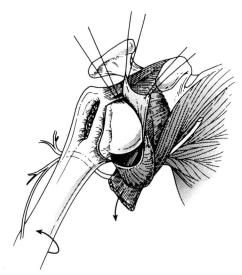

Fig. 16.4 Stay sutures are placed in the capsule as it is incised and progressive external rotation facilitates inferior dissection.

which can then be tensioned as the detached inferior capsule is shifted anteriorly.

A Fukuda ring retractor is placed, and the joint is inspected carefully. Intra-articular pathology, loose bodies and articular cartilage defects are noted. It is at this stage that special steps are added as the pathology indicates. If there is detachment of the glenohumeral ligament complex (Broca–Perthes–Bankart lesion), it is repaired. We generally prefer using sutures through drill holes in the bone but the newer suture anchors are a good alternative. Both ends of the suture are passed through the medial capsule and tied down to secure the capsule, labrum and ligaments to the roughened anterior glenoid neck. If there is anterior glenoid bone deficiency (e.g. secondary to erosion from multiple previous dislocations or from prior fracture), involving greater than 25% of the glenoid articular surface, a bone graft may need to be performed.[1]

The capsule is then incised horizontally in a 'T' fashion. This is generally performed between the middle and inferior glenohumeral ligaments (Figure 16.5). The superior flap thus has the superior and middle glenohumeral ligaments while the inferior flap consists of the three portions of the inferior glenohumeral ligament com-

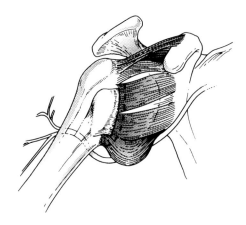

Fig. 16.3 The capsular incision is performed 5 mm medial to the lateral cuff of the subscapularis tendon as the arm is maintained in external rotation and adduction in order to avoid injury to the axillary nerve.

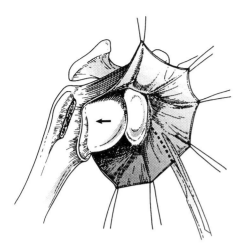

Fig. 16.5 The capsule is incised horizontally in a 'T' fashion between the middle and inferior glenohumeral ligaments.

plex. At this time the inferior capsular flap should be mobilized superiorly. The pouch should be obliterated and this can be evaluated by placing a finger inferiorly and placing traction on the sutures in a superior direction. If there is any remaining subscapularis muscle on the inferior part of the capsule, there may be difficulty mobilizing this flap superiorly. Shifting the inferior capsular flap should effectively eliminate the redundant inferior pouch and tension the posterior capsule. The bone of the humerus just lateral

to the articular margin is freshened to facilitate healing. The 'T' incision allows adjustment of medial–lateral and superior–inferior tension independently, which can be especially helpful in athletes, in whom restriction of motion needs to be avoided.

The capsule is repaired in general with the arm in approximately 25° of external rotation and 20° of abduction. This is modified based on the individual patient. The capsules of dominant shoulders in throwers should be repaired with the arm in relatively more external rotation and abduction. The repair is now performed beginning with the inferior flap, which is shifted superiorly (Figure 16.6). The sutures are placed in a simple interrupted manner progressing superiorly, repairing the inferior flap to the lateral stump of capsular insertion. If there is insufficient capsular tissue laterally to secure a sound repair, suture anchors placed medial to the biceps tendon groove provide another alternative for capsular fixation. If a Bankart lesion is present, the sutures placed through the inferior flap are now tied down. Next the superior cleft is repaired in a simple interrupted manner, closing the enlarged rotator interval. The superior capsular flap is then shifted inferiorly and repaired (Figure 16.6).

The subscapularis muscle is reattached to its insertion in an anatomical manner. It is not

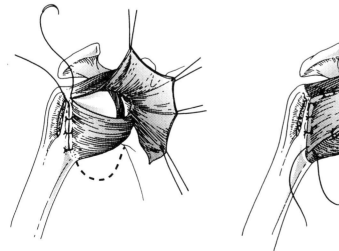

Fig. 16.6 Left, the inferior flap is shifted superiorly, reducing the inferior pouch, and is sutured to the lateral cuff of capsular tissue. Right, after closure of the superior cleft between the superior and middle glenohumeral ligaments (the rotator interval), the superior flap is shifted inferiorly. It overlaps the inferior flap in cruciate fashion.

transferred laterally. If the pectoralis major insertion has been partially released, it is repaired using non-absorbable sutures. The deltopectoral interval is closed with absorbable sutures in an interrupted simple manner and the skin is closed in a running subcuticular fashion.

POSTERIOR APPROACH

The majority of inferior capsular shift procedures for the treatment of multidirectional instability are performed from an anterior approach, and therefore posterior repairs are performed less frequently. The patient is placed in the lateral decubitus position with the back of the table raised approximately 10–15°. The arm is draped for free manipulation. An oblique skin incision, measuring 10–12 cm, is made directed approximately 60° from the scapular spine (Figure 16.7).

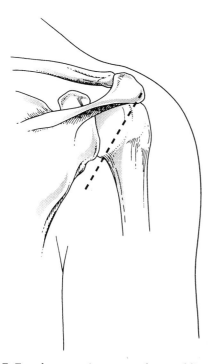

Fig. 16.7 For the posterior approach, an oblique skin incision is used, directed 60° from the scapular spine, starting at the posterolateral corner of the acromion. The incision provides a more cosmetically pleasing scar than a transverse incision over the scapular spine.

Scars have a tendency to spread on the posterior aspect of the shoulder, and an oblique incision follows Langer's lines more closely, which will result in a more pleasing scar. The incision starts at the posterolateral aspect of the acromion and proceeds distally. The incision is carried down to subcutaneous tissue, and once again a needle-tip electrocautery is used to maintain haemostasis. Scissors are then used to develop the skin flaps superiorly, inferiorly, medially and laterally. This allows for adequate exposure of the large deltoid muscle. It should be noted that the suprascapular nerve is close to the base of the scapular spine. In addition, the axillary nerve is in the quadrangular space just inferior to the teres minor muscle. As it curves to innervate the posterior deltoid muscle, it lies 7–8 cm from the posterior aspect of the acromion.

After the subcutaneous tissue is mobilized, a posterolateral raphe is identified in the deltoid. The initial incision in the deltoid muscle is made in the 'soft spot,' which is at the posterolateral corner of the acromion. The deltoid is split in the raphe for approximately 4–5 cm in line with the fibres. To provide enhanced exposure, the deltoid is also detached medially from the scapular spine for a distance of 4–5 cm, leaving a cuff of tissue on the scapular spine for later repair (Figure 16.8). If additional exposure is needed, a 'T' incision is made and 1–2 cm of deltoid muscle can be removed from the posterolateral tip of the acromion. This does not significantly weaken the deltoid muscle and the incision is easily repaired.

Retractors are then placed in the deltoid muscle, and the upper and lower borders of the infraspinatus muscle are identified. The infraspinatus muscle is a large bipennate muscle and it is important to differentiate the interval between the teres minor and the infraspinatus muscle. A small tubercle, which corresponds to the insertion of the teres minor, is often palpable on the posterior aspect of the humerus and helps in locating the proper interval. In addition, superiorly the interval between the supraspinatus and the infraspinatus muscles is identified. Using both blunt and sharp dissection, the infraspinatus muscle is carefully separated from the underlying capsule. This is frequently the tedious portion of the procedure

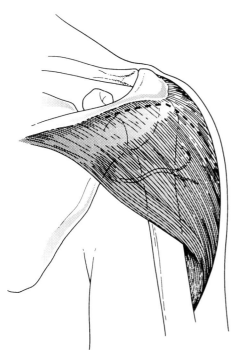

Fig. 16.8 The deltoid is split in its posterolateral raphe for a distance of ~5 cm. It is also detached from the scapular spine for several centimetres.

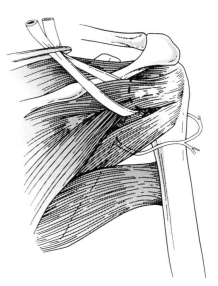

Fig. 16.9 The infraspinatus muscle is identified and then carefully dissected off the underlying capsule, medial to the glenoid rim and lateral to its insertion on the greater tuberosity.

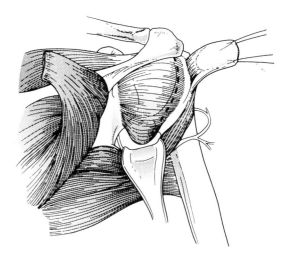

Fig. 16.10 The posteroinferior capsular pouch is seen and the capsule is incised ~1.0 cm medial to its lateral insertion, starting superiorly and proceeding inferiorly along the neck of the humerus.

as this plane is often scarred down in patients with primarily posterior instability. A penrose drain placed beneath the infraspinatus muscle will assist with retraction of the muscle from the capsule as this plane is developed medially past the glenoid rim and laterally to its insertion on the greater tuberosity (Figure 16.9). The infraspinatus muscle is then incised obliquely, starting medially in a superficial plane and proceeding laterally and deeply, thus creating two tendon flaps. However, if the tendon is too thin to allow such an oblique transection, it is incised vertically ~1.0 cm from its insertion. The tendon flaps are then tagged with nylon sutures.

The full superior and inferior extent of the capsule should then be identified. It is important to place a retractor beneath the teres minor muscle to expose the inferior capsule and protect the axillary nerve, which lies on the inferior aspect of the capsule. As in the anterior approach, here again the capsule must be freed from the overlying muscle to prevent it from being tethered. The posterior capsule is then incised 1.0 cm medial to

its lateral insertion on the humerus, beginning superiorly and proceeding inferiorly (Figure 16.10). Great care must be taken to leave enough capsular tissue on the humerus for later reattachment of the flaps. As the dissection proceeds inferiorly, a blunt Darrah retractor is placed deep

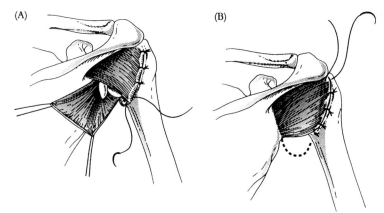

Fig. 16.11 (A) The superior capsular flap is first shifted inferolaterally and is repaired to the lateral cuff of capsular tissue. (B) The inferior flap is then shifted superolaterally. This reduces the inferior pouch and reinforces the repair.

to the teres minor, thus facilitating exposure of the capsule and also protecting the axillary nerve. In addition, it is best to use scissors and cut the capsule from inside out on the humeral neck. The arm is progressively extended and internally rotated, and the capsule is dissected off the humeral neck as far inferiorly as is needed to allow reduction of the inferior capsular redundancy. As with the anterior approach, the extent of this dissection inferiorly will depend on the location and degree of the capsular redundancy.

When the capsular dissection has been deemed sufficient, again by pulling up on the flap to obliterate the inferior pouch, the insertion of the capsule on to the glenoid is carefully examined for detachment. It is much less common to see posterior labral detachment in these cases than it is to find anterior labral detachment in cases of predominantly anterior instability. However, in ~10% of cases, such posterior labral detachment will be encountered, and the labrum must be repaired to the glenoid rim. For this purpose, we use non-absorbable braided nylon sutures through drill holes in bone.

The posterior capsule is then split in a 'T' fashion at the mid-glenoid region, thus creating two capsular flaps. The superior flap is shifted inferolaterally and is repaired to the cuff of capsular tissue left on the lateral aspect of the humeral neck (Figure 16.11). The inferior flap is then shifted superolaterally, thus reducing the inferior pouch and reinforcing the repair in

cruciate fashion (Figure 16.11). This repair gives two good layers of capsule where previously there was only one floppy layer of redundant tissue. During tensioning of these flaps, the arm is held in ~15° of abduction and 5–10° of external rotation. The infraspinatus muscle is then repaired by placing the laterally based flap deep, adjacent to the capsule, and the medially based flap is reattached anatomically to the humerus in a superficial position. If this cannot be performed because the infraspinatus tendon is too short, then the infraspinatus is repaired directly and overlapped approximately 1 cm. The deltoid is repaired to the scapular spine using the soft-tissue cuff that is left, and the split in the posterolateral raphe is also repaired. The skin is then closed with a subcuticular suture.

REHABILITATION

For those patients with classic multidirectional instability and a significant degree of posterior instability, a special brace that holds the arm in a slightly abducted position with neutral rotation is used. The arm is immobilized in this brace for 6 weeks, allowing only gentle isometric exercises and supervised elbow range of motion during that time. At 6 weeks the brace is discontinued, and range of motion exercises are gradually introduced. Isometric and progressive resistive strengthening exercises are introduced as tolerated.

Those patients with 'bidirectional' (anterior and inferior) instability, without a significant posterior component, are protected in a sling for 6 weeks, but after 10 days, the arm is removed from the sling for exercises, including isometrics and external rotation to 10° and forward elevation to 90°. From 2 to 4 weeks, external rotation is increased to 30° and forward elevation to 140°, and isometric strengthening is added. From 4 to 6 weeks, external rotation is increased to 40° and forward elevation to approximately 160°, and resistive exercises are begun. After 6 weeks external rotation is increased to 50° and forward elevation to 180°. After 3 months, external rotation may be progressed. Strengthening begins with the arm in neutral below 90°.

Patients who undergo an anterior inferior capsular shift procedure for concomitant anterior and posterior instability require special considerations regarding postoperative management. These patients must be immobilized after the operation in the neutral position of rotation for 6 weeks, usually in a lightweight brace. This will prevent posterior capsular stretching and possibly even subluxation which may occur with the arm adducted and internally rotated across the chest. After this 6-week period of time, range of motion and strengthening are restored as described above.

These are general protocols and are modified on an individual basis as indicated. For example, the dominant shoulder of throwers would be progressed more quickly, particularly with reference to external rotation. The objective is to regain motion over several months, as progression that is too quick may lead to recurrent instability. This is especially true in patients with some degree of generalized ligamentous laxity and in younger patients in late adolescence. Careful and frequent postoperative follow-up is necessary, as patients who are not progressing quickly enough may need an accelerated programme, while those who are regaining motion too quickly may need to be slowed down. Return to contact sports is generally restricted until 9–12 months have elapsed.

DISCUSSION

Since Neer's initial report[19] in 1980, several authors have reported successful treatment of multidirectional instability with use of the inferior capsular shift.[1–3,17,18,35–37] In Neer's series of 32 patients, there was only one unsatisfactory result.[19] One decade later he reported 'more than one hundred additional inferior capsular shifts have been done with similar satisfactory results'.[1] We have reported preliminary results following 75 inferior capsular shifts performed in young athletes.[18] Eighty-nine per cent were able to return to their major sport and 73% maintained the same level of competitiveness. Seven patients (9.3%) reported a single episode of probable subluxation that was not followed by recurrent instability and did not affect the final result while two patients (2.7%) dislocated after the operation. Both of these cases were associated with a traumatic episode. The average loss of external rotation was 7°.[18]

Altchek and Warren[22] reported their results following a T-plasty modification of the Bankart procedure for multidirectional instability in 42 shoulders. The patient population differed somewhat in that 38 of the 42 cases had a Bankart lesion or detachment of the labrum and glenohumeral ligament complex. Patient satisfaction was rated excellent for 40 (95%) of the shoulders. The average loss of external rotation was 5°. They noted that throwing athletes found they were unable to throw a ball with as much speed as before the operation. In addition 7 of 42 shoulders (17%) demonstrated 2+ or greater posterior instability after surgery. There were four cases of symptomatic recurrent instability, one anterior and three posterior, while one patient required a posterior stabilization 2 years after the operation.

Cooper and Brems[34] reviewed their series of 43 shoulders in 38 patients with a minimum 2-year follow-up after inferior capsular shift: 39 of 43 shoulders (91%) were rated by the patient as satisfactory with no recurrent instability. Postoperative recurrent symptomatic instability developed in four patients (9%). Two of these patients required subsequent revision inferior capsular shifts and one of those went on to a humeral head replacement for arthritis of dislocation. The latter patient had had a prior Bristow procedure. They concluded that the inferior capsular shift procedure provides satisfactory objective and subjective results. Failures and recurrences of symptomatic instability generally occurred in the early postoperative period less than 2 years after surgery. Their findings did not demonstrate a deterioration of results with follow–up to 6 years.

We recently reported our results after inferior capsular shift for classic multidirectional instability in 52 shoulders.[39] Thirty-six shoulders were approached from the anterior side and 16 from the posterior. All were completely immobilized in a brace for 6 weeks after the operation. Forty-nine shoulders were followed from 2 to 11 years (average, 5 years). Satisfactory results were achieved in 94% of cases.

Turkel and co-workers[40] demonstrated that anterior glenohumeral stability is provided by varying regions of the capsule depending on arm position. Similarly, Warner and co-workers[29] have demonstrated that inferior humeral translation is restrained by the anterosuperior capsule and ligaments with the arm at the side, and by the inferior capsule and ligaments with the arm in abduction. This is consistent with the clinical findings of Neer and Foster,[19] who described inferior humeral translation with the arm at the side and with the arm in abduction in patients with multidirectional instability, and emphasized reducing redundant capsular volume on all sides at the time of surgical reconstruction. The capsular shift procedure eliminates laxity in the rotator interval, anterosuperior capsule and anteroinferior capsule. It can be continued around the humeral neck to reduce as much laxity in the posteroinferior and posterior capsule as needed and is thus a highly versatile procedure, allowing precise soft tissue balancing. Owing to the shifting of load between different capsular regions as shown by Turkel et al,[40] the capsular shift affords stability in varying functional positions while preserving motion, and is especially useful in the reconstruction of the unstable athletic shoulder.

There is a confusing tendency in the literature to attempt to draw a distinction between 'laxity' and 'instability'. For example, some have suggested that a shoulder that is lax posteriorly, inferiorly and anteriorly but has an anterior labral tear seen at arthroscopy should be classified as 'traumatic anterior instability'.[41] Given that many loose shoulders are pain-free, the quest for understanding why the instability hurts, and especially for understanding which direction or directions of laxity are causing pain, would seem a complex undertaking. Furthermore, there is no current evidence that any of these criteria for distinguishing laxity from instability in a symptomatically unstable shoulder improve clinical treatment, while there is clear evidence that unidirectional operations on shoulders with multidirectional instability can lead to failure. Thus, when surgery is indicated and a repair is planned, the surgeon should address all components (anterior, inferior, and posterior) of instability that are actually found at surgery, rather than engaging in an analysis of which components are important. Another way of looking at this is to say that the issue is not necessarily how much posterior excursion is 'normal'; it is that a shoulder with excessive posterior (and inferior) laxity will not react well to a repair that tightens only the anterior side of the joint.

In summary, the inferior capsular shift procedure is a versatile and reliable treatment for patients with multidirectional shoulder instability. It allows for the correction of excessive capsular laxity and can be tailored according to the degree and location of the capsular pathology. By performing the vertical aspect of the capsulorrhaphy on the humeral side of the joint, by virtue of the funnel-shaped geometry of the capsule, more tissue can be shifted superiorly to obliterate the redundant inferior pouch seen in patients with multidirectional instability. In addition, when a labral detachment is found, the glenohumeral ligaments are reattached to the medial glenoid rim to anchor the capsule before shifting the capsular flaps. The repair then addresses both elements of capsular damage: labral detachment and excessive laxity. It corrects the pathology encountered without distorting the surrounding normal anatomy, thus facilitating return of full motion and function. Finally, this procedure can be performed with reliable results using either an anterior or a posterior approach, depending on the major direction of the glenohumeral instability.

REFERENCES

1. Neer, C.S., II (1990) *Shoulder Reconstruction*, pp. 273–341. Philadelphia: W.B. Saunders.
2. Neer, C.S., II (1985) Involuntary inferior and multi-directional instability of the shoulder: etiology, recognition, and treatment. *Instr. Course Lect.* **34:** 232–238.
3. Welsh, R.P. & Trimmings, N. (1987) Multidirectional instability of the shoulder. *Orthop. Trans.* **11:** 231.
4. Hawkins, R.H. & Hawkins, R.J. (1985) Failed anterior reconstruction for shoulder instability. *J. Bone Joint Surg.* **67B:** 709–714.
5. Neer, C.S. II, Perez-Sanz, J.R. & Ogawa, K. Causes of failure in repairs for recurrent anterior dislocations. Presented at New York Orthopaedic Hospital Alumni Annual Meeting, 1983, as cited in Neer, C.S. II (1990) *Shoulder Reconstruction*, p. 279. Philadelphia: W.B. Saunders.
6. Norris, T.R. & Bigliani, L.U. (1984) Analysis of failed repair for shoulder instability. A preliminary report. In Bateman, J.E. & Welsh, R.P. (eds) *Surgery of the Shoulder.* Philadelphia: Decker.
7. Rockwood, C.A. & Gerber, C. (1985) Analysis of failed surgical procedures for anterior shoulder instability. *Orthop. Trans.* **9:** 48.
8. Rowe, C.R., Zarins, B. & Ciullo, J.V. (1984) Recurrent anterior dislocation of the shoulder after surgical repair. Apparent causes of failure and treatment. *J. Bone Joint Surg.* **66A:** 159–168.
9. Samilson, R.L. & Prieto, V. (1983) Dislocation arthropathy of the shoulder. *J. Bone Joint Surg.* **65A:** 456–460.
10. Steinmann, S.R., Flatow, E.L., Pollock, R.G., Glasgow, M.D. & Bigliani, L.U. (1992) Evaluation and surgical treatment of failed shoulder instability repairs. *Orthop. Trans.* **16:** 727.
11. Young, D.C. & Rockwood, C.A. (1991) Complications of a failed Bristow procedure and their management. *J. Bone Joint Surg.* **73A:** 969–981.
12. O'Driscoll, S.W. & Evans, D.C. (1993) Long term results of staple capsulorrhaphy for anterior instability of the shoulder. *J. Bone Joint Surg.* **75A:** 249–258.
13. Hawkins, R.J. & Angelo, R.L. (1990) Glenohumeral osteoarthrosis. *J. Bone Joint Surg.* **72A:** 1193–1197.
14. Altchek, D.W., Warren, R.F., Skyhar, M.J. & Ortiz, G. (1989) T-plasty: a technique for treating multidirectional instability in the athlete. *Orthop. Trans.* **13:** 561–569.
15. Bigliani, L.U., Pollock, R.G., Soslowsky, L.J. et al. (1992) The tensile properties of the inferior glenohumeral ligament. *J. Orthop. Res.* **10:** 187–197.
16. Speer, K.P., Deng, X., Borrero, S., Torzilli, P.A., Altcheck, D.A. & Warren, R.F. (1994) Biomechanical evaluation of a simulated Bankart lesion. *J. Bone Joint Surg.* **76A:** 1819–1826.
17. O'Brien, S.J., Neves, M.C., Arnockzky, S.P., Rozbruck, S.R., DiCarlo, E.F., Warren, R.F., Schwartz, R. & Wickiewicz, T.L. (1990) The anatomy and histology of the inferior glenohumeral ligament complex of the shoulder. *Am. J. Sports Med.* **18:** 449–456.
18. Bigliani, L.U., Kurzweil, P.R., Schwartzbach, C.C., Flatow, E.L. & Wolfe, I. (1994) Inferior capsular shift procedure for anterior inferior shoulder instability in athletes. *Am. J. Sports Med.* **22:** 578–584.
19. Neer, C.S. II & Foster, C.R. (1980) Inferior capsular shift for involuntary inferior and multidirectional instability of the shoulder. A preliminary report. *J. Bone Joint Surg.* **62A:** 897–908.
20. Hawkins, R.J. & Bokor, D.J. (1990) Clinical evaluation of shoulder problems. In C.A. Rockwood & Matsen, F.A. (eds), *The Shoulder,* 1st edn, pp. 167–171. Philadelphia: W.B. Saunders.
21. Endo, H., Takigawa, T., Takata, K. & Miyoshi, S. (1971) A method of diagnosis and treatment for loose shoulder (in Japanese). *Cent. Jpn. J. Orthop. Surg. Traumat.* **14:** 630–632.
22. Harryman, D.T., Sidles, J.A., Harris, S.L. & Matsen, F.A. (1992) Laxity of the normal glenohumeral joint: a quantitative *in vivo* assessment. *J. Shoulder Elbow Surg.* **1:** 66–76.
23. Friedman, R.J., Bonutti, P.M., Genez, B. & Norfray, J.F. (1993) Cine magnetic resonance imaging of the glenohumeral joint. Presented at the American Academy of Orthopaedic Surgeons, Sixtieth Annual Meeting, San Francisco, California.
24. Burkhead, W.Z. & Rockwood, C.A. (1992) Treatment of instability of the shoulder with an exercise program. *J. Bone Joint Surg.* **74A:** 890.
25. Rowe, C.R., Fierce, D.S. & Clark, J.G. (1973) Voluntary dislocation of the shoulder. A preliminary report on a clinical, electromyographic, and psychiatric study of twenty-six patients. *J. Bone Joint Surg.* **55A:** 445–460.
26. Thompson, F.R., Moga, J.J. & Fielding, J.W. (1965) Unusual habitual shoulder dislocations. Combined operative repair. Audio-visual Presentation at the Annual Meeting of the American Academy of Orthopaedic Surgeons, New York, N.Y.
27. Beall, M.S., Jr., Diefenbach, G. & Allen, A. (1987) Electromyographic biofeedback in the treatment of voluntary posterior instability of the shoulder. *Am. J. Sports Med.* **15:** 175–178.
28. Bigliani, L.U. (1989) Anterior and posterior capsular shift for multidirectional instability. *Techniques Orthop.* **3:** 36–45.
29. Warner, J.P., Deng, X.H., Warren, R.F. & Torzilli, P.A. (1992) Static capsuloligamentous restraints to superior-inferior translation of the glenohumeral joint. *Am. J. Sports Med.* **20:** 675–685.

30. Leslie, J.T., Jr. and Ryan, T.J. (1962) The anterior axillary incision to approach the shoulder joint. *J. Bone Joint Surg.* **44A:** 1193–1196.

31. Hinton, M.A., Parker, A.W., Drez, D. & Altcheck, D. (1994) An anatomic study of the subscapularis tendon and myotendinous junction. *J. Shoulder Elbow Surg.* **3:** 224–229.

32. Steinmann, S.R., Gaccione, D.R., McGee, T.H., Higgins, D.L., Cammarata, A.C. & Hughes, S.S. (1994) Effect of anterior shoulder reconstruction on humeral head vascularity. Read at the Annual Meeting of the American Academy of Orthopaedic Surgeons, New Orleans, Louisiana.

33. Flatow, E.L. & Bigliani, L.U. (1992) Locating and protecting the axillary nerve in shoulder surgery: the tug test. *Orthop. Rev.* **21:** 503–505.

34. Cooper, R.A. & Brems, J.J. (1992) The inferior capsular shift procedure for multidirectional instability of the shoulder. *J. Bone Joint Surg.* **74A:** 1516–1521.

35. Hawkins, R.J., Abrams, J.S. & Schutte, J. (1987) Multidirectional instability of the shoulder – an approach to diagnosis. *Orthop. Trans.* **11:** 246.

36. Mitzuno, K., Itakura, Y. & Muratso, H. (1992) Inferior capsular shift for inferior and multidirectional instability of the shoulder in young children: report of two cases. *J. Shoulder Elbow Surg.* **1:** 200–206.

37. Neer, C.S. II, Fithian, T.F., Hansen, P.E., Ogawa, K. & Brems, J.J. (1985) Reinforced cruciate repair for anterior dislocations of the shoulder. *Orthop. Trans.* **9:** 44.

38. Bigliani, L.U., Pollock, R.G., Owens, J.M., McIlveen, S.J. & Flatow, E.L. (1993–1994) The inferior capsular shift procedure for multidirectional instability of the shoulder. *Orthop. Trans.* **17:** 576.

39. Pollock, R.G., Owens, J.M., Nicholson, G.P., McIlveen, S.J., Flatow, E.L. & Bigliani, L.U. (1993) Anterior inferior capsular shift procedure for anterior glenohumeral instability: long term results. Presented at the 60th Annual Meeting of the American Academy of Orthopaedic Surgeons, San Francisco, CA.

40. Turkel, S.J., Panio, M.W., Marshall, J.L. et al. (1981) Stabilizing mechanisms preventing anterior dislocation of the glenohumeral joint. *J. Bone Joint Surg.* **63A:** 1208.

41. Mok, D.W.H., Fogg, A.J.B., Hokar, R. et al. (1990) The diagnostic value of arthroscopy in glenohumeral instability. *J. Bone Joint Surg.* **72B:** 698–700.

17

Pathophysiology of Impingement

P Duke and WA Wallace

DEFINITION

Pathophysiology is defined as an alteration of normal function. Impingement syndrome is defined as a painful condition resulting from impingement of the rotator cuff under the corocoacromial arch.[1] It is a diagnosis made by history and examination with investigations contributing very little. The pain is described as an ache localized to the anterolateral border of the acromion and radiating to the upper arm. It is made worse by overhead activity or repetitive work in any plane. It commonly causes a typical 'painful arc' on elevation of the arm. It can be made worse by sleeping on the affected side and is often worse at night.[2]

CLASSIFICATION

In an aetiological classification scheme, two basic causes of impingement syndrome are commonly recognized, primary and secondary.[2]

Primary

This results from (a) a lack of space for the passage of the cuff under the arch or (b) intrinsic degeneration of the cuff tendons.

Secondary

This results from a decrease in available space for the rotator cuff caused by a number of factors including a tight posterior capsule of the glenohumeral joint, glenohumeral instability, scapulothoracic muscle imbalance and weakness of the rotator cuff muscles. The net effect is an anterosuperior translation of the humeral head causing impingement of the cuff against the coracoacromial arch.

Whatever the cause, there is a common pathological pathway resulting in tendinitis and degeneration of the rotator cuff.[2] There is a good case for renaming the syndrome rotator cuff tendinitis syndrome.

STRUCTURES INVOLVED

1. Muscles
   (a) Scapulothoracic
   (b) Rotator cuff
2. Tendons
   (a) Rotator cuff
   (b) Long head of biceps
3. Subacromial bursa
4. Corocoacromial ligament
5. Glenohumeral joint
   (a) Capsule
   (b) Ligaments

There are many structures which may have altered function in impingement syndrome. These include the scapulothoracic and rotator cuff muscles, the rotator cuff and long head of biceps tendons, the subacromial bursa, the coracoacromial ligament, the glenohumeral joint capsule and the glenohumeral joint ligaments.

Bones, joints, tendons and muscles about the shoulder may all be involved in the production or prolongation of impingement. We will discuss each of these and their contribution to impingement in turn.

Each of the structures will be discussed in two sections: first the normal function will be reviewed, and then the abnormal function with respect to its role in impingement.

Muscles

Scapulothoracic muscles

Normal function. The muscles involved in control of the scapulothoracic articulation are as follows: serratus anterior, levator scapulae, trapezius, rhomboids, latissimus dorsi and pectoralis major and minor. These muscles combine to control the position of the scapula on the chest wall. They act independently and in concert as a force couple to produce the various movements of the scapula. The scapulothoracic articulation is not a true joint and therefore lacks passive joint stabilizers. There is only one true skeletal attachment of the shoulder complex to the axial skeleton, the sternoclavicular joint. The chest wall anatomically restrains the gross movements of the scapula such that it can only move in one plane, the so-called scapular plane which is at 45° to the coronal and sagittal planes. The scapula cannot rotate about the vertical axis at all but in the scapular plane it can protract, retract, rotate and be depressed or elevated. The muscles provide the necessary stability to maintain the scapula in its normal position.

When the arm is elevated, the necessary glenohumeral movement is accompanied by scapulothoracic movement. The movements are not isolated and occur in a smooth co-ordinated fashion. The scapulothoracic movements are controlled by a complex combination of all of the above muscles. The smooth co-ordinated movement is commonly referred to as scapulohumeral rhythm.

The scapulothoracic movement serves a number of functions. First, it provides a stable base for the humerus by moving the glenoid to keep it under the humeral head as the arm elevates. It also positions the scapula to maintain the optimal length of the muscles acting directly on the humeral head enabling these muscles to work at maximum efficiency.

With full elevation of the arm the glenohumeral joint will contribute two-thirds of the range of movement and the scapulothoracic one-third. This 2:1 ratio occurs at the same rate all the way through the arc of elevation.[3] As well as rotation, the scapula undergoes protraction and elevation to maintain its optimal position in relation to the humerus.

It is plain that the scapulothoracic muscles perform three main functions: they provide stability to the scapulothoracic articulation; they maintain the scapula in its normal resting position; they provide the scapula and the humerus with a smooth rhythm in the movement of elevation. Weakness of any of the muscles involved, be it actual or relative, will cause pathology of one or more of these functions.

Abnormal function. Numerous authors have demonstrated that patients with impingement have weakness of the muscles of the scapulothoracic group.[2,4-6] There is also good evidence that weakness of the scapulothoracic group can actually cause impingement or prolong the course once it has started. This problem is seen particularly in sportsmen who use the arm in a highly repetitive fashion such as swimmers or throwing athletes. The resulting alteration in scapular position or in scapulohumeral rhythm may be the sole cause of the impingement syndrome. It should be re-emphasized at this point that any of the seven muscles concerned may be at fault.

The dynamic effect of muscle weakness on the scapula is best seen with involvement of the serratus anterior. Whatever the cause of the weakness the result is a problem with protraction of the scapula. The inability to protract the scapula gives rise to winging of the scapula when the arm is raised. The patient may also lose full elevation of the arm due to loss of the scapulothoracic contribution to elevation. This is not a common cause of impingement, but serves to demonstrate the effect that loss of only one muscle can have on the stability and position of the scapula. The weak or unbalanced scapular muscles do not normally cause a gross clinical effect but they do alter the scapulohumeral rhythm and put a greater strain on the glenohumeral articulation resulting in secondary impingement of the rotator cuff.

They also cause 'pseudo-winging' of the scapula, seen by observing elevation from behind and carefully watching the movements of the scapula. The scapula will be seen to 'wing' as the arm moves from full elevation to neutral. This is not a true weakness of the serratus anterior but is an alteration of the normal scapulothoracic rhythm caused by the pain of impingement.

There are two groups of athletes who are commonly affected with an alteration in the physiology of the scapulothoracic articulation. They are swimmers and throwing athletes, particularly baseball pitchers.[6-8] Extensive analysis of the biomechanics of the shoulder has been carried out in both these groups of athletes and it has been found that quite often the basis of the problem is weakness of one or more of the scapulothoracic muscles. This led to a successful treatment programme which involved strengthening of the weak muscles.

In the throwing athlete a simple test has been proposed to determine if weakness of the scapular retractors can be demonstrated. This is called the lateral scapular slide and it looks at the distance between the medial border of the scapula and the spinous process. A symptomatic group was seen to have an increase in this distance indicating relative weakness of these muscles which responded to a strengthening programme.[4]

Pain from impingement has a negative feedback effect: it will cause reflex inhibition of the involved muscles – the rotator cuff as well as the scapulothoracic muscles. This effect is best known at the knee joint when wasting of the quadriceps is seen very quickly after the knee is injured.

In summary, the net effect of weakness of scapulothoracic muscles is to cause either an alteration in position of the scapula or disharmony in the scapulohumeral rhythm. This then causes an impingement of the rotator cuff due to increased stresses on the glenohumeral joint. The humerus is pushed in a superior direction during elevation of the arm thus resulting in a secondary extrinsic impingement.

Rotator cuff muscles

Normal function. The subscapularis, supraspinatus, infraspinatus and teres minor muscles contribute tendons to the rotator cuff, which blend to form a hood which envelops the head of the humerus. They all contribute to elevation of the arm, humeral head depression and centring of the humeral head during elevation of the arm. All have a prime function as well, such as external rotation, internal rotation or abduction.[3,9,10]

Cadaver work has shown that the supraspinatus is the strongest of the group, contributing 50% of the power of the rotator cuff. It is a very important depressor of the humeral head as well as contributing 50% of the power of abduction of the arm.[10]

The rotator cuff muscles are important dynamic stabilizers of the glenohumeral joint. Electromyographic (EMG) analysis shows that they are all active throughout the act of elevation.[11]

The upwards shear force produced by the contraction of the deltoid is counteracted largely by the contraction of all of the rotator cuff. This is particularly important in the early phase of elevation when there is a high vertical component produced by the upward pull of the deltoid.

Abnormal function (weakness of the muscles). As the rotator cuff muscles function as dynamic stabilizers of the glenohumeral joint, any weakness or relative weakness of the rotator cuff muscles will manifest as instability in the direction of the strongest deforming force. Impingement of the cuff tendons, particularly supraspinatus, will result when the upward force generated by the deltoid is no longer balanced by the downward force generated by the cuff muscles. Pain caused by the impingement may in addition propagate the weakness by reflex inhibition of the muscles and wasting in the same fashion that the quadriceps become weak and wasted as a result of a painful knee.

In the athlete relative weakness is important. It is caused at first by fatigue of the cuff muscles.

Muscle imbalance can then occur which causes impingement as a result of the relative weakness of the humeral head depressors. Tennis players, water polo players and wheelchair athletes are three groups that have been extensively studied.[6,9,12,13] All were shown to develop muscle imbalance as a result of either their training or their sport. They were more prone to developing impingement syndrome when they had proven muscular imbalance. When the imbalance was addressed with a remedial training regimen the impingement often resolved.

Tendons: rotator cuff and long head of biceps

Normal function

The long head of biceps and the rotator cuff tendons are intimately associated and any disease process will usually involve both structures. We will consider them separately.

Rotator cuff. The four tendons of the rotator cuff blend as they near their insertion and the fibres show histological interlacing. The interlacing and blending of the subscapularis and supraspinatus also functions as part of the stabilizing mechanism for the biceps tendon as it runs in its groove.

The main functions of the tendons are to bear tensile load while gliding smoothly between two hard surfaces. The humeral head has the cuff tendons between it and the undersurface of the coracoacromial arch. They also function to provide some of the static restraints to anterior stability of the joint.[14]

Long head of biceps. The long head of biceps is thought to act as a weak head depressor and to function as a rudder on which the head of the humerus can glide when elevation of the arm is occurring. It acts as a passive superior check to humeral head migration.[5] It has a synovial lining in the bony groove which is continuous with the synovium of the glenohumeral joint. It is seen to be active in the cocking phase of throwing and may have a role in stability during this action.

Abnormal function

Rotator cuff. The rotator cuff tendons have been shown to undergo a progressive degenerative process with increasing age.[16–18] It is well known that most ruptures do not occur within the tendon proper.[18] The failure points in the muscle–tendon–bone unit are usually at the muscle–tendon junction or at the tendon–bone insertion. Bony avulsions will also occur and are seen about the shoulder involving the rotator cuff tendons. Impingement syndrome has a well-known association with rotator cuff rupture and it is thought that the tendonitis and degeneration caused by impingement syndrome will weaken the tendon and allow rupture to occur, both in the intratendinous portion and more commonly at the tendon–bone interface.

Microrupture is cited as a cause of rotator cuff tendinitis.[19] As high tensile loads are placed on the cuff, individual fibres rupture, leading to inflammatory changes and swelling of the tendon. This may lead to impingement as well as placing greater stress on the remaining tendon fibres.

These changes seen in the rotator cuff tendons are also seen in other tendons which suffer 'spontaneous' rupture. These include the achilles tendon, tibialis posterior, biceps brachii, extensor pollicus longus and the quadriceps tendon.[20] Histologically these tendons show signs of degeneration and proliferation but relatively little inflammation.[17]

Partial tears occur on the joint side of the cuff more commonly than the acromial side; there are usually no acromial changes associated with joint side tears. This lends weight to Codman's proposal[21] that there must be an alteration in the cuff physiology probably related to decreased blood supply and primary cuff degeneration as the common aetiology for cuff pathology.

In summary, the tendons of the rotator cuff become weaker, thinner and stiffer as a result of degeneration and chronic overload, resulting in impingement and eventual failure.

Long head of biceps. The main early influence of the biceps tendon on impingement is via inflammation of the surrounding synovium.[22] The tendon does not tend to become enlarged until the cuff has ruptured and when the cuff ruptures the tendon then tends to hypertrophy indicating better nutrition and a better ability to heal itself.

The inflamed synovium is more bulky and less compliant thus creating more friction and propagating the inflammation. Because of the close association of the biceps and the cuff this inflammation will easily involve the cuff.

The tendon itself seems more resilient than the rotator cuff and will often survive when the cuff has ruptured. Again this points to intrinsic factors as a cause of impingement and cuff degeneration as the same compressive forces are applied to the biceps as to the cuff. Any primary mechanical effect as proposed by Neer[1,23] would be expected to compress the biceps as well.

The subacromial bursa

Normal function

Bursae will form in any situation where repetitive gliding of two structures over each other occurs.[24] This is how the superficial bursae of the body form after birth. The deep bursae form along with the joint spaces *in utero* in response to movement of the structures concerned. There is potential for bursae to re-form from pluripotential cells if they are excised.

They have the same lining as synovial lining and function to allow gliding to occur with little friction. The subacromial bursa lies under the acromion, but it also lies under the anterolateral deltoid, thus covering any of the cuff and tuberosity that will pass under the acromion during elevation. It is normally quite thin and has no fluid in the potential space.

Abnormal function

The subacromial bursa is commonly thought of as a culprit in the pain of impingement. At operation it is often found to be densely adherent to the deltoid and the underlying cuff. It is often seen to be inflamed and swollen. It is also common to see a cuff rupture covered by thick bursal tissue which to the uninitiated can resemble the rotator cuff

itself. It is rare to see an effusion in the bursal space.

Histological investigation of the bursa by Sarkar & Uhthoff[25] showed no true acute inflammatory changes in the bursa of patients with impingement. However, the bursa was shown to be subject to degenerative and proliferative changes. These can lead to thickening of the bursa thus increasing the friction of the gliding when the arm is elevated. It is thought that changes seen in the bursa are secondary to changes in the tendons.

The coracoacromial ligament

Normal function

This ligament forms part of the coracoacromial arch which has the rotator cuff, biceps tendon and the greater tuberosity running underneath in close proximity. The arch functions as a mechanical block to upward movement of the humeral head. It normally plays only a supporting role when the humeral head depressors are functioning well. The ligament is a dynamic structure and functions as a tension band between the two bony prominences. It has properties such as elasticity and tensile strength which aid in its role as a flexible band supporting two mobile bony prominences.[26] The mobility of the coracoid and the acromion is not marked but is present. The movements that occur are analogous to the movements detected in steel beams which are obviously flexible when consisting of long pieces but are apparently rigid when consisting of short pieces.

As the humeral head moves beneath the arch there is a strain upon the structures involved, resulting in an increase in ligament length.[26] This stretching of the ligament allows absorption of some of the upward force directed through the humerus by the deltoid contraction.

In summary, the coracoacromial ligament forms part of a flexible superior block which has some 'give' in it, thus allowing for some variation in the amount of upward movement of the humerus without being an unyielding 'block' which would be more likely to impinge upon the structures passing underneath.

Abnormal function

In patients with cuff tears or chronic impingement syndrome, the ligament is known to undergo changes in its mechanical properties as well as changes in physical appearance.[27-29] The ligaments are shown to be stiffer than normal as well as shorter and thicker. They also have significant alterations in histological and ultrastructural appearance. These alterations either result from or result in impingement; it is difficult to prove which comes first.

A stiff and unyielding ligament has a decreased ability to absorb energy or deal with alterations in the amount of stress applied by the humeral head. This would increase the pressures reached in the subacromial space resulting in impingement on the structures passing below. The fact that it is also .shorter would be likely to place greater pressure on the cuff tendons and tuberosities as they move under the arch.

While it is not clear whether the stiff shorter ligament is a result or a cause of impingement, there is a definite alteration in the physiology of the arch which has an adverse effect on the nearby structures.

Capsule and glenohumeral ligaments

Normal function

The capsule of the glenohumeral joint is normally quite capacious to allow the necessary large range of movement. To act as static restraints to subluxation or dislocation there are thickenings in the capsule known as the glenohumeral ligaments. They become taut and therefore functional at different positions of the joint, as does the capsule. There are three named ligaments, superior, middle and inferior, and their complex anatomy has been clearly described by Turkel *et al.* The illustration in Figure 17.1 demonstrates these ligaments.

In the position of external rotation and abduction which is assumed when cocking to throw, there are three main static restraints to anterior dislocation. The capsule becomes taut, the anteroinferior labrum acts as a buffer and the anteroinferior glenohumeral ligament becomes taut. This

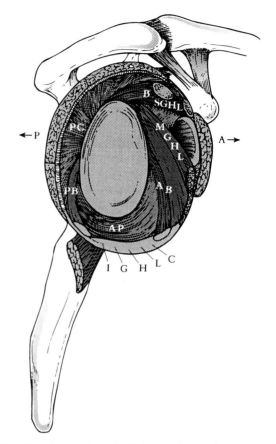

Fig. 17.1 Anatomical depiction of the glenohumeral ligaments. IGHLC, inferior glenohumeral ligament complex; P, posterior; A, anterior; SGHL, superior glenohumeral ligament; MGHL, middle glenohumeral ligament. Reproduced with permission from O'Brien, S.J., Arnoczky, S.P., Warren, R.F. & Rosbruch, S.R. (1990) Developmental anatomy of the shoulder and anatomy of the glenohumeral joint. In C.A. Rockwood, Jr. & F.A. Matsen III (eds), *The Shoulder*, p. 26. Philadelphia: W.B. Saunders.

position is the one most commonly associated with the development of anterior instability and these static restraints are therefore important when the dynamic restraints are compromised by injury or fatigue.

Abnormal function

There are two mechanisms by which these structures can cause impingement: (1) loss of posterior capsular elasticity; (2) attenuation of anterior static restraints.

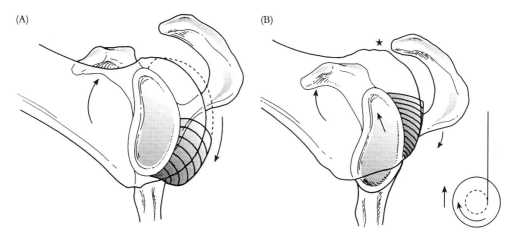

Fig. 17.2 Tightness in the posterior capsule. (A) A normally lax posterior capsule allows the humeral head to remain centred in the glenoid on shoulder flexion antero-inferior. (B) Stiffness of the posterior glenohumeral capsule aggravates the impingement process by forcing the humeral head upward against the anteroinferior acromion as the shoulder is flexed. The upward translation in association with rotation is analogous to the action of a spinning yo-yo climbing a string. Reproduced with permission from Matsen, F.A. & Arntz, C.A. (1990) Subacromial impingement. In C.A. Rockwood Jr & F.A. Matsen III (eds), *The Shoulder*, p. 628. Philadelphia: W.B. Saunders.

(1) Tightness of the posterior capsule will cause impingement when the shoulder is flexed. The tight and inelastic posterior capsule forces the head to ride up with flexion of the arm thus causing or aggravating the impingement (Figure 17.2). This is then a form of secondary impingement. Tightness of the posterior capsule is a form of pathophysiology which may result from disuse in a painful shoulder. If the pain is from impingement, it then forms a vicious circle of propagation of the impingement. Stretching of the posterior capsule by the patient will often alleviate the impingement pain. As part of the routine shoulder examination, testing of cross-body adduction will often cause pain in the acromioclavicular joint if it is the cause of the pain. This test will also reveal a tightness of the posterior capsule and aggravate the impingement pain if the posterior capsule is tight and causing impingement.

(2) The anterior static restraints are subject to increased loads in the athlete. The dynamic restraints are subject to fatigue; in the chronic situation this will lead to stretching and attenuation of the static restraints as they are subject to overuse. In the normal shoulder the position of external rotation in abduction will cause a translation posteriorly of the humeral head.[30] The mechanism of this translation is tightening of the anterior structures including the capsule and the glenohumeral ligaments as the position is attained. Once the static anterior restraints are stretched and the dynamic restraints are either weak or fatigued, a situation arises where the humeral head can translate anteriorly when the arm is abducted and externally rotated. The shoulder now has anterior instability and this causes impingement of the rotator cuff on the coracoacromial arch.[31,32] The result is a secondary impingement which may become self-propagating. This form of pathophysiology may occur naturally in the patient with lax ligaments and multidirectional instability. It will often cause impingement in the same fashion.

REFERENCES

1 Neer, C.S. II (1983) Impingement lesions. *Clin. Orthop.* **173**: 70–77.
2 Fu, F.H., Hamer, C.D. & Klien, A.H. (1991) Shoulder impingement syndrome. *Clin. Orthop.* **269**: 162–173.
3 Wallace, W.A. (1982) The dynamic study of shoulder movements. In I. Bayley & L. Kessel (eds), *Shoulder Surgery*, pp. 139–143. Berlin: Springer-Verlag.
4 Kamkar, A., Irrgang, J.J. & Whitney, S.L. (1993) Non-operative management of secondary shoulder impingement syndrome. *J. Sports Physiotherapy* **17**: 212–224.
5 Kibler, W.B. & Chandler, T.J. (1989) Functional scap-

ular instability in throwing athletes. *American Orthopedic Society for Sports Medicine 15th Annual Meeting, Traverse City, Michigan,* June 19–22.

6 McMaster, W.C., Long, S.C. & Ciaozzo, V.J. (1991) Isokinetic torque imbalances in the rotator cuff of the elite water polo player. *Am. J. Sports Med.* **19:** 72–75.

7 Richardson, A.B., Jobe, F.W. & Collins, H.R. (1980) The shoulder in competitive swimming. *Am. J. Sports Med.* **8:** 159–163.

8 Jobe, F.W., Moynes, D.R., Tibone, J.E. & Perry J. (1984) An EMG analysis of the shoulder in pitching: a second report. *Am. J. Sports Med.* **12:** 218–220.

9 Burnham, R.S., May, L., Nelson, E., Steadward, R. & Reid, D.C. (1993) Shoulder pain in wheelchair athletes (the role of muscle imbalance). *Am. J. Sports Med.* **21:** 238–242.

10 Keating, J.F., Waterworth, P., Shaw-Dunn, J. & Crossan, J. (1993) The relative strengths of the rotator cuff muscles. A cadaver study. *J. Bone Joint Surg.* **75B:** 137–140.

11 Matsen, F.A. III & Arntz, C.T. (1990) Subacromial impingement. In Rockwood, C.A. Jr & Matsen, F.A. III (eds) *The Shoulder,* lst edn, pp. 623–646. Philadelphia: W.B. Saunders.

12 Mont, M.A., Cohen, D.B., Campbell, K.R., Gravare, K. & Mathur, S.K. (1994) Isokinetic concentric versus eccentric training of shoulder rotators with functional evaluation of performance enhancement in elite tennis players. *Am. J. Sports Med.* **22:** 513–517.

13 Kennedy, J. & Kennedy, R. (1990) Patterns of flexibilty, laxity, and strength in normal shoulders. *Am. J. Sports Med.* **18:** 366-375.

14 Symeomides, P.P. (1972) The significance of the subscapularis muscle in the pathogenesis of recurrent anterior dislocation of the shoulder. *J. Bone Joint Surg.* **54B:** 476-483.

15 Burkhead, W.Z. (1990) The biceps tendon. In C.A. Rockwood, Jr. & F.A. Matscn III (cds) *The Shoulder,* 1st edn, pp. 791–836. Philadelphia: W.B. Saunders.

16 Nakajima, T., Rokuuma, N., Hamada, K., Tomatsu, T. & Fukuda, H. (1994) Histological and biomechanical characteristics of the supraspinatus tendon: reference to rotator cuff tearing. *J. Shoulder Elbow Surg.* **3:** 79-87.

17 Ozaki, J., Fujimoto, S., Nakagawa, Y., Masuhara, K. & Tamai, S. (1988) Tears of the rotator cuff of the shoulder associated with pathological changes of the acromion: a study of cadavera. *J. Bone Joint Surg* **70A:** 1224.

18 Cofield, R.H. (1985) Current concepts review. Rotator cuff disease of the shoulder. *J. Bone Joint Surg.* **67A:** 974–979.

19 Nirschl, R.P. (1989) Rotator cuff tendinitis: basic concepts of pathoetiology. *Instr. Course Lect.* **38:** 439–446.

20 Kannus, P. & Jozsa, L. (1991) Histopathological changes preceding spontaneous rupture of a tendon. *J. Bone Joint Surg.* **73A:** 1507–1525.

21 Codman, E.A. (1984) The pathology of the subacromial bursa and of the supraspinatus tendon. In *The Shoulder,* p. 65. Malabar, FL: Robert E. Kreiger Publishing Company.

22 Neviaser, T.J. (1987) The role of the biceps tendon in the impingement syndrome. *Orthop. Clin. North Am.* **18:** 383–386.

23 Neer, C.S. II (1972) Anterior acromioplasty for the chronic impingement syndrome in the shoulder. A preliminary report. *J. Bone Joint Surg.* **54A:** 41.

24 Canoso, J.J. (1991) Bursae, tendons and ligaments. *Clin. Rheum. Dis.* **7:** 189–221.

25 Sarkar, K. & Uhthoff, H.K. (1983) Ultrastructure of the subacromial bursa in painful shoulder syndromes. *Virchows Arch. A Pathol. Anat. Histopathol.* **400:** 107–117.

26 Burn, W.C. & Whipple, T.L. (1993) Anatomic relationships in the shoulder impingement syndrome. *Clin. Orthop.* ; **294:** 96–102.

27 Soslowsky, L.J., Ann, C.H., Johnson, S.P. & Carpenter, J.P. (1994) Geometric and mechanical properties of the coracoacromial ligament and their relationship to rotator cuff disease. *Clin. Orthop.* **304:** 10–17.

28 Sarkar, K., Taine, W. & Uhthoff, H.K. (1990) The ultrastucture of the coracoacromial ligament in patients with chronic impingement syndrome. *Clin. Orthop.* **254:** 49.

29 Turkel, S.J,, Paniom M.W., Marshall, J.L. & Girgis F.G. (1981) Stabilising mechanisms preventing anterior dislocation of the glenohumeral joint. *J. Bone Joint Surg.* **63A:** 1208–1217.

30 Harryman, D.T., Sidles, J.A., Clark, J.M., McQuade, J.A., Gibb, T.D. & Matsen, F.A. (1990) Translation of the humeral head on the glenoid with passive glenohumeral motion. *J. Bone Joint Surg.* **72A:** 1334–1343.

31 Jobe, F.W. (1989) Impingement problems in the athlete. *Instr. course Lect.* **38:** 205–209.

32 Kvitne, R.S. & Jobe, F.W. (1993) The diagnosis and treatment of anterior instability in the throwing athlete. *Clin. Orthop.* **291:** 107–123.

18

Open Decompression

P Duke, WA Wallace and SP Frostick

INDICATIONS

The patient who is suitable for open or arthroscopic decompression should have a definite diagnosis of primary subacromial impingement syndrome which has failed to respond to an adequate course of non-operative treatment for at least 6 months. The surgeon should consider carefully the differential diagnosis, and, particularly in a younger patient or an athlete, the diagnosis of occult instability should be considered. Other diagnoses to be considered are glenohumeral or acromioclavicular joint degenerative disease, early frozen shoulder and the possibility of cervical spondylosis as a cause of the pain.[1]

Confirmation of the diagnosis may be obtained by performing the Neer test: an injection of 5 ml of local anaesthetic into the subacromial space. If the pain is eliminated or significantly decreased, one can infer that the pain is originating in the subacromial space or the tendons of the rotator cuff.[1] Neer recommended non-operative management for a period of 9 months in his 1972 paper.[2] Some authors have recommended periods of as little as 3 months while others will wait at least 1 year to 18 months before offering surgery.[3] The patient may have a chronic tendinitis which needs an extended period of conservative management to settle down. One should be cautious when interpreting the published results of decompression as the recovery period following surgery is significant, lasting from 4 to 12 months.[3]

It is essential to ensure that adequate non-operative treatment has actually occurred and that if physiotherapy was used as a treatment modality that this was correctly undertaken.[1,4-6] The correct non-operative management must include strengthening and stretching exercises as well as avoidance of painful activity and the prescription of non-steroid anti-inflammatory drugs (NSAIDs) or other analgesics. Supervision of the programme by a trained physiotherapist is essential. The use of subacromial injections of steroids such as triamcinolone in combination with local anaesthetic is also a useful treatment tool.[7,8] Up to three separate injections can be given over a period of 1 year before worrying about damage to the tendon from the trophic effects of the steroid.[6,9]

The other indication for open decompression is as a routine when performing a repair of the rotator cuff.[1,10]

INVESTIGATION

The use of various imaging techniques is essential to aid in the assessment of the state of the rotator cuff. They are also useful to rule out conditions that may mimic impingement or cause impingement. Such conditions as calcific tendinitis, degenerative disease of the acromioclavicular joint or glenohumeral joint or changes in the undersurface of the acromion will all be seen on plain X-ray of the shoulder.[6]

X-ray

An AP radiograph in the plane of the scapula and an axial view of the involved shoulder should always be obtained. Both of these views require a radiographer with special skills. To assess the subacromial space and to obtain an adequate view of the cuff, the AP view should be taken with a 30° downward tilt and should be repeated in internal and external rotation. The supraspinatus outlet view is also useful in outlining the subacromial space and in looking at the undersurface of the coracoacromial arch. To look at the acromioclavicular joint the X–ray beam should be angled 20° upwards on the AP view. These techniques are described in great detail in relevant chapters of *The Shoulder*.[6,11]

Ultrasound scan

If there is a clinical suspicion of a tear of the rotator cuff, then an ultrasound scan is a good method of assessment. It is only reliable if the person performing and reporting on the scan is keen and experienced. There is a long learning curve and the reliability of the report is very operator-dependent.[12–15]

Magnetic resonance imaging (MRI)

The reliability of MRI in the assessment of rotator cuff disease continues to change, as do the techniques used. With a radiologist who is competent in the interpretation of shoulder MRI scans this is a reliable method of assessment of the state of the rotator cuff.[12]

POSITION OF PATIENT

Most shoulder surgery is carried out with the patient in the beach chair position. Figure 18.1 shows this position which will be fully discussed in the following paragraphs. This position enables all forms of shoulder surgery to be carried out including arthroscopy.

The operating table

Ideally this should have the capacity to break in the middle and at the lower end, forming an open W, as well as the ability to tilt in either direction.

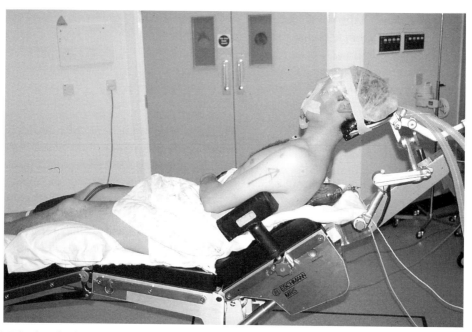

Fig. 18.1 The beach chair position. There is easy access to the shoulder from all directions. The arm can be fully extended and the scapula is prevented from moving posteriorly by a 500 ml bag of fluid.

Control of the head and access to the shoulder

This is made easier by the use of a Mayfield neurosurgical head rest. This device enables the head and neck to be placed in any position as well as enabling removal of that part of the table immediately behind the shoulder. This gives easy access to the posterior part of the shoulder. If the Mayfield head rest is not available then a dough-nut head ring should be used.

Lateralizing the patient

This is essential to allow the arm to be fully extended over the edge of the operating table. In the case of an open decompression, it is difficult to visualize fully the rotator cuff which is mainly achieved by moving the arm and not the wound.

Stability of the scapula

Stabilizing the scapula is not absolutely essential for this operation but it helps. To obtain stability of the scapula a 500 ml bag of saline is placed under and medial to the medial border of the scapula. This will project the scapula forwards and significantly stabilize it there.

Protection of the nerves

The ulnar nerve at the elbow on the contralateral side can be injured by lying the arm beside the abdomen for a prolonged period of time. The ulnar nerve should always be protected by lying the elbow on a soft roll. The common peroneal nerve is also in danger if the legs are allowed to roll laterally on to the nerves as they pass around the neck of the fibula. They are more susceptible to injury if the knees are kept extended, thus placing a stretching force on the sciatic nerve as well as the common peroneal. It is therefore wise to place a pillow under the knees to flex the knees and provide protection of the common peroneal nerve.

Lateral stability

To ensure that the assistant does not pull the patient off the operating table, one should always have some form of lateral support. This may take the form of a standard pelvic support plate but this will often have a bar that projects laterally into the surgeon's abdomen or interferes with the movement of the arm of the patient. As is shown in Figure 18.1, the use of a custom-made device will eliminate this problem; the device shown here has a direct attachment to the table and has no need to be adjustable so the troublesome bar has been removed.

How much can the patient be sat up?

The patient should be placed in a sitting position at 45–60° from the horizontal. This will initially alarm the uninitiated anaesthetist, particularly if the patient is elderly and has compromised cerebral circulation. However, it is very uncommon for patients to suffer from this position and most patients can tolerate this amount of elevation. With the patient in this position the access to the shoulder is easier and the patient position is more anatomical.

TECHNIQUE

Anaesthesia

Operations on the shoulder can be carried out under either regional or general anaesthesia. Regional blockade is the best way to avoid the use of a general anaesthetic. In the day case setting, it is much quicker to use a general anaesthetic and to supplement this with a regional block if the anaesthetist is familiar with the technique.[16] Most shoulder surgery in our unit is performed under general anaesthetic for both day case and inpatient surgery. The use of an interscalene block is quite successful in a day case setting.[17]

Incision

For open acromioplasty, two incisions are currently in regular use: (a) the bra-strap incision;

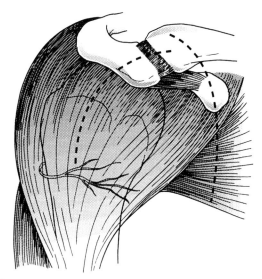

Fig. 18.2 Skin incisions: the bra-strap incision is cosmetically more acceptable while the coronal incision is easier to use.

(b) a coronal incision based over the anterior acromion. These two incisions are shown in Figure 18.2.

Bra-strap incision

This is a very good cosmetic incision. If necessary one can mark the position of the bra strap before the operation to ensure that the incision is in the correct place. It is hidden from view by the bra-strap of ladies if correctly placed. However, it does mean that extensive mobilization of the lateral skin flap is necessary to gain access to the lateral acromion and to split the deltoid. It therefore takes slightly longer. The dissection may often divide the supraclavicular branches of the cervical plexus and the patients will often complain of a numb patch lateral to the wound. However, with reassurance and the passage of time patients do not seem to have a long-term problem with this.

Coronal plane incision

This is the incision we currently use in most male patients. It is quick and gives good access to the acromioclavicular joint and the acromion. It does

not have the same problem with injury to the superficial nerves. It is easier to extend the exposure if necessary to repair the rotator cuff. It gives a less cosmetically acceptable result than the bra-strap incision but most men do not seem to be concerned about this.

Approach to the acromion

The aim of the approach is to gain access to the inferior aspect of the anterolateral part of the acromion. This can be through a simple deltoid split but this does make adequate resection more difficult, although it does leave the deltoid well attached. We prefer to use the 'deltoid on' approach popularized by Rockwood.[6] This is illustrated in Figure 18.3. This approach gives excellent exposure of the acromion and the coracoacromial ligament while allowing acromioclavicular joint surgery to be incorporated when necessary. The deltoid is taken off only the leading edge of the acromion and is split where the anterior part meets the middle part of the deltoid. This is at the anterolateral acromion and there is a fibrous raphe to be found here. This is where the split in the deltoid should be made as it leaves good tissue to be repaired.

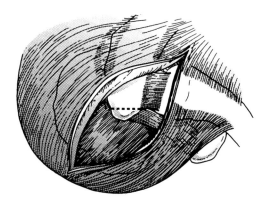

Fig. 18.3 The 'deltoid on' approach to the undersurface of the acromion. The deltoid is peeled off the acromion starting at the anterior flap back from the edge of the acromion to give a good cuff of tissue to be repaired. The extension to incorporate the acromioclavicular joint is only made when there is a need to expose this joint to resect it. The dotted line indicates the extent of the acromion to be removed.

Coracoacromial ligament

This ligament forms an important part of the superior coracoacromial arch of the shoulder complex. In the impingement syndrome it is often shorter and thicker, forming part of the secondary impinging structures.[18] It should be released and partly resected in the treatment of impingement, either as a isolated procedure or along with bony decompression.

It is our current practice to preserve the coracoacromial ligament in total shoulder arthroplasty as we believe that it forms an important superior support structure. It is actually divided for the purpose of exposure but is repaired at the end. Other shoulder surgeons are now reporting the reattachment of the ligament as a part of routine cuff repair surgery.[19] This is easily achieved if the ligament is detached from its insertion to the front and undersurface of the acromion as one and then retracted along with the overlying deltoid. This usually gives it enough length to be reattached along with the deltoid to the front of the acromion. Most commonly at present this ligament is routinely divided and partly resected as part of the acromioplasty.

The acromial resection

Taking the right amount of acromion is vital to the success of this operation. Taking too much can cause problems with the deltoid attachment thus weakening the shoulder. Radical or complete acromionectomy has few proponents[20] and in our opinion as well as others is thought to be a bad operation with poor results long term.[21] Our unit has treated a group of patients who have required reconstruction of the acromion following an excessive acromioplasty. These patients all had ongoing pain and disability. Acromioplasty – undercutting of the acromion – was originally popularized by Neer in 1972.[2] He proposed that the anterolateral part of the acromion was the offending portion and that this portion should be resected. We currently follow the practice of Rockwood who proposed the 'deltoid on' approach. He recommends that the anterior 'pro-

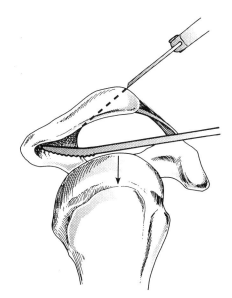

Fig. 18.4 Acromial resection. A sagittal saw is used to cut the acromion accurately. The actual amount taken varies depending on the thickness of the acromion and the amount of 'hook' that is present. Enough should be taken for the cuff to run smoothly under the acromion after any thickened bursa has been removed and any adhesions have been freed up.

jection' of the acromion be removed with a saw; this usually entails removing no more than 0.5–1.0 cm of the acromion. The saw is directed obliquely to make an angled cut to remove the anteroinferior part with a small amount of the inferolateral part of the acromion. Once again a small piece of bone is removed; the saw should be aimed at the posteroinferior part of the acromion and the fingers can be used to judge how much of the acromion has been taken (Figure 18.4).

The acromioclavicular joint

When should the acromioclavicular joint be removed? This joint does have a role in the production of pain around the shoulder and is often the site of osteoarthritis. It may in fact have a role in the production of impingement pain via pressure on the cuff by inferiorly projecting osteophytes. It can be difficult to decide whether the acromioclavicular joint is the source of enough pain to warrant its resection. This joint should be removed if it is thought to be the source of impingement or pain.

Assessment of the joint is an important part of patient assessment before operation. Pain from the acromioclavicular joint is often made worse by cross-body adduction, the last 30° of elevation and by forced internal rotation. The pain is localized to the joint or slightly more posterior or more medial. The joint may be tender to palpation. Radiographic evaluation may reveal significant degeneration.

During the acromioplasty the inferior part of the acromioclavicular joint should be palpated to ascertain the presence of any inferior projecting osteophytes. These can be removed with the saw if the joint is to be preserved or the joint can be 'excised' by taking out the lateral 1 cm of the clavicle.

In summary, the acromioclavicular joint should be removed if it is a cause of symptoms, as assessed by a combination of clinical, radiographic and operative findings.

Assessment of the need for a drain

We feel that there is no need for the routine use of a drain. There is no dead space in the subacromial area for the blood to collect if all layers are securely closed. This practice also has the benefit of allowing the routine use of an epidural catheter in the subacromial space for the delivery of local anaesthetic for postoperative pain relief.

Deltoid reattachment

It is vital to obtain a good reattachment of the deltoid to the acromion. The use of heavy absorbable sutures is recommended; a no. 1 Vicryl suture is currently used in this unit. The suture can usually be passed through the bone of the anterior cut edge of the acromion to give an excellent hold. Good bites of the deltoid are also essential and the thin fascial envelope of the deltoid should be included.

POSTOPERATIVE MANAGEMENT

Postoperative pain relief

With the current push for increased efficiency in health-delivery systems worldwide, there is an increase in the use of day surgery facilities. Open acromioplasty without cuff repair is suitable for day case surgery. It does warrant the use of narcotic analgesia after surgery if a regional or local anaesthetic agent is not used in addition to the general anaesthetic. Even for inpatients the use of these methods will speed up the recovery and provide additional comfort. It is recommended that the routine use of regional blockade in the form of a scalene block should be employed. For those who are treated as inpatients we currently use a local infiltration of 10 ml Marcain (bupivacaine) 0.25% via an epidural catheter, with delivery to the subacromial space every 4 h.

If the necessary staff are not available to supervise the continuous or intermittent flow of local anaesthetic, then we use a one-off dose of local anaesthetic into the wound at the time of closure, again using Marcain 0.25%. Ice packs are commonly used by many surgeons as a means of decreasing pain in the first postoperative days. Rockwood routinely uses ice packs applied in the recovery room along with local anaesthetic to manage pain after total shoulder replacement.

Interscalene blocks are safe to use in the day case setting and they have been shown to decrease the hospitalization rate.[17] When it is working well, it allows the physiotherapist to begin passive range of movement exercises in the immediate postoperative period. This is an essential part of the rehabilitation for this procedure.

Rehabilitation

One of the most important facets of a successful decompression is adequate rehabilitation. If this phase is not performed properly, then even the best operation will be of no benefit or may leave the patient worse off. When the cuff is intact, the therapist can proceed with no fear of injury to it. This means using a passive range and then an active assisted range when the effect of any anaesthetic has worn off.

The initial full elevation is performed supine, and gradual progression is made to full elevation while the patient is sitting then standing. Pendulum exercises are particularly useful. After the wound has healed and the initial swelling and pain has settled 2 weeks after surgery, the therapist will begin active exercises and begin to stretch the end of range. With increasing confidence and decreased pain at 4–6 weeks, the phase of building up strength in the cuff muscles can begin with resisted active exercises.

The patient should be familiar with the regimen from their preoperative programme of non-operative treatment.

COMPLICATIONS

Patient positioning

Cerebral perfusion

There are no reported instances of significant problems with cerebral perfusion in the beach chair position. It is often a cause for concern with the elderly patient who is receiving prolonged anaesthesia in the upright beach chair position with some hypotensive element to the anaesthetic. Ultimately it is the anaesthetist who is responsible for the well-being of the patient during the operation and it should be left to their discretion to put the patient into a lower position if they are at all concerned about perfusion of the brain.

Cervical spine

Patients with either a stiff cervical spine from spondylosis or an unstable cervical spine from rheumatoid arthritis require extra care in positioning. It is the combined responsibility of the surgeon and the anaesthetist to ensure that no complications such as a ligamentous strain or cord injury occur from poor positioning of the patient's neck.

Pressure injury to nerves and soft tissues

The responsibility for this is primarily that of the anaesthetist but also to a lesser extent that of the surgeon. The complications are not specific to the beach chair position, and they relate to unprotected nerves and pressure areas. The common problems seen with nerves involve the ulnar nerve on the opposite side and the common peroneal nerves on both sides. These nerves should be safe if properly padded during the operation. The pressure areas that need to be considered are the sacrum and the heels.

Operative neural injury

The deltoid-splitting surgical approach can injure the axillary nerve if the split is taken further than 5 cm from the edge of the acromion. While it is safe if the split remains at 5 cm, it is easy to propagate the split if care is not taken during the operation. Some surgeons recommend that a stay suture be placed at the end of the split to stop this from occurring.

Infection

This a rare occurrence in shoulder surgery, particularly with simple operations like a subacromial decompression. The shoulder area has an excellent blood supply, resembling that of the face, and is therefore relatively resistant to infection. Skin flap necrosis and infection are very uncommon. Because the risk of infection is so small, there is no indication for the use of prophylactic antibiotics in the routine open acromioplasty.

Haematoma

Our unit does not routinely use a drain. There is little dead space when the wound is closed in layers and haematomas are rare. Some large blood vessels are commonly divided when the coracoacromial ligament is divided, and these should always be cauterized.

Shoulder stiffness

Stiffness of the shoulder is a disabling but often

avoidable problem in shoulder surgery. It can arise very quickly after any form of shoulder surgery and open decompression is no exception. Adequate postoperative mobilization must follow decompression. This involves supervision of the therapy by the surgeon or a physiotherapist. Ideally the patient is taught the postoperative exercise programme before the operation and is closely supervised by the therapist until a good range of movement is acquired.

Scar cosmesis

Use of the coronal plane incision which crosses Langer's lines will give rise to a less cosmetically acceptable scar than the bra-strap incision. In those prone to keloid formation, this is even more of a problem. Although the bra-strap incision is slightly more difficult to use than the coronal plane incision, its use is recommended, particularly in females. Actual bra-strap pressure does not usually cause a problem with the wound or scar long term but patients often prefer to wear their bra-straps crossed over for the 6 months immediately after surgery.

Skin sensory loss

This can occasionally be a problem after the use of the bra-strap incision when by necessity some of the small superficial branches of the supraclavicular nerves are divided. The skin lateral to the incision will often be numb but this is seldom a long-term problem for the patient.

Deltoid detachment

As part of the 'deltoid on' approach the deltoid is actually detached from a small part of the acromion anteriorly. It is subsequently reattached to the acromial edge and usually heals to this with little trouble. However, it can become detached if not secured properly at the end of the operation or if large amounts of the deltoid are detached from the lateral acromion during the operation.

Deltoid detachment is a cosmetic and functional problem. Cosmetically it leaves the patient with an obvious defect in the deltoid – particularly noticeable when the arm is elevated. Functionally it is a very real problem when combined with a rotator cuff deficiency. This leads to a decrease in active elevation and painful impingement. It can be avoided by meticulous repair of the soft tissues.

Technical tips

1. Always mark the side that the operation is on with an indelible felt pen during the preoperative visit on the ward. This will reassure the patient that care is taken and help avoid operating on the wrong side.
2. Infiltrate the operative site with Marcain and adrenaline before making the incision. This will decrease the amount of bleeding.
3. Make a bold initial incision and insert a self retaining retractor before attempting to control the many small bleeding points. This will temporarily stop a lot of the small bleeding points which will then become haemostatic during the operation.
4. Use a no. 15 blade for the subperiosteal dissection of the deltoid off the bone of the anterior acromion. Change the blade regularly during the operation as it rapidly becomes blunt on bone.
5. There will always be a large vessel cut as you take the deltoid and coracoacromial ligament off the front of the acromion. This is the deltoid branch of the thoracoacromial trunk. Control this vessel by having adequate exposure and using a sucker to allow you to see it, then obtain haemostasis with the use of diathermy.
6. The coracoacromial ligament attaches to the front and to the undersurface of the anterior acromion. To divide it without cutting the rotator cuff tendons, slide the no. 15 blade firstly down the front then under the acromion to release the ligament.
7. The deltoid is often stuck to the underlying bursa and can be difficult to peel off with blunt finger dissection in the early part of the release. This is made a lot easier by using sharp dissection, either with a knife or scissors, to free up a plane between the deltoid and the bursa.

8. Use a Bristow periosteal dissector as a lever to hold the humeral head down when making the cut in the acromion. It should be slid through to the back of the acromion and then this point is used as the fulcrum to lever the head down, thus creating a gap.
9. When reattaching the deltoid to the acromion make sure you have a secure hold in the acromion by using a no. 1 Vicryl suture and put the suture through bone. If the suture needle will not pass easily in a young patient, then use a sharp towel clip to create a passage for the suture.

REFERENCES

1. Neer, C.S. (1983) Impingement lesions. *Clin. Orthop.* **173:** 70–77.
2. Neer, C.S., II (1972) Anterior acromioplasty for the chronic impingement syndrome in the shoulder. A preliminary report. *J. Bone Joint Surg.* **54A:** 41.
3. Bartolozzi, A., Andreychik, D. & Ahmad, S. (1994) Determinants of outcome in the treatment of rotator cuff disease. *Clin. Orthop.* **308:** 90–97.
4. Fu, F.H., Harner, C.D. & Klien, A.H. (1991) Shoulder impingement syndrome. *Clin. Orthop.* **269:** 162–173.
5. Jobe, F.W. & Moyes, D.R. (1982) Delineation of diagnostic criteria and a rehabilitation programme for rotator cuff injuries. *Am. J. Sports Med.* **10:** 336–339.
6. Matsen, F.A., III & Arntz, C.T. (1990) Subacromial impingement. In C.A. Rockwood, Jr. & F.A. Matsen, III (eds), *The Shoulder*, 1st edn, pp. 623–646. Philadelphia: W.B. Saunders.
7. Hollingworth, G.R., Ellis, R.M. & Hattersley, T.H. (1983) Comparison of injection techniques for shoulder pain: results of a double blind, randomised study. *Br. Med. J.* **287:** 1339–1341.
8. Kessel, L. & Watson, M. (1977) The painful arc syndrome. *J. Bone Joint Surg.* **59B:** 166–172.
9. Kapetanos, G. (1982) The effect of the local corticosteroids on the healing and biomechanical properties of the partially injured tendon. *Clin. Orthop.* **163:** 170–179.
10. Cofield, R.H. (1985) Current concepts review. Rotator cuff disease of the shoulder. *J. Bone Joint Surg.* **67A:** 974–979.
11. Rockwood, C.A., Jr., Szalay, E.A., Curtis, R.J., Young, C.D. & Kay, S.P. (1990) X-ray evaluation of shoulder problems. In: Rockwood, C.A., Jr. & Matsen, F.A., III (eds) *The Shoulder*, 1st edn, pp. 178–207. Philadelphia: W.B. Saunders.
12. Sonnabend, D.H., Hughes, J.S., Guiffre, B.M. & Farrell, R. (1993) Ultrasound assessment of shoulder pathology. In M. Vastamaki & P. Jalovaara (eds) *Surgery of the Shoulder*, pp. 13–17. Amsterdam: Elsevier.
13. Nelson, M.C., Leather, G.P. et al. (1991) Evaluation of the painful shoulder. *J. Bone Joint Surg.* **73A:** 707–716.
14. Paavolainen, P. & Ahovuo, J. (1994) Ultrasonography and arthrography in the diagnosis of tears of the rotator cuff. *J. Bone Joint Surg.* **76A:** 335–340.
15. Collins, R.A., Gristina, A.G., Carter, R.E. et al. (1987) Ultrasonography of the shoulder. *Orthop. Clin. North Am.* **18:** 351.
16. Conn, R.A., Cofield, R.H. & Byer, D.E. (1987) Interscalene block anaesthesia for shoulder surgery. *Clin. Orthop.* **216:** 94–98.
17. Kinnard, P., Truchon, R., St-Pierre, A. & Montreuil, J. (1994) Interscalene block for pain relief after shoulder surgery. *Clin. Orthop.* **304:** 22–24.
18. Soslowsky, L.J., Ann, C.H., Johnston, S.P. & Carpenter, J.P. (1994) Geometric and mechanical properties of the coracoacromial ligament and their relationship to rotator cuff disease. *Clin. Orthop.* **304:** 10–17.
19. Flatow, E.L., Rodosky, M.W., Yamaguchi, K., Self, E.B., Pollock, G.R. & Bigliani, L.U. Coracoacromial ligament preservation in rotator cuff surgery. *Abstracts 6th International Congress on Surgery of the Shoulder. J. Shoulder Elbow Surgery.* In Press.
20. Bosley, R.C. (1991) Total acromionectomy. *J. Bone Joint Surg.* **73A:** 961–968.
21. Neer, C.S., II & Marberry, T.A. (1981) On the disadvantages of radical acromionectomy. *J. Bone Joint Surg.* **63A:** 416.

19

Open Repair of Instability

L Neumann and WA Wallace

INTRODUCTION

Since Hippocrates treated recurrent shoulder dislocation by cauterization with a red-hot iron, numerous procedures have been devised to deal with this common problem. As even recreational sports are often carried out at a fairly high level, shoulder instability today often requires surgical stabilization to allow the individual to return to leisure activities at the previous level. The demands put on the shoulder joint in the throwing sports, racquet sports and swimming, where hypermobile and thus fragile shoulder joints tend to predominate, or in the contact sports, where injuries frequently cause instability, often require the joint to be surgically repaired after an injury.

Shoulder instability is not one single pathology, and it is very important that the surgeon treating these shoulders is able to make a detailed diagnosis and has enough experience to be able to restore the joint to its normal asymptomatic state.

As patients in 1996 expect a normal shoulder after surgery, several procedures used in the past should today be considered obsolete as they have short-term or long-term morbidity that is no longer acceptable. Even though reports with very good results exist for many of these procedures, many of the studies were carried out a number of years ago when success was defined as 'no recurrence of dislocation' and parameters such as late arthritis or reduced external rotation were often not assessed.

With the increasing use of the arthroscope, not only for diagnostic procedures but also for surgical reconstruction, the future need for open stabiliza-

tion procedures has been questioned. We believe open stabilization is still the 'gold standard'. The recurrence rate is lower for the open procedures, and the arthroscopic procedures do not guarantee a normal range of motion (ROM) and only seem to be successful when carried out by very experienced surgeons. The postoperative course after arthroscopic surgery is as long as for an open one. There is some evidence that arthroscopic procedures do best in first-time dislocators operated on very early after the injury. In most clinics this will be an unusual scenario because of waiting lists etc. If cosmesis is not considered by the patient to be of major importance, a carefully performed open procedure will provide a predictable good result with low morbidity, and will still be the first choice in most patients, especially the very demanding athletes who cannot afford a recurrence or loss of movement.

PATHOLOGICAL ANATOMY

The Bankart lesion (also called Perthe's pocket) is the typical finding in the unstable shoulder. It is almost always seen after traumatic anterior instability, but also frequently after posterior instability. At the time of the dislocation the shoulder structures appear to undergo three stages of injury: stage 1, the head subluxes forward and stretching of the anterior capsule and the middle and inferior glenohumeral ligaments occur; stage 2, a Bankart lesion (pocket) is created on the anterior inferior glenoid rim as a result of the glenoid labrum being pulled off its insertion together with the glenohumeral ligaments and capsule; stage 3, the humeral head is physically dislocated and pulls the periosteum and soft tissues off the front of the scapular neck. The Bankart lesion or pocket so created shows little or no tendency to heal back on to the bone, probably because the synovial fluid filling it prevents healing taking place. Speer and collaborators[1] showed that a Bankart lesion alone is not enough to create recurrent instability of the shoulder; the capsular stretching is a necessary component of the pathology. The Hill–Sachs lesion (sometimes called the Broca and Hartmann lesion) is a compression fracture occurring in the humeral head when the head is impacted on to the glenoid rim during the dislocation. In an anterior dislocation the lesion is in the back of the humeral head, and in a posterior dislocation the lesion is in the front of the head – a reverse Hill–Sachs lesion. After the initial dislocation, the presence of these intra-articular lesions makes recurrence likely because when the arm is brought into the critical position of external rotation in abduction, the impression fracture engages the glenoid rim and causes a further dislocation to occur. With the elongation of the ligaments caused by stretching and as a result of the Bankart lesion present, the shoulder has lost its soft tissue stability. In the presence of a humeral head defect, the articulating surface area of the head is reduced and re-dislocations occur more and more easily. A deficient glenoid rim increases the risk of re-dislocation even more (Figure 19.1). In patients above the age of 40 damage to the rotator cuff becomes more common with shoulder dislocations. This can be either a pure tendinous lesion not visible on X-ray film or it can be a bony cuff lesion, i.e. an avulsion of fragments of the tuberosities.

The close relation of the brachial plexus to the humeral head when this is anteriorly dislocated or the risk of traction being applied to the plexus during the dislocation and the subsequent reduction makes nerve lesions an important complication associated with shoulder dislocations. Isolated lesions to nerves around the shoulder, mainly the axillary nerve and the musculocutaneous nerve, may be seen both in relation to the dislocation, and also as a complication to stabilization proce-

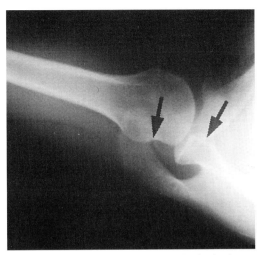

Fig. 19.1 Severe bone deficiency on both the humeral and the glenoid side means that this shoulder is almost dislocating as the two defects engage.

dures. In the posterior surgical procedures the suprascapular nerve and its branch to the infraspinatus muscle is at risk.

INDICATIONS FOR AN OPEN STABILIZATION OPERATION

The history is extremely important in establishing the correct diagnosis as very often the patient, by clearly describing the first dislocation or symptoms, gives a very strong indication of the likely pathology.

The most frequent type of dislocation is the traumatic anterior. This is a unidirectional instability, usually with a very typical history of a traumatic episode after which a previously asymptomatic shoulder becomes symptomatic. Typically the trauma occurs with the shoulder abducted and externally rotated. Recurrences are frequently seen, occurring more and more easily, eventually just by taking the arm above shoulder level. The patient becomes very apprehensive and develops a very protective attitude to prevent recurrences. The clinical findings are typical: a positive apprehension test, positive Jobe's relocation test (Figure 19.2) and sometimes a positive drawer test and sulcus sign.

(A)

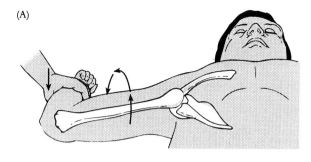

(B)

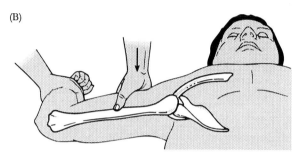

(C)

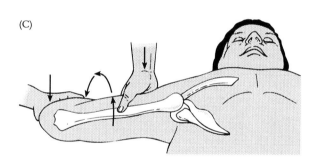

(D)

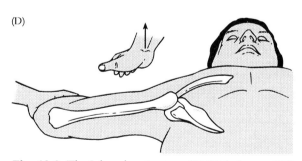

Fig. 19.2 The Jobe relocation test. (A) With the arm 90° of abduction, the humerus is externally rotated to the point of pain. (B) Firm pressure is applied to the humeral neck which reduces the joint and relieves the pain. (C) While maintaining this pressure, further external rotation can be achieved, until another point of pain is reached. (D) When the pressure on the humeral neck is suddenly removed, the patient experiences a sudden increase in pain.

In these patients we base our diagnosis mainly on the clinical findings. A set of radiographs (AP shoulder in the plane of the glenoid surface and an axillary view) are standard to allow any bony lesions to be detected.

We do not expect the patient to 'earn' the right to a stabilization procedure by proving a certain number of dislocations. A large number of patients seem to stabilize their shoulders with time,[2] but in top athletes or patients depending on good shoulder function in their job, we are prepared to carry out a stabilizing operation even after one dislocation.

If an operative stabilization is decided upon, as a routine, we always carry out an examination under anaesthesia (EUA) and a shoulder arthroscopy to assess in detail the direction and degree of instability and the intra-articular damage. This is performed in the same session as the open procedure with the patient in the beach chair position. One can therefore proceed to the open repair without needing to reposition the patient.

In this type of instability we use the Bankart repair as described by Rowe,[3] but adapted to use Mitek suture anchors. These anchors shorten the operation time considerably, provide an excellent hold, and can be inserted without the need to take sutures through the joint surface, which was necessary with the original Bankart procedure and which could cause some damage to the glenoid surface.

If the history or the preoperative clinical examination gives rise to suspicion of a posterior or an inferior instability, or both, combined with the anterior instability and the arthroscopy does not show any Bankart lesion or capsular damage, the preferred operation is the inferior capsular shift procedure as described by Neer & Foster.[4] These patients have multidirectional instablity, often not associated with trauma. Characteristically they often have similar clinical findings in the opposite shoulder even though it may be asymptomatic. Operating on these patients is very difficult and requires some experience to balance the capsule during the 'shift'. Overtightening may lead to either reduced ROM or to accentuation of the instability in the direction 'away' from the repair.

An undertightening may lead to recurrence of the instability.

If the instability is multidirectional but mainly posterior, the capsular shift can be carried out through a posterior approach. This is somewhat more difficult as the posterior capsular tissues are thinner and less solid than the anterior ones.

The clinical findings may show both a multi-directional instability and a true Bankart lesion. In these cases we do the capsular shift on the glenoid side of the joint and combine it with a repair of the Bankart lesion with suture anchors. A similar procedure can also be carried out posteriorly.

If the radiographs suggest major damage to the glenoid rim anteriorly, during the surgical approach we prepare for an eventual Bristow repair by taking off a slightly larger tip of the coracoid process which we routinely osteotomize during our Bankart repairs. The Bankart repair can then be reinforced with the coracoid transfer if necessary. If there is a suspicion of a major bony Bankart lesion the patient will have been con-sented and informed of the risk of loss of rotation if a Bristow procedure needs to be carried out. The authors reserve this method for use in patients for whom a minor loss of external rotation is not crucial and who have a bony Bankart lesion with a deficient anterior rim reducing the surface area of the glenoid. This is usually due to either wear of the rim by repeated dislocations or to a fracture. It is a 'compensatory' procedure, as anatomical repair is not possible, and we only use it in cases where the bony and capsular damage is considered to be too extensive to be addressed by a Bankart repair only.

In patients with major bone loss to the glenoid or in epileptics who suffer very forceful disloca-tions during fits, we perform the bone buttress procedure. This procedure has the disadvantage of reducing the rotation somewhat, but in these difficult patients it provides excellent restoration of stability and function.

The use of any kind of metal staples or screws to reattach the capsule to the scapular neck or to the humeral head should now be avoided. The risk of migration of these implants is very high and this may cause severe complications such as pre-mature arthritis or neurovascular injuries. Even

the Bristow screw has been reported to break and migrate. In our view the screw in the Bristow procedure is the only acceptable exception to the rule, as there is no better alternative.

The Mitek anchors are deeply embedded in bone and there are currently no reports of them migrating or causing intra-articular problems if correctly inserted. During discussions of whether anchors should be used and what type is the best, arguments of pull-out strength are often used. We prefer the Mitek G–II anchor as it is very simple, with a small instrumentation set and its pull–out strength exceeds by far the strength of the sutures attached to it.

A very special group of patients are those with instability and degenerative changes in the joint caused by either failed surgery in the past or 'post-dislocation arthropathy'. There might be an indi-cation to perform a hemiarthroplasty but their instability must be adequately addressed either in a separate procedure before the arthroplasty or in the same session as the joint replacement, other-wise the instability may return after the hemiar-throplasty. Reappearance of instability after hemiarthroplasty presents a very difficult problem, which is discussed further in Chapter 26.

Generally, a Bankart lesion should be treated with a Bankart repair, while a stretched or defi-cient capsule should be treated with a capsular shift.

It has to be remembered that patients with no confirmed dislocations can suffer from subluxa-tions. Symptoms caused by these subluxations can be very disabling, with shooting pain down the arm (the dead arm syndrome) and the develop-ment of very protective attitudes to avoid the symptoms. We consider subluxations to be a relative indication for a stabilization procedure, and often, even though no clear-cut instability is found during EUA, a Bankart lesion may be present in these patients.

In elderly patients, a rotator cuff tear may be present after dislocation of the shoulder. In these patients, once the tear has been confirmed by arthrography, ultrasound, magnetic resonance imaging (MRI) or arthroscopy, stability can usually be achieved by repairing the tear prefer-ably at an early stage. Formal stabilization procedures are very rarely required in these patients, and should not be carried out before the effect of the cuff repair has been assessed.

Impingement pain is often a symptom of instability in a superior direction. In a hypermobile or a multidirectional unstable shoulder we would not carry out subacromial decompression before the shoulder has been stabilized by either conservative or surgical means. The impingement is secondary to the instability and removal of a few millimetres of the undersurface of the acromion will just allow the humerus to drift proximally a little further until the impingement recurs.

FURTHER EXAMINATIONS

We base almost all our diagnoses on clinical findings and plain X-ray films, but occasionally additional examinations are of value.

Radiographs

Conventional radiographs are mandatory in the acute situation to clarify the direction of the dislocation and even more importantly to reveal any associated fractures or avulsions. Radiographs are also very useful in the elective situation, as secondary changes to bone can often be seen. Usually, an AP view in the plane of the glenoid surface and an axillary view are sufficient. Sometimes films of the opposite normal shoulder can be useful for comparison. If previous dislocations have damaged the glenoid rim, fragments can often be seen sitting adjacent to the glenoid rim or as loose bodies within the joint. Calcification within the joint capsule may also be detectable. With repeated dislocations, abrasion of the glenoid rim can be detected on the axillary view. This lesion can very often also be identified on the AP view as a defect in the condensed line representing the normal anterior glenoid rim (Figure 19.3). The Hill–Sachs lesion is often visible on the axillary view, as an impression in the humeral head found posteriorly in shoulders with anterior instability and anteriorly in shoulders with posterior instability. We believe the size of the Hill–Sachs lesion is important. If it is very large, conventional surgical procedures may not be sufficient to restore stability. Although the Hill–Sachs lesion can be better imaged using the Stryker view or the West Point view, we do not use these views as a routine.

Detailed information about dysplastic changes of the glenoid can usually not be obtained from plain films.

The pain in a dislocated or recently reduced

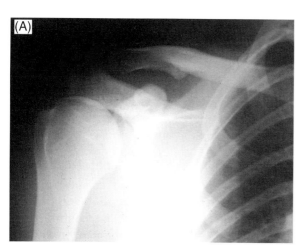
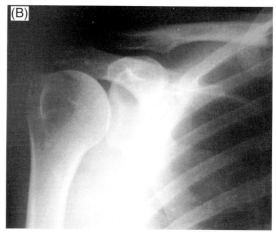

Fig. 19.3 (A) Anteroposterior view, the condensed line normally indicating the location of the anterior glenoid rim is missing. For comparison a normal shoulder is shown in (B). If this line is missing, it is strongly indicative of a glenoid rim defect.

shoulder or the presence of a sling may prevent the radiologist from obtaining a conventional axillary view. This view is, however, of great importance, as it reveals not only the direction of the dislocation, but very often also shows associated lesions not visible on the AP view. In such patients, we use the modified axillary view – the Nottingham view[5] (Figure 19.4).

In the acute state, X-ray views in two planes are mandatory. The posterior dislocation in particular is easily missed if only an AP view is obtained (Figure 19.5).

(A)

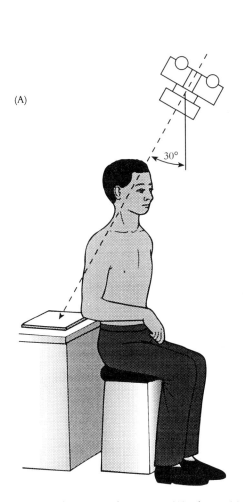

(B)

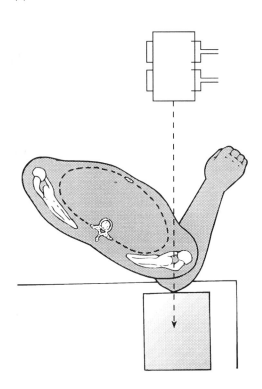

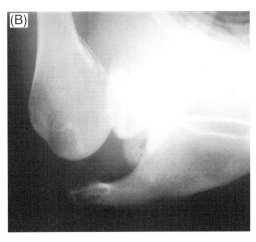

Fig. 19.4 The Nottingham view. (A) The positioning of the patient and X-ray equipment for the modified axillary view of the shoulder; (B) even in a Gilchrist-type of sling a clear view of the relation of the humeral head to the glenoid and of any humeral head and glenoid rim defects can be obtained.

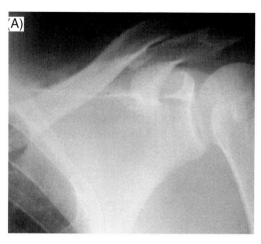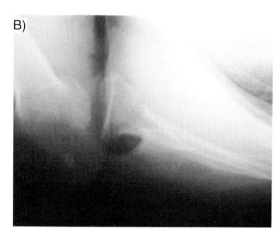

Fig. 19.5 (A) Anteroposterior view, this shoulder appears normal, but an axillary view (B) shows a posterior dislocation.

Computed tomography (CT) scan

A CT scan provides excellent and very detailed information about the osseous structures in the shoulder, and is the examination of choice if dysplastic changes such as retroversion of the glenoid are expected, or to assess the extent of fractures of the glenoid or humeral head. As the 'slices' will usually include the opposite shoulder, comparison of the pathological with the normal shoulder is easy.

MRI scan

The MRI scan is valuable in identifying labral tears. In most clinics, MRI is expensive and access to this investigation is limited. It has not yet established itself as a routine investigation in these patients.

Arthrogram – conventional and with CT scan

A conventional double-contrast arthrogram can be of use, especially if additional cuff pathology is suspected. However, if detailed information about the soft tissues is required, a CT–arthrogram is the investigation which gives most detail not only of the cuff but also of the labrum and its

relation to the glenoid rim and of bony lesions of the glenoid and humeral head. CT–arthrography is very sensitive in identifying pathological lesions.

Examination under anaesthesia (EUA)

We have found this examination to be important and of value in assessing shoulder instability. With the patient asleep the shoulder is put into the positions in which it is most likely to be unstable, and 'stressed' while in these postions. For anterior instability, abduction of 40–140° and external rotation with axial loading will cause the shoulder to anteriorly sublux or dislocate. For posterior instability, flexion of 90–120° and slight adduction and internal rotation with axial loading will cause the shoulder to sublux or dislocate. This is discussed in more detail in Chapter 6.

Arthroscopy

A diagnostic arthroscopy carried out in conjunction with an EUA is a must in the assessment of any shoulder instability and will clarify its exact nature and the associated intra-articular lesions. This allows good preoperative planning and choice of the correct procedure.

POSITIONING

For anterior procedures we use the beach chair position. The patient sits on the operating table at a 45° angle to the floor. The head is either supported in a neurosurgical head rest (which allows excellent access to the shoulder region) or rested on a head ring on the table. To prevent the patient from sliding distally during the procedure, the hips are flexed to at least 60° leaving the femurs tilted up at a 15° angle to the floor. Ideally, the knees should be flexed 10–15° leaving the lower legs horizontal. The patient is placed with the shoulder to be operated on as close as possible to the edge of the table. The shoulder blade is supported by a 500 ml infusion bag of the Viaflex® type which is soft, and as it tends to stick to the skin it remains stable during the procedure. This bag tilts the patient some 10–15° away from the surgeon and thereby provides a better view of the glenoid rim and surface. It also stabilizes the shoulder blade, and at arthroscopy it eases the access. To protect the patient from sliding sideways off the table, a specially designed side-post clamped on to the table on the same side as the operated shoulder is used. This support is thin (20 cm long and 15 cm high), slightly concave and padded to avoid pressure problems. As it has no protruding parts it does not hamper the free movement of the arm alongside the table. It should be positioned about 6–8 cm below the axilla to allow sufficient antiseptic prepping.

The whole forequarter up to the mandible is prepped inclusive of the hand, and a disposable draping set with an elastic plastic hole, as used in knee surgery, is used to cover the patient. The arm up to the mid-humerus level is covered with a stockinette. If arthroscopy is performed, no further draping is needed at this stage. If surgery is carried out, an adhesive drape should be added to help to control the position of the drapes. With the patient in this position, diagnostic and therapeutic arthroscopy as well as open procedures can be carried out.

For posterior procedures the patient is placed in the lateral position. A firm support, i.e. a rolled-up drape, is placed under the opposite axilla to relieve pressure on the arm on which the patient is lying. Supports are applied at the level of the lower thoracic spine posteriorly and at the lower ribs anteriorly. This allows the upper trunk to roll slightly forwards, positioning the posterior operative field almost horizontally. The forequarter is prepped to include the neck and hand, and the same drapes as in the anterior approach are used. If an arthroscopy is carried out in conjunction with the operation, it is performed with the patient in the lateral position also. In both positions, free movement of the arm is mandatory to allow good access during the procedures.

SURGICAL PROCEDURES

Many of the procedures devised for shoulder stabilization do not aim to repair the damage inflicted on the shoulder. Instead, they aim to compensate for the deficiency of capsule and bone by preventing the Hill–Sachs lesion from engaging the glenoid rim by tightening the anterior structures of the shoulder. These methods include the Putti–Platt, the Magnusson–Stack and the Boytchev procedures. Although often effective in preventing further dislocations, the price can be a moderate to severe loss of external rotation. These methods produce almost the same anatomical changes as did Hippocrates with his red-hot irons. The ideal procedure today is a reparative and reconstructive one that will leave the patient with a normal or near-normal ROM and allow return to predislocation activities. However, as the entity shoulder instability consists of a number of different conditions, it is obvious that it is necessary for the surgeon to have a number of procedures available to be able to treat each individual case in the most appropriate way.

In our clinic we have limited ourselves to a selection of procedures that allow us to address the different pathologies responsible for shoulder instability. These have been selected because we think they are the most conservative reparative procedures which, when carried out carefully, will restore the shoulder to the same ROM, power and stability as before the occurrence of the instability symptoms.

The Bankart operation

The Bankart procedure was described by Blundell Bankart in 1938.[6] It is a true reparative procedure aiming to make good the damage inflicted on the joint at the time of the dislocation. The goal is to restore a normal or almost normal joint. It is most suited to the treatment of traumatic anterior dislocations, but, if a posterior capsular avulsion has been diagnosed, a 'reversed' repair can be carried out posteriorly.

The use of sutures through drill holes in the glenoid rim allows the avulsed labrum and capsule to be taken back to where it was torn off. It is always logical to treat a disability by eliminating the pathological lesion, in this case the Bankart lesion. However, the procedure, as originally described by Bankart[6] and modified by Carter Rowe,[3] was complicated and difficult to perform, and many surgeons have tended to use other less complicated methods. With the introduction of suture anchors, some of the difficult and time-consuming details of the operation have been eliminated, and it is now gaining wide acceptance. Another advantage of the use of anchors is that they are placed in the glenoid rim at the margin of the cartilage. The glenoid joint surface, which may already have been slightly reduced in size due to wear during dislocations or due to fracture of the rim, is not additionally reduced in size by sutures taken through it. This was necessary in the original operative procedure.

Using suture anchors instead of sutures taken through drill holes, the Bankart procedure is our method of choice for patients with traumatic dislocations, but this operation may be combined with other procedures such as a capsular shift or even a Bristow procedure. Reports of a recurrence rate of 3.5% or less have been published. The most important advantage of the Bankart operation is that reduction of external rotation after the operation is minimal. Rowe[3] found normal external rotation in 69% of the shoulders he re-examined.

The surgical approach is through a vertical 6 cm incision from just below the tip of the coracoid in the direction of the anterior axillary fold. In women, the operation should be carried out through a bra-strap incision for cosmetic reasons. Locating the deltopectoral groove can sometimes be difficult, but it is usually identified by the presence of a fat stripe, within which the cephalic vein is found. If there is no obvious fat stripe, the vein can most easily be found distally in the operating field. The deltopectoral groove is then opened, and the cephalic vein is protected and retracted *medially* after division of the branches coming from the deltoid muscle. We prefer to retract the vein medially as it provides options of extending the incision proximally if neccessary.

The coracoid process is drilled and tapped for a 4.0 mm half-threaded cancellous screw. As the shape of the coracoid is curved, we recommend palpation in the direction of the process before drilling to be able to pass the drill exactly in the long axis of the coracoid to achieve a good purchase in the bone. Usually a 35-mm long screw is used and it should be completely contained within the bone when tightened. With an oscillating saw, the coracoid is then osteotomized 1 cm from its tip. If a bony defect to the anterior glenoid rim is expected, a bigger fragment of the coracoid may be taken to allow an alternative Bristow repair to be used.

The conjoined tendons are reflected medially and inferiorly, taking care not to damage the musculocutaneous nerve which enters the muscles on the medial side usually 3–5 cm below the coracoid. However, no attempt is made to mobilize the conjoined tendons distally, and traction or dissection injuries to the musculocutaneous nerve should therefore be avoided.

The subscapularis muscle is now well exposed, and, with the arm in external rotation, two strong stay sutures are taken through the muscle as medially as possible under vision. Care should be taken not to take the stay sutures so deep that they engage the capsule. This will prevent the muscle from being released from the capsule later during the aproach.

The brachial plexus is quite near – only 2–3 cm medial to the area where the stay sutures are introduced – and the stay sutures act as protectors of the plexus during the operation until the muscle is later repaired. As long as surgery is performed lateral to these stay sutures there will be no risk of involving the brachial plexus or the large vessels in this area in the repair. The stays are also helpful in retrieving the medial part of the muscle when it is repaired during closure. Any surgeon who has tried to find a retracted subscapularis muscle behind the brachial plexus will never want to do that again!

The subscapularis is divided vertically 2 cm medially to its insertion on the lesser tuberosity just medial to the musculotendinous junction. Proximally it is divided all the way up to the base of the coracoid process, and distally a small portion of the muscle can be left to give protection to the axillary nerve at the point where it travels posteriorly below the distal pole of the glenoid. Usually a couple of horizontally orientated vessels mark the lower margin of the division, and these vessels should be coagulated. While dividing the muscle it is important to remember the orientation of the blade of the scapula and that the patient is tilted somewhat away from the surgeon. Thus care must be taken not to enter the muscle in a tangential direction. Ideally the direction into the muscle should be towards the centre of the humeral head. The superior part of the tendon is solid and contains a lot of strong fibrous tissue and must be completely divided to allow the muscle to be retracted medially. With careful gradual division of the muscle and tendon with small strokes of the diathermy, the white joint capsule gradually presents itself in the depth of the split. The capsule must not be damaged. If this happens, the defect thus created should be repaired before the medial capsulotomy is carried out. Using blunt dissection (a Bristow elevator is useful) the muscle is scraped off the capsule. Laterally the capsule and muscle blend together, whereas more medially there is an obvious plane through which the muscle can easily be separated from the capsule.

Once the muscle has been retracted, the capsule is inspected for defects. Often these are present superiorly, and, if found, should be repaired at this stage. The capsule is then opened at the level of the glenoid rim, with as much capsule as possible lateral to the capsulotomy retained. If there is a Bankart lesion present, the capsulotomy can be made on the rim itself opening the soft tissues medial to the level of their insertion. This leaves plenty of soft tissue for the subsequent reattachment and allows the tension of the capsule to be balanced. Using this approach rather than a more lateral capsulotomy and an inside repair as advocated by others has the advantage of not leaving any 'working portals' to be closed after the labrum has been reattached, and therefore there is less risk of producing capsular shortening. It is crucial not to go too far laterally with the capsulotomy as this will cause shortening of the capsule after the repair and consequent loss of external rotation. If the capsulotomy is carried out too laterally, the surgeon has to use this approach as a working portal and perform an inside repair. Under no circumstances should another capsular incision be attempted more medial and parallel to the first one, as this will leave the patient with a 'sliced' capsule which is almost impossible to repair without causing marked shortening.

The medial capsule with the avulsed labrum is then retracted to expose the glenoid rim. A Bankart's skid is introduced into the joint to retract the humeral head and expose the glenoid surface, and, if necesary, a Homann's retractor can be placed medially on the scapular neck deep to the subscapularis muscle to retract the medial structures. The glenoid rim is prepared by removing any fibrous tissues and then creating a rough bony surface, care being taken not to remove any glenoid bone.

The suture anchors – usually three – are then inserted with the entry point of the drillholes on the glenoid rim just next to the free margin of the cartilage. The sutures should be inserted as far apart as possible to allow all detached capsule to be securely fixed to bone. The lower anchor should be introduced as close to the inferior glenoid pole (the 6 o'clock position) as possible, and the remaining two a minimum of 1–1.5 cm apart. The majority of the anterior rim will be encompassed by the anchors which should ideally be positioned as seen in Figure 19.6. The direction of

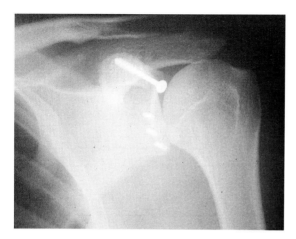

Fig. 19.6 Ideal position of three Mitek G-II anchors along the anterior glenoid rim, with the lower anchor almost at the lower pole of the glenoid. The entry point of the drill holes for the anchors are just on the glenoid rim into the body of the scapular neck.

the drill should be into the body of the scapular neck. For the most inferior anchor there is a risk of drilling the hole through the posterior cortex and thus placing the anchor extraosseous with poor hold. The drill may therefore be directed slightly upwards when the inferior hole is drilled. We use Ethibond no. 2 sutures in the anchor and after insertion into the drill hole, we tie one knot to lock the suture in the hole of the anchor. Both strands of sutures from each anchor are then taken on a Mayo needle inside out in the rim of the lateral capsule. It is important not to shift the capsule distally, and the sutures from the distal anchor should therefore be taken through the capsule at a corresponding level to the drill hole in the glenoid rim or slightly distal to it to allow for some shift in proximal direction. By tying single strands of sutures from adjacent anchors together, a strong suture line is created on the glenoid rim holding the capsule firmly down on to the roughened bone. Before tying the knots the surgeon should check that there is at least 45° of external rotation present with the elbow at the patient's side or the repair has been made too tight. Common causes for this are either that too little capsule has been left laterally because the capsulotomy has been made lateral to the glenoid

rim, or because too large a bite of the rim of the capsule has been taken by the sutures when performing the reattachment. The medial part of the capsulotomy can often be elevated from the bone and brought laterally on top of the capsular reattachment for reinforcement using the sutures attached to the anchors once more. Figure 19.7 shows the different steps of the capsular reattachment.

The subscapularis is repaired with Vicryl no. 1 mattress sutures, and the repair is completed with a running suture in the anterior fascia. The repair must be carried out without shortening to avoid reducing external rotation. If the rotator interval is found to be widened, this too should be closed. The coracoid is reattached with a screw, and the wound is closed. For cosmetic reasons it is important to put one or two loose resorbable sutures across the deltopectoral interval as in some patients a persistent visible separation of the two muscles may occur. Of course these sutures should not include the cephalic vein!

We use a subcuticular nylon suture (Prolene 2-0) to the skin in an attempt to make the scar as narrow as possible. This region is well known to produce keloid scars particularly in younger patients, but the suture marks should at least be avoided.

If a large bony defect is found in the anterior glenoid rim, the coracoid can be transferred to the anterior scapular neck. A combination of a Bristow-type repair as described below and a Bankart procedure above the transferred coracoid will provide the necessary stability in these patients.

The posterior Bankart operation

In posterior traumatic dislocations, we use an approach through a vertical skin incision just medial to the location of the joint, extending from just cranial to the spine of the scapula and about 8 cm distally. The medial margin of the deltoid can be very difficult to identify, and is often much further medial than first expected and there is no definite landmark like the cephalic vein for the anterior approach. The posterior third of the deltoid is detached from the scapula spine preferably with subperiosteal dissection to retain

(A)

(B)

(C)

(D)

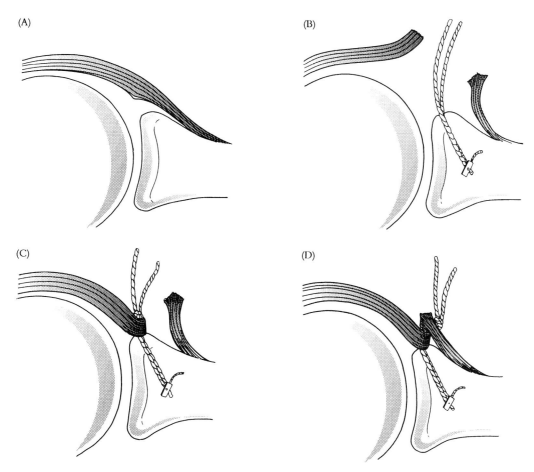

Fig. 19.7 Bankart repair with Mitek anchors. (A) A Bankart lesion. The anterior labrum is detached from the glenoid rim, and the capsular attachment and periosteum is stripped from the anterior scapular neck. (B) The capsule is opened just next to the glenoid rim, and the suture anchors are inserted in drill holes on the rim. (C) The lateral capsule is taken down on to the glenoid rim with the sutures attached to the anchors. (D) Using the same sutures, the medial flap reinforces the repair.

good tissue facilitating its subsequent repair. The muscle can then be reflected laterally to expose the underlying muscles. For this purpose a stay suture in the medial margin of the detached muscle is helpful. The infraspinatus and the teres minor muscles are now visible. Characteristically the infraspinatus consists of two muscle bellies almost of the same size, the teres minor below being clearly identifiable and separate from the infraspinatus. The musculotendinous junction of the infraspinatus is quite lateral and the muscle can be divided in a similar way to that used with the subscapularis in the anterior procedure. It is advised to use stay sutures in the medial part, and usually with advantage also in the lateral part. The direction of the division should be towards the centre of the humeral head to avoid a tangential division of the muscle. At this stage the suprascapular nerve is very close as it passes around the lateral margin of the scapular spine in the spino-glenoid notch and utmost care should be taken when using the diathermy and during the dissection. When the muscle has been divided the nerve is often directly visible. The posterior shoulder capsule is very thin compared with the anterior capsule and this makes the repair more difficult to perform and more fragile in the postoperative period.

The repair itself is carried out in a quite similar way to the anterior repair. Again it is important to spread the anchors along the whole glenoid rim with a minimum of 1–1.5 cm between the drill holes, and the inferior anchor should be placed as close to the inferior pole of the glenoid as possible. The infraspinatus is repaired with a number of mattress sutures and a continuous fascial suture to smoothen the repair. Some slight shortening of the infraspinatus will not leave any permanent loss of mobility and might be an advantage in the rehabilitation of these patients. The deltoid is reattached with sutures through drill holes in the scapular spine, and eventually a continuous suture closing the fascia overlying the deltoid and the trapezius.

The Bristow operation

This method, originally described by Helfet[7] and usually performed with the modifications introduced by May[8] has gained widespread use. Hovelius and co-workers[9] have shown that it is crucial for the success of this operation that it is carried out with extreme attention to the exact placement of the coracoid.

In some series it has a reported high success rate with recurrences of only 3%. However, it is also associated with some limitation of postoperative external rotation, and therefore it is not the method of choice for athletes carrying out overhead activities. The loss of ROM in external rotation with the shoulder abducted is usually no more than 10°, but as a full ROM in this position is crucial to some athletes, even a minor loss may terminate a career at the top level.

The effect of this procedure is to create a 'dynamic sling'. After having been transposed the conjoined tendons act as a sling in front of the humeral head in the critical position of external rotation in abduction. At the same time, the transposed bone acts as a glenoid extension, preventing contact between a Hill–Sachs lesion and the anterior glenoid rim. Finally because of the position of the coracoid tip through the subscapularis muscle, the lower third of this muscle is kept inferiorly in relation to the humeral

head in external rotation in abduction, thus supporting the dynamic stabilization of the joint.

The same surgical approach as for the Bankart procedure described earlier is used. However, a larger fragment of the coracoid process should be taken off, around 1.5 cm. The subsequent preparation of the coracoid tip is made much easier if the coracoid is drilled and tapped before it is osteotomized.

When dividing the subscapularis, only the superior two-thirds is divided just medial to its musculotendinous separation (or the muscle can be split), and the joint is inspected through a capsulotomy on the glenoid rim. If a Bankart lesion is present in the area of the glenoid rim not covered by the coracoid transfer, it is repaired as described above. The coracoid is then positioned on the anterior aspect of the glenoid. The capsulotomy allows the positioning of the coracoid in relation to the joint to be carried out under vision as this positioning is extremely important. The coracoid *must* be placed below the 'equator' of the glenoid, preferably on the lower third of the scapular neck and the bone on which it is placed should be carefully cleared of all soft tissues to allow a solid bony union. The transposed bone should be positioned just next to the joint line, without causing impingement on the humeral head during movement of the arm. The screw used for fixation should be of the lag-type providing solid compression, and it should have a firm grip in the anterior and the posterior cortex of the scapular neck.

In small coracoids we usually use a 4.0 mm half-threaded AO cancellous screw for this purpose, as larger screws cause risk of fracturing the coracoid. In large individuals a 4.5 mm AO cortical screw is preferred. Figure 19.8 shows a well-positioned transposed coracoid tip.

The capsule is then repaired without shortening either using Mitek anchors or if no Bankart lesion has been found by direct closure. The subscapularis is also repaired without shortening.

The bone buttress operation

This method was originally used by us for the treatment of recurrent anterior dislocations in

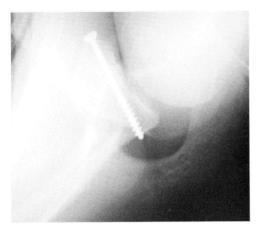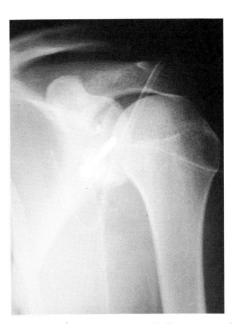

Fig. 19.8 A Bristow procedure has been carried out, and the transposed coracoid tip is ideally positioned below the equator of the glenoid and close to the joint without impinging on the humeral head.

epileptic patients who suffer shoulder dislocations during fits.[10] Because of the numerous dislocations suffered in relation to very forceful muscle contractions, extensive wear of the glenoid rim in conjunction with a large Hill–Sachs lesion is usually seen in these patients. In these patients the main aim is to achieve a stable shoulder that can be trusted by the patient in everyday use, and some loss of external rotation can be accepted. Having used this method in 18 shoulders without recurrences and with an acceptable reduction of external rotation, we now also use it in non-epileptic patients who have extensive bone defects. The positioning and approach is as for the Bankart repair. When the joint capsule has been exposed and the arthrotomy performed along the anterior glenoid rim, the bony lesion is exposed and any fibrous tissue removed to form a bed of sound bleeding bone.

Using either a 4 cm wide and 3 cm deep tricortical iliac crest graft or an allograft from a femoral head, the glenoid is then extended anteriorly by fixing the graft on to the bony lesion with two 4.5 mm cortical screws. When using an autograft, it is important to remember that the

donor site is often very painful after the operation. As the patient should be given the opportunity to rest the area by using a stick, we recommend that the graft is harvested from the same side as that on which the stabilization procedure is carried out. When solidly fixed with the screws, the graft is then trimmed down to form a glenoid extension with the same curvature as the remaining glenoid. The glenoid joint surface thus created will be slightly wider than the anatomical glenoid to prevent the Hill–Sachs lesion engaging the anterior glenoid rim. When positioning the screws, care should be taken to place them as far as possible from the 'joint' surface of the graft so that impingement on the humeral head does not occur. Once trimmed, the graft must not protrude over the level of the remaining glenoid articular surface as it is supposed to be an extension not a buffer stop (Figure 19.9).

The capsule is then held in position against the newly created 'anterior glenoid rim' by means of two no. 2 Ethibond sutures tied around the heads of the screws; eventually the capsule can be left without repair.

The remaining repair and closure is as for the Bankart procedure.

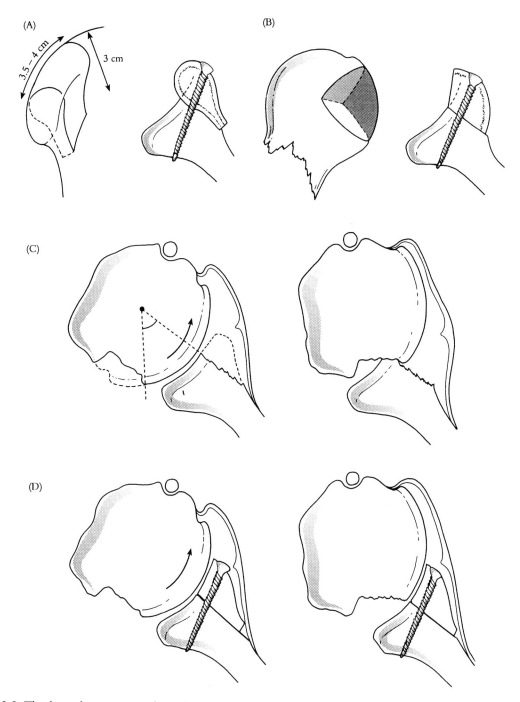

Fig. 19.9 The bone buttress procedure. (A) Autograft: donor site and position of graft on scapular neck before trimming. (B) Allograft: section to be cut from allograft femoral head and its position on the scapular neck before trimming. (C) A bony Bankart lesion and a Hill–Sachs defect engaging during external rotation. (D) The same shoulder after application of a bone buttress.

The lateral capsular shift (humeral side) operation

In 1980 Neer and Foster[4] described the capsular shift procedure for the treatment of involuntary inferior and multidirectional instability. This procedure has, in most centres, become the method of choice for surgical treatment in these difficult cases.

It is of extreme importance, before deciding on surgery in these patients to exclude voluntary dislocators, unidirectional instabilities, neural or psychological disorders and patients with bony abnormalities of the joint. In our opinion they should all be managed by alternative methods.

In patients with involuntary inferior and multidirectional instability at arthroscopy no Bankart lesion is found and therefore there is no need for reattachment of the capsule medially. The capsulotomy is thus performed laterally. Using the information obtained from the EUA, the surgeon chooses an anterior approach if the instability is mainly anterior/inferior, and a posterior aproach if the instability is mainly posterior/inferior. We would always carry out an arthroscopy before finally deciding on the surgical approach. The initial surgical approach is the same as for the Bankart procedure described above, but the coracoid osteotomy can be avoided if a lateral (humeral side) capsular shift is planned. The subscapularis division should be performed as close to the insertion on the humerus as possible, otherwise the lateral stump of the subscapularis will obstruct the view of the capsulotomy and make this very difficult. Before any capsular incision is made it is very important to make sure that any capsular deficiency is repaired first using resorbable sutures including the rotator interval gap. In these patients the capsule is usually not only thin, but defects are often present. The capsule is incised vertically close to its attachment to the humeral head extending it as far distally as possible under vision. To allow sufficient capsular mobilization, the capsulotomy must be extended well beyond the 6 o'clock position. By externally rotating the humerus, the incision can be extended into the posteroinferior attachment also, but the surgeon must always protect the axillary nerve which is in considerable danger during this procedure. A Trethowen retractor inserted on the external surface of the capsule under the muscles is useful for this purpose, and the plane for the instrument is easily identified if the instrument is introduced before the capsulotomy is performed. A horizontal incision is then made in the capsule at the level of the equator of the humeral head making the capsulotomy T-shaped. This transverse incision should be taken as far as the anterior glenoid rim. Two triangular flaps, one superiorly and one inferiorly, are now created and to control these flaps during the shift it is useful to put a stay suture into each corner. By taking the distal flap as far proximally as it will go and suturing it to the lateral stump of the capsule, the inferior recess and the inferior glenohumeral ligaments are tightened. Usually a shift of 1.5 cm can be easily achieved. However, before reattaching the capsule, it is important to test the tightness of the shift. By using the stay suture in the inferior flap and shifting the flap superiorly to the level where the attachment is expected to be performed, it should be possible to take the arm to 45° of external rotation without displacing the flap. If this is not possible, less shift should be applied and the test repeated. If any capsular defect or widened rotator interval has not been repaired before the capsulotomy and shifting, testing the tightness of the shift is much more unreliable at this satge. Once a suitable tightness has been achieved the inferior flap is sutured on to the lateral stump of the capsule and the undersurface of the subscapularis. The superior flap is then taken down to cover the inferior flap partially, thus double-breasting the repair (Figure 19.10). The horizontal part of the repair is closed with resorbable sutures. By this time the shoulder should still easily externally rotate to at least 45°. If this is not possible, the repair has been made too tight. The subscapularis is repaired in the usual way avoiding any shortening. The subsequent closure is as for the Bankart repair.

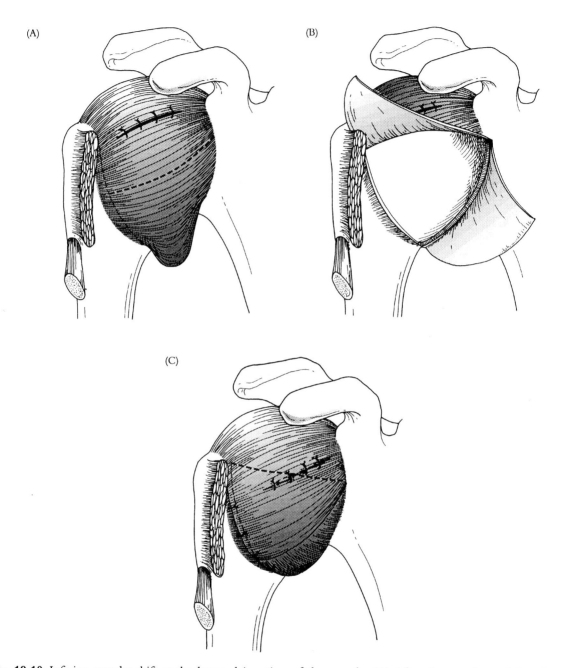

Fig. 19.10 Inferior capsular shift at the humeral insertion of the capsule. (A) After closure of any defects in the anterosuperior capsule, the capsule is cut some 3–4 mm from its insertion on the humerus and split horizontally. (B) This creates a T-shaped incision and a superior and inferior flap. (C) The inferior flap is then mobilized proximally and sutured to the lateral capsular remains. The superior flap is then taken distally to double-breast and reinforce the capsular shift.

The medial capsular shift (glenoid side) operation

This procedure was described by Altcheck and co-workers.[11] The approach for this operation is as for the Bankart procedure with coracoid osteotomy and subscapularis division. When the capsule has been exposed and any defects repaired, the muscle must as usual be separated from the capsule using a blunt instrument such as a Bristow elevator. This separation must, however, be carried out not only anteriorly, but should be extended past the 6 o'clock position inferiorly towards the posterior aspect of the joint. As long as this dissection takes place on the capsular surface the axillary nerve is protected. If sharp dissection is used or muscular division is carried out at the inferior pole, the nerve is at a higher risk of damage. The separation of the capsule from the subscapularis muscle is necessary to allow sufficient mobilization of the inferior capsular recess when performing the shift. It is usually an advantage to carry out this dissection before opening the capsule. The capsule is opened vertically at the anterior glenoid rim exactly as in a Bankart repair but the capsulotomy is extended past the lower pole of the glenoid as far posteriorly as possible. With retractors between the capsule and the muscle the axillary nerve is protected. A horizontal capsulotomy is then carried out approximately at the equator of the humeral head. The horizontal incision should be extended all the way to the insertion of the capsule on the humeral head. To allow a satisfactory view when performing this capsulotomy, a stay suture can be inserted in the lateral stump of the subscapularis to retract it laterally. The vertical part of the T-shaped caspsulotomy thus created is then extended as far distally and posteriorly as possible. Here it is also of help to insert a stay suture in the two corners of the capsular flaps. By lifting the inferior flap upwards while extending the capsular division and at the same time retracting the muscles at the inferior glenoid pole with a blunt retractor (a bone spike is useful) the capsule can usually be divided well behind the 6 o'clock position under vision. It must be made very clear that the capsulotomy in the capsular shift proce-

dures is performed very close to the axillary nerve, and this procedure should only be carried out by surgeons who are familiar with the detailed anatomy of the region.

The glenoid rim is then prepared as for a Bankart procedure, and three drill holes for Mitek anchors are made. In this procedure the inferior anchor *must* be inserted almost at the inferior pole of the glenoid to control the position of the capsule after the repair has been completed. To do this, the drill must be directed upwards and into the body of the scapular neck to avoid taking the hole through the posterior cortex of the scapula. The remaining two holes are made at aproximately the 1 and 3 o'clock positions for a right shoulder (11 and 9 o'clock for a left shoulder). If the vertical capsular division has been performed correctly and sufficient capsular tissue is available, the inferior flap can now be brought upwards and the corner that was originally at the 3 o'clock position can now be brought up to the top anchor. It is advisable before tying the sutures to test the range of external rotation with the flap held in position by hand only as correction can still be made at this stage. It is advisable to take only one of the strands of the Ethibond of the superior anchor through the corner of the flap and to tie it to the other strand from the same anchor to hold the flap in position and prevent it from sliding distally. Apart from this modification, the capsule is sutured on to the glenoid rim as in the Bankart repair. The sutures are not cut after they have been tied. Instead by taking the Mitek sutures inside out through it, the superior flap is double-breasted over the inferior flap, taking it as distally as it will go and tying the Mitek sutures over it. The horizontal overlap of the flaps is then closed using resorbable sutures (Figure 19.11).

The shoulder should now still easily externally rotate to 45°, or the repair is too tight. The surgeon has to be very critical, and even though redoing the repair at this stage is a major decision requiring new anchors to be inserted, it might be necessary to take the repair down and insert three new anchors and perform another repair with less shift if the first attempt is too tight. The closure is carried out as in the Bankart repair.

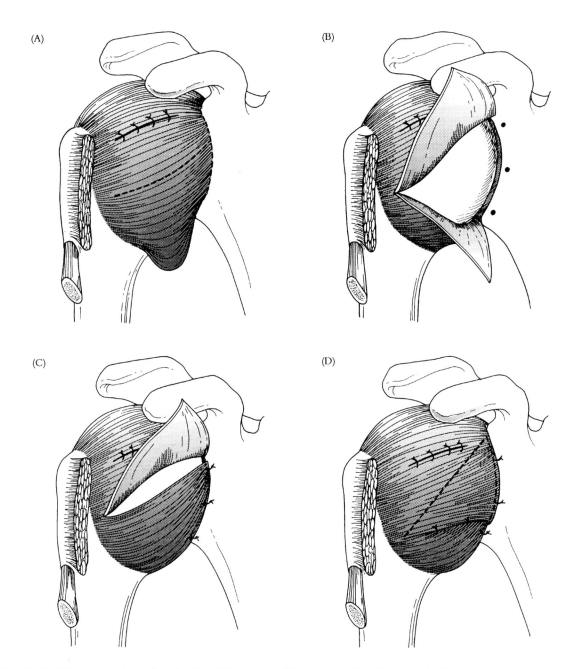

(A)

(B)

(C)

(D)

Fig. 19.11 Inferior capsular shift at the glenoid insertion of the capsule. (A) A horizontal split of the capsule in addition to the capsular opening of the conventional Bankart repair creates a T-shaped incision. Any defects of the capsule must be repaired before mobilization of the flaps. (B) A superior and an inferior flap are created, and the glenoid rim is prepared as in a Bankart repair with drill holes for the suture anchors. (C) The inferior flap is taken proximally and down on to the anterior rim with the sutures attached to the anchors. (D) The superior flap is taken distally to double breast the repair, once more using the sutures attached to the anchors.

The capsular shift operations – posterior approach

The medial and lateral capsular shifts can both be carried out through a posterior approach in cases where the instability is predominantly posterior or where a posterior Bankart lesion is found.

The posterior approach is particularly dangerous as the axillary nerve is at risk when the inferior capsule is mobilized, and similar precautions to those in the anterior procedure should be taken. The use of retractors inserted between the capsule and muscles is mandatory.

The McLaughlin operation

In dislocations with massive Hill–Sachs lesions (up to 40% of the articular surface) the McLaughlin procedure can be useful.[12] The anterior humeral head defect associated with a posterior dislocation can be obliterated by detaching the subscapularis from bone or eventually by taking the lesser tuberosity off with it and transposing it into the humeral head defect. Fixing it in this position prevents the defect engaging the glenoid rim but the procedure has the price of severely limiting internal rotation. In a few cases we have used part of an allograft femoral head to fill the humeral head defect. Fixing the graft with countersunk screws seems to provide stabilization without causing the same amount of restriction of movement.

In our practice, for patients with loss of more than 40–50% of the humeral head a hemiarthroplasty is carried out. It has to be borne in mind that if a shoulder is unstable before an arthroplasty is carried out, it is likely to remain unstable after the arthroplasty unless the instability is addressed surgically. This is a very difficult condition to treat and preferably any other factors contributing to instability should be addressed before hemiarthroplasty is considered.

Open reduction

In some cases the surgeon is faced with the difficult problem of needing to carry out an open reduction in conjunction with a stabilizing proce-

dure. In any patient with a 'locked' shoulder dislocation such procedures are a possibility. This also includes cases with associated fractures and bony avulsions.

If an open reduction turns out to be necessary, the surgeon should be prepared to meet very distorted anatomy during his approach to the shoulder joint. In the anterior approach, which is preferred for anterior dislocations, the space under the conjoined tendons will be occupied by the humeral head covered by the subscapularis muscle. The musculocutaneous nerve is very close and usually a coracoid osteotomy gives a good exposure of the subscapularis muscle and protection to the neurovascular structures. When dividing the subscapularis, it should be remembered that the humerus may be externally rotated, and care should therefore be taken to divide the muscle laterally close to the musculotendinous junction. If the humeral head does not relocate early, it might not be possible to carry out a capsulotomy on the desired location corresponding to the glenoid rim. As it is covered by the humeral head the glenoid rim cannot be palpated and the capsule should then be opened laterally to create a 'working portal'. Once the joint is opened it is usually possible to disengage the glenoid rim and the Hill–Sachs lesion and perform a stabilization procedure in the usual way.

REHABILITATION

Our after treatment for the anterior repairs – excluding the bone buttress procedure – includes 2 weeks in a broad-arm sling with limitation of external rotation. At 2 weeks the waistband of the sling is discarded and the patient is allowed to take the arm out of the sling and perform careful pendulum excercises. The sling is still used when the patient is not excercising. At 3 weeks the sling is discarded completely and the patient starts mobilizing at his own pace, taking care not to strain the repair mainly by avoiding external rotation. At 6–8 weeks it is expected that about 130° of active elevation will have been acchieved. Only at this stage, if there is less movement, do we use formal physiotherapy with careful stretching excercises. At 3 months when healing has taken place, the patient is allowed to return to non-contact sports including swimming and at 4 months contact sports such as rugby or football is allowed. It is important to abstain from pushing the rehabilitation at a early stage, as there is a considerable risk of tearing the repair apart before strong healing unites the capsule and anterior glenoid.

Our rehabilitation programme is completely controlled by the patient in more than 90% of the cases and physiotherapy is only given if the mobilization is slow. It is our experience that with early physiotherapy once the pain has gone, either the patient or the therapist tends to be too enthusiastic, and overstretching or detachment of the repair may occur.

Patients who have undergone the bone buttress operation have the arm immobilized for 3 weeks in a broad arm sling with restriction of external rotation. The sling is then discarded and the shoulder is mobilized by the patient without any formal physiotherapy as in the Bankart patients. If movement is not progressing satisfactorally at 8 weeks, physiotherapy is started, as the graft by then will be firmly seated in a fibrous pocket and some early bony union will have taken place. After the posterior approach, the arm is immobilized in a spica type splint in 20–30° of abduction and 0–10° of external rotation. It is usually easier to make a spica in the preferred position the day before the operation and bivalve it so it can be reapplied on the operating table after surgery and closed with a few layers of plaster. Off-the-shelf splints can be even easier to use, but do not always give an optimum fit.

The spica is used for 4 weeks and gentle mobilization is commenced after splint removal with pendulum excercises. A broad arm sling is used for 1–2 weeks until the patient is comfortably out of the splint. Also in these patients formal physiotherapy is only given if there is excessive stiffness and no sooner than at 6–8 weeks.

REFERENCES

1. Speer, K.P., Deng, X., Borrero, S. et al (1994) Biomechanical evaluation of a simulated Bankart lesion. *J. Bone Joint Surg.* **76A:** 1819–1826.
2. Hovelius, L., Augustini, B.S., Fredin, H. et al (1996) Primary anterion dislocation of the shoulder in the young. A prospective study on the 10-year prognosis. *J. Bone Joint Surg.* In press.
3. Rowe, C.R. (1978) The Bankart procedure. A long-term end-result study. *J. Bone Joint Surg.* **60A:** 1–16.
4. Neer, C.S. & Foster, C.R. (1980) Inferior capsular shift for involuntary inferior and multidirectional instability of the shoulder. *J. Bone Joint Surg.* **62A:** 897–908.
5. Wallace, W.A. & Hellier, M. (1983) Improving radiographs of the injured shoulder. *Radiography* **49:** 223–229.
6. Bankart, A.S.B. (1938) The pathology and treatment of recurrent dislocation of the shoulder joint. *Br. J. Surg.* **26:** 23–26.
7. Helfet, A.F. (1958) Coracoid transplantation for recurring dislocation of the shoulder. *J. Bone Joint Surg.* **40B:** 198–202.
8. May, V.R., Jr. (1970) A modified Bristow operation for anterior recurrent dislocation of the shoulder. *J. Bone Joint Surg.* **52A:** 1010–1016.
9. Hovelius, L., Körner, L., Lundberg, B. et al (1983) The coracoid transfer for recurrent dislocation of the shoulder. Technical aspects of the Bristow–Latarjet procedure. *J. Bone Joint Surg.* **65A:** 926–934.
10. Hutchinson, J.W., Neumann, L. & Wallace, W.A. (1995) The bone buttress operation for recurrent anterior shoulder dislocation in epileptic patients. *J. Bone Joint Surg.* **77B:** 928–932.
11. Altcheck, D.W., Warren, R.F., Skyhar, M.J. et al (1991) T-plasty modification of the Bankart procedure for multidirectional instability of the anterior and inferior types. *J. Bone Joint Surg.* **73A:** 105–112.
12. McLaughlin, H.L. (1952) Posterior dislocation of the shoulder. *J. Bone Joint Surg.* **34A:** 584–590.

20

Arthroscopic Stabilization of Shoulder Instability

G Declercq

INTRODUCTION

Increasing understanding of the anatomy and pathophysiology of shoulder instability has definitely improved the results of treatment of shoulder instability. The standard approach to operative treatment of the unstable shoulder has been through an open procedure. Since the recognition of the Bankart lesion as the primary cause of recurrent traumatic anterior instability, the open Bankart repair has been the 'gold standard'. To many authors it still remains the gold standard. Additional plastic deformation of the inferior glenohumeral ligament (IGHL) complex occurs probably more frequently than was previously thought. This excessive anterioinferior capsular laxity should be conected at the time of surgery, which implies that both the attachment site and tension of the IGHL should be corrected. As for multidirectional instability, these standard procedures will fail because they do not correct all the directions of instability. An inferior capsular shift procedure seems far more appropriate to correct this type of instability. According to some authors, posterior subluxation should be corrected through a posterior capsular shift in patients where a supervised rehabilitation programme has failed.

Over the last decade arthroscopic stabilization has become a fairly popular procedure, but, as for many new and exciting techniques, the initial enthusiasm was somewhat tempered by the publication of results on larger numbers at a longer follow-up. The goal of this chapter is to guide the reader through the technical details of arthroscopic stabilization of shoulder instability.

ARTHROSCOPIC STABILIZATION PROCEDURES FOR ANTERIOR STABILITY

For patient positioning and room set-up, the reader is referred to Chapter 14 on arthroscopic evaluation of shoulder instability.

General principles

Both shoulders should be tested for instability in all directions. The patient is positioned in a lateral decubitus position, using a single shoulder holder to suspend the arm in a longitudinal traction of 2– kg. A second sling is applied at the upper arm which is pulled at 90° to the chest, with a traction of 3–6 kg. This twin-traction set-up allows distraction of the shoulder in a slightly abducted and forward-flexed position. Also the shoulder can be held in an internally rotated position throughout the procedure, relaxing the anterior capsule and increasing the working space of the anterior compartment. A pump system is extremely helpful for obtaining a clear visualization throughout the procedure.

A standard posterior portal is used to visualize the glenohumeral joint for diagnostic arthroscopy. I prefer two anterior portals, as described by Wolf et al,[1] to gain a better view of the anterior glenoid rim and scapular neck during the procedure. First, the anteroinferior portal (AIP) is created by advancing the obturator and sheath through the joint (inside-out). Palpation of the coracoid process with the blunt trocar is the next step. Then the blunt tip slips off laterally and inferiorly to the coracoid process. Finally the trocar is pushed through the soft tissues, and, after skin incision, a cannula can be retrograded back into the joint over the tip of the obturator. A second anteriosuperior portal (ASP) is created with an outside-in technique, by inserting a needle at the inferior border of the coracoacromial ligament into the rotator interval. This portal is used for anterior visualization.

After completion of the arthroscopic examination through both the posterior and anterior portal and when the shoulder is judged to be a good candidate for arthroscopic stabilization, the anterior glenoid rim and scapular neck are prepared. I usually look through the ASP with the scope and instrumentation is used through the AIP. A rasp with a sharp leading edge is used to separate the labrum from the scapular neck up to the inferior border of the glenoid. Careful preparation of the scapular neck is accomplished with a full-radius resector and sometimes an abrader to create a bleeding surface. This step is essential to create a healthy environment for healing of the Bakart lesion. Also, the inferior capsulolabral complex must be mobilized far enough inferiorly and medially to allow the advancement and retensioning of the capsulolabral complex later in the procedure.

These general principles are basically the same in all arthroscopic anterior stabilization procedures since the goal is to restore the normal capsulolabral restraint to anterionferior instability.

Arthroscopic staple repair

This technique was popularized by Johnson[2] in the early 1980s, being a quick and simple method of repairing a Bankart lesion.

After preparation of the anterior glenoid rim and scapular neck, the staple is inserted through the anterior portal. The staple grasps firmly the superior band of the IGHL. The capsulolabral complex is then shifted superiorly by pulling on the capsule and rotating the staple. Finally the staple is hammered home. Careful inspection and palpation of the ligaments and the position of the staple should be performed at the end of the procedure.

This procedure has been abandoned by most surgeons because of a high recurrence rate (up to 27%) and a high complication rate. Incorrect staple placement and loose staples can induce a rapidly progressing and devastating degenerative arthritis of the shoulder. Also silent staple loosening has been reported in patients who are doing well clinically. A biodegradable staple could resolve most of these problems but no results have been published.

Arthroscopic transglenoid suture repair

After arthroscopic assessment of the Bankart lesion and ligamentous complex, the capsulolabral system should be carefully released to allow sufficient advancement. Shifting the capsule superiorly with a grasper should tighten the anterior structures. Once the tissue quality is considered to be sufficient, careful debridement of the anterior glenoid neck is performed down to bleeding bone. A suture pin is passed through the anterior portal and the sharp tip is used to spear the lower portion of the IGHL. Through a second ASP, a grasper is passed and the capsulolabral tissue can be advanced superiorly. The suture pin pieces the IGHL and is positioned approximately at the the mid–glenoid notch. The pin is drilled in a posterior and slightly downwards direction through the posterior cortex and recovered after it exits from the posterior skin (Figure 20.1). Two size 1 absorbable monofilament sutures are passed through the eye of the pin. One end of each

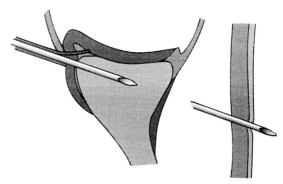

Fig. 20.1 Transglenoid drilling. The flanged cannula rests on the glenoid rim and the guide wire pierces the IGHL.

suture is held anteriorly with a haemostat, when the pin is advanced through the shoulder. A second passage of the pin is made through the cannula with two additional sutures. This pin is positioned more superior and angled through the glenoid almost parallel to the first pin. Now, there are two sets of sutures through the shoulder. Each suture is coupled with a suture from the other drill hole and tied separately in front of the joint. When a very long PDS suture is used, the end that was previously held with a haemostat in front, could be passed through the joint with the second pin passage. In that case there is no need to make a knot in front of the joint. Pulling on the two sets of sutures in the back of the shoulder should reattach and tension the capsulolabral complex in front of the joint. Through a subcutaneous tunnel at the posterior aspect of the shoulder the sutures can be joined and tied separately over the infraspinatus fascia.

Several variations to this technique have been described. Rose et al[3] use several sutures through the superior band of the IGHL and incorporate them into the horizontal mattress sutures of the Bankart repair. This technique allows better tensioning of the laxity of the anterior capsule. Also soft tissue is retracted from between the two suture pins posteriorly, before the exit of the second pin, by the use of a slotted cannula and obturator. This allows the sutures to be tied down to bone, avoiding entrapment of infraspinatus muscle belly. This seems preferable when non-absorbable sutures are used.

Caspari & Savoie[4] described a suture technique with multiple sutures using a suture punch. Up to eight sutures are passed through the prepared capsulolabral complex from low inferior to superior and passed through the glenoid with a single pin passed high on the anterior aspect of the glenoid. The suture bundle is split posteriorly in two halves and some infraspinatus fascia is caught in the knot.

Several potential complications and pitfalls are associated with the transglenoid suture technique.

1. Les flexible pins can now be used to avoid inadvertent pin migration and a flange on the cannula helps to prevent medial migration.

2. Branches of the suprascapular nerve are definitely at risk during this procedure.
3. Tying the sutures over muscle and fascia, often distended with extravasated fluid, is sometimes less than optimal.

As for results of transglenoid suture techniques we see rather divergent publications. Morgan & Bodenstab[5] reported a recurrence rate of only 5% after a 1–7-year follow-up of 175 patients. Savoie[6] reported a 9% failure rate in 161 patients, using the Caspari suture technique. In 1993 Rose et al[3] presented their results on 50 patients with a 2–6-year follow-up and the failure rate was 10%. Other reports showed far less favourable results. Mologne[7] presented his results in 1994 on the transglenoid suture technique in active military population. He obtained a 39% failure rate and noted three cases of suprascapular nerve palsy. Walch et al[8] published results on 59 patients in 1995; the recurrence rate was 49%. At my institution the results on this technique have also been analysed after a 2–6-year follow-up; 31 patients were retrospectively analysed and a combined (recurrence of dislocations and subluxations) failure rate of 45% was noted. One patient sustained a suprascapular nerve palsy. This procedure has not been used at this institution since 1992.

Arthroscopic capsulolabral reconstruction using suture anchors

After the initial success of open Bankart repair using suture anchors (Mitek), Wolf et al[1] popularized this technique under arthroscopic control, trying to avoid the potential complications of transglenoid drilling. The patient positioning is a classic lateral decubitus with a double-traction set up. The classic posterior portal is used as an outflow cannula. A double anterior portal technique, as described above, is used, with the arthroscope in the ASP position and the AIP as the working portal.

A threaded 9 mm cannula is used in the AIP position to allow easy instrumentation. The next step is the preparation of the glenoid rim and scapular neck, down to bleeding bone. The release of the capsulolabral complex is carried far

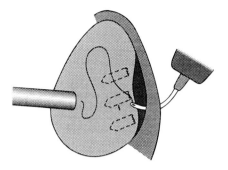

Fig. 20.2 Arthroscopic Bankart repair with suture anchors. After careful debridement of the scapular neck and predrilling of the anchor holes, the inferior portion of the IGHL is pierced with a suture book and a suture is advanced into the joint.

enough inferior and medial on the scapular neck, since advancement and shift of the capsule is an essential part of the procedure. With the special drill guide, three drill holes are made at the anterior edge of the cartilaginous edge of the glenoid. The lower drill hole is created as inferior as possible on the glenoid rim. Through the working portal the most inferior position of the detached IGHL is pierced with a suture hook, which will feed a 1 PDS into the joint (Figure 20.2). The suture hook can be withdrawn after leaving sufficient length of suture in the joint. This end of the suture can be pulled back out of the joint with a grasper through the anterior cannula. A suture anchor is mounted on the inserter and can be slid down the inside limb of the suture. The anchor is then inserted into the first drill hole, creating a sliding loop of suture anchored to bone. The loop is closed using a slip knot that is slid down the cannula, approximating the most inferior part of the IGHL (Figure 20.3).

In general, three anchors are inserted, sufficient to close the lesion completely (Figures 20.4–20.6).

In recent years several modifications to this technique have been proposed: same anchor, but with non-absorbable sutures, using a suture shuttle; other fixation devices, with or without pre-drilling; adsorbable anchors or tags. Since these techniques are relatively new, long-term follow-up results are scarce in the literature. Iserin[9] reported at the ICCS meeting in Helsinki on 182 patients with a 1–3 year follow-up; he noted 28% unsatisfactory results. We have reviewed our results on 27 patients after a minimum 2-year follow-up, using the Mitek anchor and absorbable sutures. Recurrence (dislocation and subluxation) was observed in five patients. Longer follow-up is definitely needed to obtain a complete view on this technique.

Arthroscopic repair using a biodegradable tack

To overcome the problems of transosseous drilling and the technically difficult knot tying in front of the shoulder, a cannulated absorbable fixation device was designed (Suretac; Acufex Microsurgical). The same basic arthroscopic technique is used. The glenoid neck is prepared to promote a bleeding surface for healing. Through an accessory portal the capsulolabral tissue is tensioned with a grasper. A cannulated drill bit with a guide wire is placed through the anterior portal and the inferior capsulolabral tissue is pierced with the guide wire and advanced super-

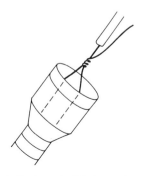

Fig. 20.3 A slip knot is slid down the cannula.

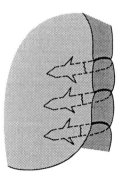

Fig. 20.4 The lesion is completely closed with three anchors and the capsulolabral complex is reconstructed.

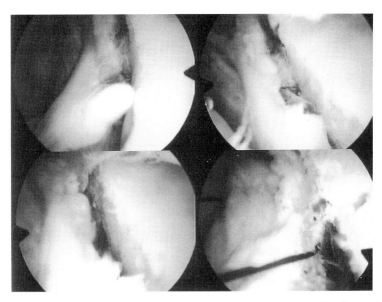

Fig. 20.5 Top: anterior views on a Bankart lesion with detachment of the capsulolabral complex. Bottom left: a view of the debrided glenoid rim and scapular neck. Bottom right: the inferior suture grasps firmly the IGHL.

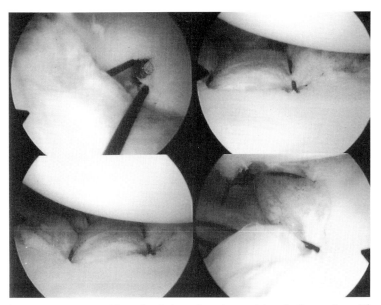

Fig. 20.6 Top left: anterior view with a loaded anchor in position before tying. The other pictures show a reconstructed anterior instability as seen through a posterior and anterior portal.

iorly up to the lower portion of the glenoid neck. The drill bit is advanced to a preset depth and retrieved, leaving the guide wire in place. The tack is then placed over the wire and gently impacted with good compression of the tissue against the glenoid rim. Usually two or three tacks are needed to complete the repair (Figures 20.7–20.9).

Recently Warner et al[10] reported on 96 patients treated with Suretac devices. Fifteen

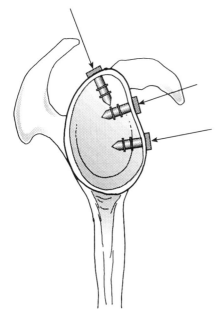

Fig. 20.7 Reconstruction of a Bankart lesion combined with a type II SLAP lesion, using three Suretac devices.

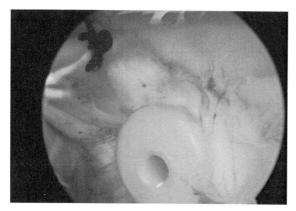

Fig. 20.8 Anterior shoulder stabilization. The inferior fixation (top left) is achieved with a suture anchor and a Suretac closes the superior half of the defect.

patients required a second-look arthroscopy for recurrent instability (seven), pain (six) or paid with stiffness (two). They stated: 'Success of the procedure might be expected to improve by selecting only patients with unidirectional, postraumatic, anterior instability who are found to have a discrete Bankart lesion and well-developed ligamentous tissue.'

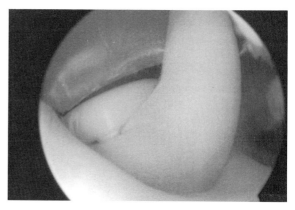

Fig. 20.9 In the same patient as in Fig. 20.8 a SLAP lesion type II was treated with an additional Suretac.

Arthroscopic technique for posterior and multidirectional instability

The management of multidirectional instability remains a difficult issue. Although most authors explicitly exclude multidirectional instability as an indication for arthroscopic reconstruction, others have extended their arthroscopic techniques to correct for excessive capsular laxity posterior, inferior and anterior.

Duncan[11] recently described the technique of superomedial shift of the capsule to correct for multidirectional instability. Through an anterior portal the capsule is divided from the 1 o'clock position, downwards and around the inferior and posterior aspect of the glenoid, up to the attachment of the posterior band of the IGHL. The glenoid neck is abraded down to bleeding bone anteriorly and inferiorly. Multiple sutures are placed, using the Caspari suture punch, into the different capsular and ligamentous structures (including the subscapularis tendon). A single transglenoid passage is created at the 1 o'clock position and all the sutures (eight to twelve) are pulled through to the posterior aspect of the shoulder. While the sutures are being tensioned, the quality of the shift is checked both arthroscopically and by translation testing. Finally, the sutures are tied over the infraspinatus fascia.

Wolf et al[1] described a capsulolabral reconstruction using a plication and suturing technique in order to reduce the capsular volume. First the area of capsule adjacent to the labrum must be abraded with a rasp or a non-aggressive shave blade to allow for capsular healing. Next multiple sutures are placed through the capsule 1 cm from the labral edge and then through the labrum. The sutures should be placed circumferentially around the glenoid in order to reduce the capsular volume in all directions.

In the case of recurrent posterior and posteroinferior instability, fairly similar techniques can be applied. When capsular redundancy is present, multiple sutures are placed through the capsule and the intact labrum to obliterate the posterior capsular sulcus. The posterior band should be shifted superiorly and the capsule itself between the suture entry and the labrum should be carefully debrided. When a posterior capsulolabral detachment is present (reverse Bankart), suture anchors can be used in combination with capsular suture and shift techniques.

CONCLUSIONS

It is widely agreed that arthroscopic repair techniques are not yet as reliable as open techniques. Although the arthroscopic procedure offers the attractive advantage of a selective and anatomic repair of the Bankart lesion with minimal soft tissue dissection, the distinct disadvantages are the higher failure rate and the technical difficulty of the procedure itself. Better patient selection will probably be the key to improving results. A patient with a traumatic unidirectional instability, not involved in contact sports and willing to follow a rehabilitation programme strictly could be a good candidate for current arthroscopic stabilization techniques. Insufficient quality of the capsular tissues or technical difficulties during the procedure should prompt the surgeon to abort the arthroscopy and move to an open repair.

REFERENCES

1. Wolf, P.M. (1991) Arthroscopic Bankart repair using suture anchors. *Oper. Tech. Orthop.* **1**: 184–191.
2. Johnson, L.L. (1993) The glenohumeral joint. In L.L. Johnson (ed.), *Diagnostic and Surgical Arthroscopy of the Shoulder,* pp. 276–364.
3. Rose, D.J. (1993) Arthroscopic suture capsulorrhaphy for anterior and anterioinferior shoulder instability, 2–6 years follow-up. Presented at 12th Arthroscopy Association of North America meeting, April, 1993, Palm Desert.
4. Caspari, R.B. & Savoie, F.M. (1991) Arthroscopic reconstruction of the shoulder Bankart repair. In J.B. McCinty (ed.), *Operative Arthroscopy*, pp. 507–515. New York: Raven Press.
5. Morgan, C. & Bodenstab, A. (1991) Arthroscopic transglenoid Bankart suture repair. *Oper. Tech. Orthap.* **1**: 171–179.
6. Savoie, F.H. (1995) Book of abstracts of 6th International Congress on Surgery of the Shoulder (ICSS). Helsinki, Stockholm. June 27–July 4, 1995.
7. Mologne, T.S. & Lapoint, J.D. (1996) Arthroscopic anterior labral reconstruction using a transglenoid suture technique: results in the active duty military patients. *Am. J. Sports Med.* **24**: 268–274.
8. Walch, G. (1995) Arthroscopic stabilisation of recurrent anterior shoulder dislocation: results of 59 cases. *Arthroscopy* **11**: 173–179.
9. Iserim, A. (1995) Book of abstracts of 6th International Congress on Surgery of the Shoulder (ICSS). Helsinki, Stockholm June 27–July 4.
10. Warner, J.P. et al (1995) Arthroscopic Bankart repair with the Suretac device. Part I: clinical observations. *Arthroscopy* **11**: 2–13.
11. Duncan, R. & Savoie, F.A. (1993) Arthroscopic inferior capsular shift for multidirectional instability of the shoulder: A preliminary report. *Arthroscopy* **9**: 24–27.

21

Arthroscopic Subacromial Decompression

SA Copeland

INTRODUCTION

Open anterior acromioplasty for the treatment of the chronic impingement syndrome was originally described by Neer in 1972.[1] Arthroscopic subacromial decompression was described by Ellman in 1985.[2] Other authors have confirmed that results comparable to the open procedure can be achieved by this technique.[3,4] The technique may be difficult to learn, but the potential advantages are worth while. It is carried out as a day case procedure and patients have less postoperative pain and return to work sooner. However, the time taken to full recovery is similar.

INDICATIONS

The indications for arthroscopic subacromial decompression are identical with those for open anterior acromioplasty.

1. Stage 2 impingement. The ideal indication is the patient that has chronic impingement syndrome without a cuff tear who has failed to respond adequately to conservative measures, including rest, non-steroidal anti-inflammatories and a physiotherapy programme to strengthen the rotator cuff and restore normal scapular humeral rhythm. It is advised that no more than three steroid injections into the subacromial space should be given during any course of treatment.
2. Selected full-thickness rotator cuff tears. In the younger patient with the full-thickness rotator cuff tear, the best treatment is repair of the tear. This has been shown to give better relief of pain and return to function and strength. However, sometimes in the elderly, those that could not cope with the rehabilitation programme after a formal rotator cuff repair, decompression alone may be considered to relieve pain. The results of this are not as predictable as repair and decompression, but may be offered as a first treatment and the majority will be improved by decompression alone.
3. Fracture of the greater tuberosity. The minimally displaced but united fracture of the greater tuberosity may cause a mechanical impingement. Subacromial decompression increases the subacromial outlet, relieving impingement.
4. Calcific tendinitis. The pain of chronic calcific tendinitis may be partly due to impingement and subacromial decompression may be added to the operation of removal of the calcific deposit to relieve symptoms.
5. Rotator cuff repair. If the patient is undergoing a rotator cuff repair, by either arthroscopic or open surgery, then arthroscopic subacromial decompression should be part of the procedure to decompress the repaired tendon. If a major rotator cuff repair is undertaken open, there is little point in attempting the decompression arthroscopically. However, if a small rotator cuff is being repaired, then the decompression may be achieved arthroscopically and then the repair done through a mini deltoid split approach.

CONTRAINDICATIONS

1. Instability. In the young patient with symptoms of impingement this may be due to an underlying instability, and decompression alone will not be adequate to relieve the symptoms. The underlying instability should be addressed.
2. Adhesive capsulitis. Minor degrees of stiffness are a frequent accompaniment of the impingement syndrome, and a full range of movement cannot be achieved before surgery, but only after the pain of impingement is relieved can full movement be regained after the operation. However, if stiffness is a major component, then it is wise to try to regain the movement before surgery by a physiotherapy regime, otherwise decompressive surgery may make the stiffness worse.

EQUIPMENT

The standard 30° fore-oblique arthroscope is used with camera and television monitor. An arthroscopic pump is most helpful, preferably one that allows variability of flow and pressure to help maintain vision (Figure 21.1). A power shaver is essential and the actual type is of critical importance. Many shavers have been developed for use in the knee and are not adequate for shoulder acromioplasty. On the undersurface of the acromion is a very odd rubbery connective tissue at insertion of the coracoacromial ligament. This can be difficult to penetrate with some shavers and it can block most. Two separate blades may be required, one soft tissue resector and one bony burr, although now specific acriomoplasty blades are available which may do both. This is important as the blades are reusable and this halves the cost. Bleeding may be a problem with the procedure and diathermy can be very helpful. Initially the use of diathermy was difficult because the inflow fluid had to be changed from saline to either water or glycine. However, commercially available point source diathermy probes are avail-

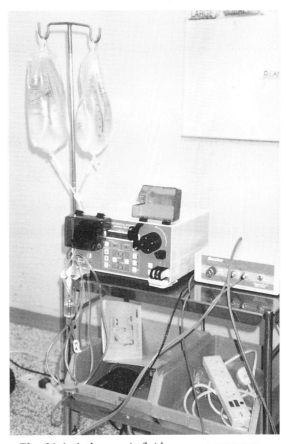

Fig. 21.1 Arthroscopic fluid management pump.

able that do not require change of fluid and can be used in the presence of saline.

POSITION OF PATIENT

The patient is placed in the lateral position with the arm abducted 30° and forward-flexed 20° on 10 lb of balanced traction.

TECHNIQUE

Following a standard glenohumeral arthroscopy via the posterior portal, the subacromial bursa is entered. The bursa should be fully inspected and the bursal surface of the cuff assessed. Partial

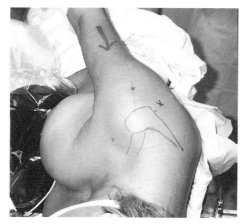

Fig. 21.2 Posterior and lateral portals marked.

bursectomy may be required to achieve this. Attention is then turned to the undersurface of the acromion and the coracoacromial ligament where the 'kissing lesion' of abrasion will be found. The undersurface of the acromion and coracoacromial ligament may be inflamed and roughened. The presence of these findings confirms the diagnosis of impingement and hence the surgeon can proceed to acromioplasty.

The shaver is passed into the bursa via the lateral portal (Figure 21.2). This is placed 5 cm laterally from the anterior edge of the acromion and 1 cm posteriorly. A 5 mm skin incision is made and the shaver pushed through the subcutaneous tissues obliquely into the bursa to be visualized by the scope (Figure 21.3). The

circumflex nerve is not endangered by this approach, because, although the nerve runs approximately 5 cm from the lateral point of the acromion, the shaver is aimed always more proximally and obliquely through the tissues and never directly on to the humerus. At this stage a partial bursectomy may be required to gain adequate visualization of the undersurface of the acromion. By direct vision and feel, any hooking or spur formation on the undersurface of the acromion may be assessed. The attachment of the coracoacromial ligament to the whole undersurface of the anterior aspect of the acromion is seen. If there is any doubt as to the bony landmarks, then a percutaneous needle passed medial and lateral to the acromion can be helpful in orientation. First, the undersurface of the acromion is palpated with the shaver not rotating, then the undersurface of the acromion bone itself must be adequately visualized by removing all the soft tissue and peeling off the undersurface of the coracoacromial ligament by stroking the shaver from posterior to anterior, to finally detach the ligament from the anterior aspect of the acromion (Figure 21.4).

Having exposed the undersurface of the acromion to at least 2 cm posteriorly from the anterior lip, burring of the bone may then begin. Initially, burring is started from lateral to medial (Figure 21.5) to take off the full depth of the acromion anteriorly and across to the acromioclavicular

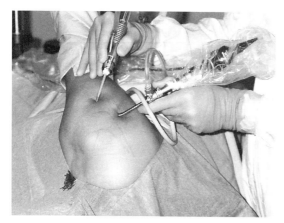

Fig. 21.3 The athroscope is in the posterior portal, and the shaver in the lateral portal.

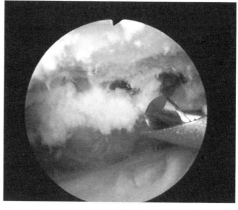

Fig. 21.4 The coracoacromial ligament is being peeled off the undersurface of the right acromion.

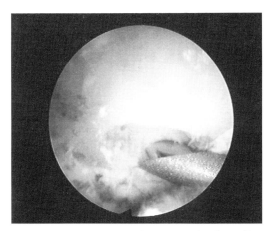

Fig. 21.5 Commencing bone resection laterally.

ASSESSING ADEQUACY OF ACROMIONECTOMY

There is no doubt that successful assessment of adequacy of bone removal depends upon experience. However, certain measurements can be applied. First, the diameter of the shaver tip is known and this can be used to obtain an absolute measurement of the depth and width of the bone excised. The width of the resection can be verified by exactly delineating the origin of the coracoacromial ligament by working from lateral to medial. If the acromioclavicular joint is reached, then by definition this must be the full width of the acromion. To assess whether the undersurface of the acromion is left as a straight line now that the hook has been removed, the straight edge of the shaver can be used to check that a straight line has been achieved by pressing this against the undersurface of the acromion. The arm may be removed from traction and taken up into the impingement position to make sure there is no mechanical impingement still present. At the end of the procedure the bursa should be thoroughly irrigated to remove all possible traces of bone dust. The incidence of new bone formation is greater using a burr than using an awl type blade because the bone debris is removed immediately

On completion of the bony excision, the coracoacromial ligament itself must be excised back towards the coracoid, removing at least half its length. This can be achieved by using the soft tissue resector. At this stage all bleeding points are touched with the diathermy if necessary. The scope and shaver are removed, no sutures are used for closure of the wound but the irrigation fluid is allowed to leak out.[5] A padded dressing is applied over the wound and the arm placed in a sling. At the end of the procedure the shoulder may be swollen and tense depending on the length of the procedure and the pressure of inflow fluid. Both these factors should always be kept to a minimum, although no compartment syndrome has yet been described following this procedure. The intramuscular fluid pressure returns to normal very quickly.[6]

joint, and all bone is removed which lies anterior to the acromioclavicular joint. Again, if there is any doubt as to where the joint lies, a needle passed through the joint into the bursa can be helpful for orientation. Some resection of the medial fat pad may need to be undertaken at this stage.

The second stage is to obliquely remove the undersurface of the anterior third of the acromion, shaping the bone from full-thickness resection at the front and graduating back to the undersurface of the acromion posteriorly. The aim is to provide a straight undersurface to the acromion without any anterior hooking or bowing. This is best achieved by working from lateral to medial. If the medial portion is left intact, then this can be used as a measure of the amount of bone that has already been removed. Having completed the lateral half of the removal, then the medial half is completed across to the acromioclavicular joint. Another reason for working from lateral to medial is that the main bleeding points that may be encountered tend to lie in the medial border of the coracoacromial ligament and hence the majority of the work can be carried out before any major bleeding. If any osteophytosis is apparent on the undersurface of the lateral end of the clavicle, this may also be removed at this stage so that the whole undersurface of the clavicle through to the acromion is a gentle curve which is parallel to the humeral head in the AP plane.

POSTOPERATIVE MANAGEMENT

Patients are encouraged to move the arm from the earliest opportunity and are told that no harm may be done by moving the shoulder, even though it may hurt. They are asked to discard the sling as soon as possible. In practice the majority of patients get rid of the sling within the first 3–4 days. They are shown mobilizing exercises and are seen again at 2 weeks when they have a reasonable range of movements, up to and above shoulder height. Repetitive movements at this stage above shoulder height are still uncomfortable. Patients are told that approximately 80% improvement will occur by 3 months after surgery, but improvement will continue for several months after that. As with most forms of shoulder surgery the prediction of pain is extremely variable; the majority of patients have very little pain, but a few do have considerable pain. Strenuous and repetitive overhead activities are avoided for 6–12 weeks.

COMPLICATIONS

Preoperative stiffness delays recovery after the operation and all efforts should be made to regain movement before surgery. If some degree of stiffness was present before, then these patients require a more aggressive postoperative physiotherapy programme. Patients with partial-thickness tears may have a less than satisfactory recovery and take longer to improve.

The final result of decompression should not be judged until at least 6 months after the operation. Causes of failure of the arthroscopic procedure may be similar to those of open acromioplasty. In every published series there is a percentage of failure. Some of these failures are due to an unrecognized improper diagnosis, some pre-existing osteoarthritic change, or chondromalacia of the humeral head and associated with long head of biceps tears. If a long head of biceps tear of more than two-thirds of the width of the tendon is seen, then it may be

wiser to go to immediate biceps tenodesis. Occasionally removal of pain from the subacromial impingement may reveal an underlying early osteoarthritic change in the acromioclavicular joint which can cause persistent problems. If this occurs then the patient may require an additional acromioclavicular joint excision arthroplasty.

Technical causes of failure decrease with experience, but the most common is inadequate removal of bone. The commonest area for inadequate removal of bone appears to be the very lateral margin of the acromion. Also medially any bulbous enlargement of the lateral end of the clavicle should be flattened and level with the acromion. If the coracoacromial ligament is just divided rather than removed, then this can reheal and cause further impingement. The ligament must be removed rather than divided. Occasionally the patients with the best early results do less well later, as they resume strenuous activity far too early. The patients are told not to resume sport too early, but to carry out strengthening exercises within the pain-free range and pure stretching exercises to gain motion.

RESULTS

Ellman & Kay[7] have reported at 2 years that patients with intact or only partially torn rotator cuffs achieved an 88.5% satisfactory result. In those with a full-thickness rotator cuff tear, only 55% gained a satisfactory result, the size of the tear having a bearing on the functional outcome.

REFERENCES

1. Neer, C.S. (1972) Anterior acromioplasty for the chronic impingement syndrome in the shoulder: a preliminary report. *J. Bone Joint Surg.* **54A:** 41.
2. Ellman, H. (1985) Arthroscopic subacromial decompression: a preliminary report. *Orthop. Trans.* **9:** 49.
3. Gartsman, G.M. (1990) Arthroscopic acromioplasty for lesions of rotator cuff. *J. Bone Joint Surg.* **72A:** 169.
4. Mendoza, F.X., Nicholas, J.A. & Rubenstein, M.P.

(1988) Arthroscopic treatment of stage 2 subacromial impingement. *Orthop. Trans.* **12:** 732.

5. Copeland, S.A. & Williamson, D. (1988) Suturing of arthroscopy wound. *J. Bone Joint Surg.* **18:** 145.

6. Ogilvie-Harris, D.J. & Boynton, E. (1990) Arthroscopic acromioplasty. Extravasation of fluid into the deltoid muscle. *Arthroscopy* **6:** 52.

7. Ellman, H. & Kay, S.P. (1991) Arthroscopic subacromial decompression for chronic impingement; 2–5 year results: *J. Bone Joint Surg.* **73B:** 395.

22

Arthroscopic Excision Arthroplasty of the Acromioclavicular Joint

SA Copeland

INTRODUCTION

The acromioclavicular (AC) joint is a common site of painful shoulder disorders and open resection arthroplasty of this joint has been a reliable treatment for cases not responding to conservative treatment.[1] Traditionally via an open approach the outer 1.5–2 cm of clavicle is removed and any osteophyte on the acromial side is also trimmed. However, this open approach violates the capsule of the AC joint and can result in an irritating horizontal instability causing continuing symptoms. Using arthroscopy the arthroplasty may be kept as an intracapsular approach hence maintaining stability of the joint in all directions. As with most arthroscopic procedures the initial morbidity is less, the patient requires less analgesia, a shorter stay in hospital and an easier rehabilitation programme, and there is improved cosmesis. In the open procedure, if the superior ligamentous structures are not carefully reconstructed at the time of excision arthroplasty in the young, then an aching instability may ensue, after repetitive use above shoulder height. This problem, however, is less noticeable in those over 45 years of age.

INDICATIONS

The indications for arthroscopic excision of the AC joint are the same as for open excision arthroplasty.

1. Symptomatic AC osteoarthritis that does not respond to conservative therapy.
2. Rotator cuff impingement secondary to degenerative change in the AC joint with large inferior osteophytosis causing secondary impingement.
3. Osteolysis of the distal clavicle. This is sometimes encountered in the young weight lifter or after minor trauma.

CONTRAINDICATION

Arthroscopic resection is not indicated in grade 3 AC dislocation as the symptoms are not really due to bony abutment, but instability. In patients with grade 2 subluxation, arthroscopic excision arthroplasty is certainly possible but the results are less favourable. The symptoms from bony abutment are relieved but instability remains.

PREOPERATIVE INVESTIGATION

The diagnosis is clinical. Pain is well localized to the AC joint and on examination the patient has a high and increasingly painful arc of elevation beyond 130° and pain induced by stress in the AC joint with forced adduction. All this pain may be relieved by local anaesthetic injected into the joint itself.

POSITION OF PATIENT

The lateral position is used with the arm on traction as for glenohumeral arthroscopy but the patient is rolled towards the operator who is standing on the posterior aspect of the patient. This allows manoeuvrability of the shaver anteriorly during resection of the joint.

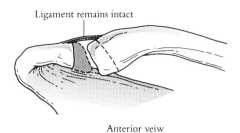

Ligament remains intact

Anterior veiw

Fig. 22.1 Bony resection remains intracapsular so that the superior AC ligament remains intact.

TECHNIQUE

The arthroscope is inserted through the standard posterior portal and a routine glenohumeral arthroscopy is made to exclude any other source of shoulder pain and pathology. The subacromial bursa is then inspected and any coexisting impingement noted. An anterolateral portal is then made 4 cm inferior to the joint and 2 cm lateral. The shaver is then passed through this anterior portal into the subacromial bursa and directly visualized with the arthroscope. Initially the undersurface of the AC joint may not be seen, but resection of the medial fat pad must be undertaken. The position of the AC joint may now be ascertained by three helpful manoeuvres.

1. Direct palpation of the shaver pushing up on the outer end of the clavicle which can be palpated on the skin surface.
2. The passage of the needle directly through the AC joint and into the fat pad.
3. By pressure on the outer end of the clavicle the joint line may be seen. Then bone is identified on the medial side of the acromion and resected with the notchplasty.

Arthroscopic arthroplasty of the AC joint involves removal of bone from both the clavicular side and the acromial side to remain intracapsular. Removal of bone from the acromial side also aids direct vision from the posterior portal. Approximately 4 mm of bone, i.e. one width of the shaver, is removed from the acromial side; the whole of the lateral end of the clavicle is then visualized directly. Again one shaver's width of bone, i.e. 4 mm, is removed from the outer end of

the clavicle. It is easier to do this full resection inferiorly first so that the amount of bone removed can be readily identified by the bone remaining. Having completed the resection on the inferior half, the superior half is then resected leaving the superior AC ligament intact (Figures 22.1–22.4).

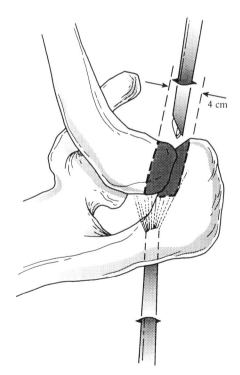

Right shoulder viewed from above

4 cm

Fig. 22.2 The AC joint is viewed with the scope in the posterior portal and the shaver through an accessory portal anterior to the AC joint.

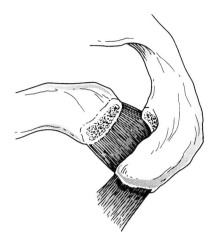

Fig. 22.3 The completed operation shows bone removed from the clavicular and acromial sides with the superior ligament remaining intact.

(A)

(B)

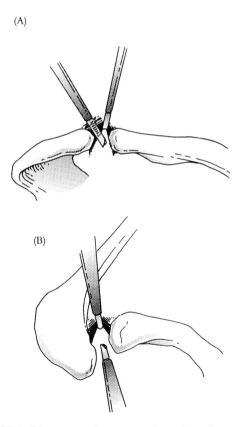

Fig. 22.4 Direct superior approach with arthroscope and shaver passed directly into the AC joint. Anterior (A) and superior (B) view of instruments in the joint.

AC ARTHROPLASTY IN CONJUNCTION WITH ACROMIOPLASTY

Excision arthroplasty of the AC joint is often required in conjunction with acromioplasty to decompress the anterior rotator cuff. The posterior portal is made first, glenohumeral joint inspected and then the scope passed into the bursa via the posterior portal. A direct lateral portal is made initially as described in Chapter 21, and the power shaver used to complete the acromioplasty. When the acromioplasty is completed the AC joint is easily delineated as the most medial margin of the acromion. With the power shaver still in the lateral portal, the inferior half of the lateral end of the clavicle is removed. Complete resection of the lateral end of the clavicle, however, cannot usually be completed from that direct lateral portal, but may be facilitated by downward pressure on the outward end of the clavicle during shaving. Usually a further third portal must be made anterolaterally as described in the preceding section (Figure 22.5). The shaver is then passed into the subacromial bursa under direct vision and the resection of the superior part of the clavicle completed. Figure 22.6 shows the arthroscopic view of the completed excision arthroplasty.

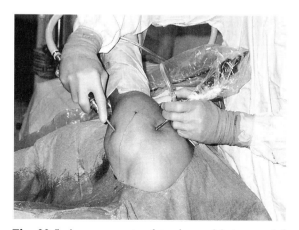

Fig. 22.5 Accessory anterolateral portal being used for AC joint excision arthroplasty.

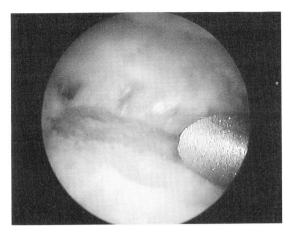

Fig. 22.6 Arthroscopic view of completed excision arthroplasty.

ALTERNATIVE METHOD USING DIRECT SUPERIOR APPROACH

Johnson[2] described the superior approach to the AC joint in which the arthroscope and instruments are inserted directly into the AC joint allowing direct visualization of the joint surfaces. Flatow et al[3] have used this approach for AC joint resection. This has the advantages of leaving the subacromial bursa unviolated and the capsule almost completely intact.

Technique

The procedure is performed with the patient in the beach chair position. Diagnostic glenohumeral and subacromial examinations are not routinely performed but only when clinically indicated. Depalma[4] and Petersson[5] have demonstrated that an age-related narrowing of the AC joint exists and that variability of the inclination of the joint line is present. It is important to determine this inclination exactly using through-and-through needles. The joint is then insufflated with normal saline solution. The anterosuperior portal is placed in line with the AC joint and 1 cm anterior to it. The posterior portal is placed in line with the joint and 1 cm posterior to it. The portals are injected with 1%

xylocaine with adrenaline to decrease skin bleeding. Initially a 2.7 mm wrist arthroscope is used from the posterosuperior portal. A 2 mm shaver is then passed from the anterior portal under direct vision to debride the meniscal remnant and joint debris. This procedure exposes the articular surfaces. The acromial side is usually avoided as small burrs beginning with the 2 mm burr are used to resect the distal clavicle to widen the joint space. The standard 4 mm arthroscope is then used. Electrocautery can be used to shell out the distal clavicle from the surrounding soft tissues. The capsule and ligaments are not incised but are subperiosteally elevated to expose the bone. This elevation provides visualization of the distal clavicle and allows precise resection. A 4 mm burr is used to complete the resection of the distal clavicle. The burr is switched from the anterosuperior to the posterosuperior portal and the arthroscope switched vice versa to facilitate uniform resection anteriorly and posteriorly.

POSTOPERATIVE MANAGEMENT

Patients are put in a sling for pain relief but told that they can do no harm by moving the arm and are encouraged to do so as soon after the operation as possible. Most patients get rid of the sling within a few days but are told they will still have discomfort in the shoulder for some weeks. At 3 weeks they have a reasonable range of movement and are told that it takes approximately 3 months to achieve 80% improvement. Strenuous activity above shoulder height is avoided for 6 weeks. Return to golf, etc. can usually be achieved after 6 weeks.

COMPLICATIONS

The most common cause of failure is incomplete resection of bone leaving a small bridge of bone anteriorly or posteriorly. Hence it is mandatory to see the whole circumference of the clavicle at the time of resection and to remove equal bone anteriorly and posteriorly. Persisting symptoms after adequate removal may indicate some pre-existing unrecognized instability and certainly explains the lower success rate in grade 2 AC separations.

ASSESSING ADEQUACY OF EXCISION

For the open procedure most authors have recommended excision of up to 2 cm or even 2.5 cm of the distal clavicle.[6-8] Failure of distal clavicle resection when less bone is removed has been reported because of abutment of the distal clavicle against the acromion with arm motion.[9] The abutment of the clavicle against the acromion results more from destabilization of the AC joint from trauma (grade 2 injury), or surgery (open resection of the distal clavicle) than from inadequate bone removal.[3] Arthroscopic resection of the distal clavicle preserves the ligamentous envelope of the AC joint. Flatow et al[3] have shown that resections of as little as 5 mm are successful in relieving symptoms and leaving the AC joint stable.

REFERENCES

1. Copeland, S.A. (1986) Primary osteo-arthritis of the acromioclavicular joint – results of excision arthroplasty. 128–130 of The Shoulder. Professional post-graduate service Tokyo 1986. *In* Proceedings of the Third International Conference on Surgery of the Shoulder. N. Takagishi (Ed.) Fukuora, Japan.
2. Johnson, S.L. (1981) *Diagnostic and Surgical Arthroscopy*. St. Louis: C.V. Mosby.
3. Flatow, E.L., Xavier, A.D., Gregory, P., Nicholson, P., Pollock, R.G. & Bigliani, L.U. (1995) Arthroscopic resection of the distal clavicle with the superior approach. *J. Shoulder Elbow Surg.* **4:** 41–49.
4. Depalma, A.F. (1957) *Degenerative Changes of the Sternoclavicular Joint and Acromioclavicular Joints in Various Decades*. Springfield, IL: C.C. Thomas.
5. Petersson, C.J. (1983) Degeneration of the acromioclavicular joint: a morphological study. *Acta Orthop. Scand.* **54:** 434–438.
6. Gartsman, G.M. (1993) Arthroscopic resection of the acromioclavicular joint. *Am. J. Sports Med.* **21:** 71–77.
7. Gurd, F.B. (1941) The treatment of complete dislocation of the outer end of the clavicle: a hitherto undescribed operation. *Ann. Surg.* **63:** 1094–1098.
8. Mumford, E.B. (1941) Acromioclavicular dislocation a new operative treatment. *J. Bone Joint Surg.* **23:** 799–801.
9. Rockwood, C.A. & Young, D.C. (1990) Disorders of the acromioclavicular joint. In C.A. Rockwood & F.A. Matsen (eds) *The Shoulder*, pp. 413–476. Philadelphia: W.B. Saunders.

23

Rotator Cuff Repair

PM Connor and LU Bigliani

INTRODUCTION

The first rotator cuff tear was described in 1834 by J.G. Smith,[1] an English anatomist. Ernest A. Codman, however, has been given the distinction of being the person who performed the first rotator cuff repair. His initial report[2] on repair of the rotator cuff was in 1911 and was followed by his classic book *The Shoulder*,[3] in 1934. Wilson[4] in 1931 introduced the concept of reinserting the torn rotator cuff tendon edge into a 'bony trench' in the anatomic neck of the humerus, and Bosworth[5] later modified this technique by altering the position of the trough more proximally. McLaughlin[6–8] wrote on the pathogenesis and treatment of rotator cuff tears over the next 30 years, including his report of 100 consecutive patients who underwent rotator cuff repair and were followed for an average of 3 years.[6] Since that time operative treatment of rotator cuff tears has become a common shoulder procedure, with many different techniques described.[5–11] Initially, however, results were not ideal with several series reporting a significant number of unsatisfactory results (26–46%).[3–5,12]

The results of open rotator cuff repair improved significantly after Neer's report[13] on anterior acromioplasty in combination with cuff mobilization and repair in 1972. More recent studies[14–19] have reported predictably satisfactory results in both pain relief and function with the use of this approach, which is the gold standard for operative treatment of rotator cuff tears. Over the last several years, however, shoulder arthroscopy has had a profound impact on the evaluation and treatment of rotator cuff disease.[20–22] New information has resulted from the ability to visualize glenohumeral pathology during procedures previously carried out through an open approach confined to the subacromial space. This information, as well as that available from improved imaging technology, has led to improved understanding in some areas and increased controversy in others. Treatment options have also been revolutionized as arthroscopically assisted rotator cuff repair is now widely used and arthroscopic repair is evolving. Not surprisingly, the arthroscope has worked most effectively in the hands of those surgeons who have treated it as one additional tool to be used according to principles established in the open treatment of rotator cuff disease.

INDICATIONS

The mere presence of a rotator cuff tear is not necessarily in and of itself an indication for operative repair. Cadaver studies have shown an incidence of full-thickness tears of the rotator cuff approaching 60%, with partial-thickness tears being even more common. More recently, magnetic resonance imaging (MRI) studies[23,24] have shown rotator cuff tears in up to 33% of asymptomatic shoulders, with an increased incidence with age. Sher et al[24] found that 54% of asymptomatic volunteers over 60 years of age had a tear of the rotator cuff as diagnosed by MRI. The question of why some rotator cuff tears are well tolerated by patients and others are disabling is one of great debate, the answer to which is most certainly multifactorial.

The supraspinatus insertion on the greater tuberosity must repeatedly pass underneath the coracoacromial arch when the arm is used for vigorous overhead activity. Subacromial bursitis as well as rotator cuff tendinitis and tears are common disorders in the shoulder, and can result in pain, weakness and difficulties with activities of daily living.[25,26] Many factors have been implicated in rotator cuff pathology, including extrinsic tendon injury due to compression from an abnormal coracoacromial arch[13,27–30] (Figure 23.1), abutment against the glenoid rim,[31] tendon and bursal swelling in a confined space,[32] tensile overload[33] or altered glenohumeral kinematics (e.g. instability)[33] and intrinsic tendon injury from tendinitis,[32] altered vascularity[34] or shear between different fibre bundles.[35,36]

Whether a primary factory or secondary effect, subacromial impingement is thought by many investigators to be an ongoing cause of tendon injury by the time surgical intervention is considered. Neer[13] proposed that variation in acromial slope and morphology were clinically relevant, and Bigliani et al[27] demonstrated a

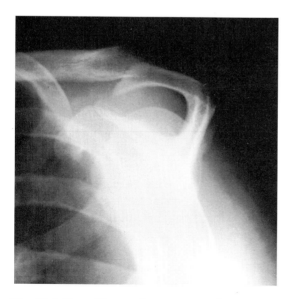

Fig. 23.1 Type III acromion as seen on the supraspinatus outlet radiograph, which has been associated with full-thickness tears of the rotator cuff.[27]

relationship between acromial morphology and the incidence of rotator cuff tears in cadavers. Flatow et al[38] performed contact studies on the subacromial space, and found that contact was centred on the supraspinatus insertion, where cuff tears generally initiate, and involve the anteroinferior acromion, supporting the removal of that region (anterior acromioplasty) in the treatment of rotator cuff impingement.[29]

Thus the indication for surgical intervention in rotator cuff disease is the presence of pain and/or functional deficits which interfere with activities and have not been successfully managed with conservative treatment. The rationale includes decompressing impingement, debriding non-viable or inflamed tissue and thus presumably stimulating healing, repairing tendon defects, treating any associated pathology, and carefully staging and supervising a comprehensive rehabilitation programme.

TECHNIQUE

The repair of a rotator cuff tear can be divided into four distinct phases: the approach, the decompression, the repair of the cuff tear, and postoperative rehabilitation. We currently perform the procedure using interscalene block anaesthesia with intravenous sedation, thereby avoiding the use of a general anaesthetic. This has been a tremendous advantage as it enables the elimination of many complications associated with general anaesthesia. Also, the analgesic effect of 0.5% bupivacaine will last for an extended period of time (8–10 h), so that the patient does not have significant pain in the immediate postoperative period.

Approach

The patient is placed in a modified beach chair position with the torso angled approximately 60° from the horizontal plane. A head rest is used which allows access to the superior and posterior aspects of the shoulder. The arm is draped free allowing shoulder rotation, extension and elevation. If an endotracheal tube is used, it should be taped to the opposite side of the mouth. A broad-spectrum antibiotic is administered before the skin incision and is continued for 24 h in the post-operative period.

A 10–12 cm skin incision is made in the superoanterior aspect of the shoulder in Langer's skin lines. The incision extends from the lateral aspect of the anterior third of the acromion inferiorly to the lateral aspect of the coracoid. It is placed perpendicular to the longitudinal orientation of the deltoid fibres. The incision is then deepened to the subcutaneous layer, and self-retaining Gelpi skin retractors are used to aid in exposure of the subcutaneous tissues. Mayo scissors or needle-tip electrocautery are used to expose the fascial layer of the deltoid. The needle-tip electrocautery is preferred as it significantly decreases bleeding. Subcutaneous flaps to the level of the deltoid fascia are then raised to allow access to the acromioclavicular joint and the lateral aspect of the acromion. At this point, it is important to identify the precise location of both

the lateral tip of the acromion and the acromio-clavicular joint in preparation for the split in the deltoid.

The incision in the deltoid is started just anterior to the acromioclavicular joint and extends laterally to the lateral edge of the acro-mion where it curves slightly posteriorly (Figure 23.2). This will take the incision into the fibres of the middle deltoid, centring the split over the greater tuberosity. The deltoid origin is preserved as a 5–10 mm cuff of strong tissue is left on the anterior aspect of the acromion and the acromio-clavicular joint to facilitate closure of this split. The incision is usually extended 3 or 4 cm past the lateral tip of the acromion. A stay suture is then placed at the distal end of the split to avoid injury to the axillary nerve which generally runs 4–5 cm from the tip of the lateral acromion. If more exposure is needed for a larger tear, the split can be carefully extended to 5 cm past the lateral tip of the acromion. The split is then deepened down to the area of the bursa using the needle-tip electro-cautery. At this stage, the superior aspect of the

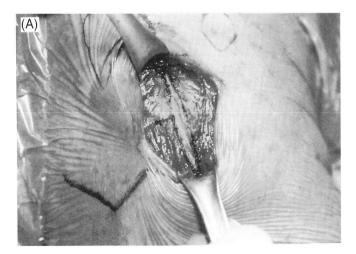
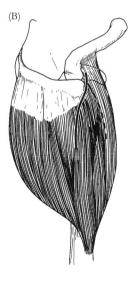

Fig. 23.2 (A) Deltoid incision starting just anterior to the acromioclavicular joint and extending laterally to the lateral edge of the acromion where it curves slightly posteriorly ending about 3–4 cm lateral to the lateral acromial edge. (B) The posterior curve of the deltoid incision allows the exposure to be centred over the greater tuberosity for better access to the cuff. The dotted line demonstrates the less desirable anterior exposure provided by the older and more anterior type of deltoid incision.

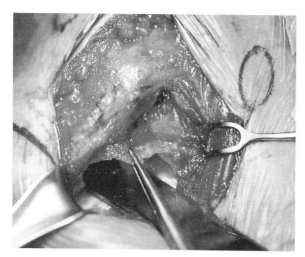

Fig. 23.3 The coracoacromial ligament is identified as it inserts into the undersurface of the anterolateral aspect of the acromion.

bursa is carefully opened and the lateral edge of the coracoacromial ligament is defined (Figure 23.3). The entire coracoacromial ligament should then be identified. The superior part of the bursa lateral to the ligament should be removed. Before the ligament is subperiosteally dissected off of the acromion, an attempt should be made to cauterize the artery which often bleeds in this portion of the approach, the acromial branch of the thoraco-acromial trunk. A wide flat retractor can then be placed underneath the acromion in the sub-acromial space and the humeral head can be levered inferiorly so that adequate exposure of the acromion and coracoacromial ligament can be achieved.

Using this approach, the split in the deltoid is centered more posteriorly over the greater tuberosity. This enables access to the entire rotator cuff by manoeuvring the arm in flexion, extension, internal and external rotation. Furthermore, the anterolateral aspect of the deltoid is anterior to the incision and does not block access to the posterior cuff.

Decompression

Subacromial impingment has been described by Neer as an important factor in the aetiology of full-thickness rotator cuff tears.[13,17,38] Imping-

ment can occur at the coracoacromial ligament, anterior acromion and/or the acromioclavicular joint. To perform an adequate decompression, the coracoacromial ligament is released and the anterior acromial 'spur' is excised. The undersurface of the acromioclavicular joint should also be examined for excrescences which may extend into the subacromial space. These can be easily removed with a ronguer or high-speed burr. The entire acromioclavicular joint is only removed when there is preoperative tenderness and arthrosis, which has occurred in roughly 10–15 % of our cases.

In preparation for the anterior acromioplasty, the lateral edge of the coracoacromial ligament is identified and subperiosteally removed from the undersurface of the acromion. It must be remembered that the ligament starts on the lateral aspect of the acromion and extends anteriorly and inferiorly to the coracoid. We have recently modified our management of the coracoacromial ligament in patients with larger cuff tears.[40,41] The coracoacromial arch has a passive buffering function against superior humeral translation. If the dynamic head-depressing function of the cuff is lost, and then the arch overly resected, the head may translate superiorly to a subcutaneous position. Thus, in repairs of massive tears with associated superior migration of the humeral head, we have recently reported on the repair of the coracoacromial ligament back to the acromion in a more medial position after performing a conservative acromioplasty, to preserve this soft-tissue buffer.[40,41] If the coracoacromial ligament is not going to be preserved and reattached, it can then be excised close to the coracoid. The remaining cuff of strong deltoid insertion tissue is then meticulously elevated in a superior direction from the anterior part of the acromion and the acromioclavicular joint.

The undersurface of the acromion is cleared of bursal and/or rotator cuff tissue which is often adherent. A thin sharp bevelled osteotome is then used to perform the anterior acromioplasty. The bevel is placed upwards to prevent removal of too much bone. A mallet is used to cut the wedge while an assistant gently provides counterpressure by pressing on the posterior aspect of the acromion. Traditionally, the amount of acromion removed has been approximately 7–8 mm in thickness and should extend posteriorly approximately one-quarter to one-third the length of the acromion. Recent work in our laboratory, however, suggests that this may be too much bone and that only 4–5 mm of bone resection is necessary. The emphasis should be on contouring a smooth undersurface of the acromion for contact. The wedge of bone excised should, however, consist of the full width of the acromion from the medial to the lateral border and it is then cut free of the attached soft tissue by sharp dissection. The thickness of the acromion can then be palpated between the index finger and thumb. A double-action laminectomy ronguer, rasp or burr can be used to smooth the undersurface of the remaining acromion and remove any remaining uneven ridges of bone. In most cases, a properly performed acromioplasty removes a portion of the acromial aspect of the acromioclavicular joint, often leaving the undersurface of the distal clavicle quite prominent; these rough edges should then be smoothed with a rasp. This completes the modified acromioclavicular arthroplasty which widens the subacromial space medially. If the entire distal clavicle needs to be removed, this can be performed from underneath with a burr or ronguer. Approaching the acromioclavicular joint from below prevents violation of the superior acromioclavicular ligaments, helping to preserve stability of the joint.

It is important to re-emphasize that lateral or radical acromionectomy should be avoided.[42–44] This procedure deforms the deltoid by removing its site of origin. Without this normal site of attachment, the deltoid is weakened and shoulder function is severely compromised. Transacromial approaches can also weaken the deltoid or result in non-union and are not recommended. In addition, decompression is technically difficult to perform from this approach.

Rotator cuff repair

Attention is now turned towards mobilizing the torn rotator cuff tissue. The biceps tendon is inspected to see whether it is intact, frayed or torn. The oblique course of the biceps tendon runs just beneath the rotator interval tissue which is formed by the junction of the supraspinatus and subscapularis tendons. If intact, the biceps is left in its groove and not transposed posteriorly. In rare situations, the intact tendon can be incorporated into the rotator cuff repair to help provide additional tissue coverage. If the biceps tendon is torn, the proximal stump can sometimes be used in the repair and the distal stump is tenodesed in the groove if it has not fully retracted distally into the arm.

The leading edge of the rotator cuff tear is then identified and sutures are placed into the medial aspect of the tear. Zero or no. 1 non-absorbable sutures are used. An elevator is then used to sweep the superficial aspect of the bursa beneath the coracoid in the area of the subscapularis. It is important to remove only the superficial bursa, as the deep bursa may provide blood flow to the edges of the torn rotator cuff. Minimal tissue is debrided from the leading edge of the tear, as it has been shown that this tissue does have blood supply.[45,46]

The cuff is then mobilized from anterior to posterior in a sequential fashion. Multiple stay sutures are placed at the visible edge of the torn tendons. Internal rotation and extension of the free arm help to provide access to the posterior tissues. The posterior aspect of the cuff is also more accessible because of the 'more posteriorly' placed deltoid split. Attention is initially turned towards the bursal surface of the cuff. A periosteal elevator or scissors can be used to mobilize the cuff and its associated bursa from the undersurface of the acromion. It is important to emphasize that the undersurface of the acromion is a common location for cuff and bursal adhesions and this area should be released before the acromioplasty to prevent inadvertent extension of the tear. Generally, though, these adhesions are underneath the posterolateral aspect of the acromion and the deltoid muscle, and become more apparent after the acromioplasty is performed. The stay sutures previously placed are used to advance the torn edge of the rotator cuff anteriorly. To gain additional posterior exposure, the humeral head can be depressed with a blunt retractor while in a position of internal rotation and extension. After complete bursal surface release and exposure, the posterior tissues are assessed to determine the full extent of the tear. Usually a portion of the infraspinatus and/or the teres minor remain attached to the humeral head. The surgeon should be careful not to remove these during attempts at mobilization and release of surrounding adhesions.

Attention is then turned towards mobilization and release of the undersurface of the rotator cuff. The undersurface is commonly scarred to the glenoid rim and base of the coracoid. Undersurface release is generally carried out bluntly with an elevator. Sharp dissection may be carried out with scissors, but this should be performed with caution. If scissors are used, spreading is more advisable than cutting in the posterior aspect of the cuff, especially near the base of the scapular spine in the vicinity of the suprascapular nerve. After a complete and systematic release of the undersurface of the cuff from posterior to anterior, the excursion of the torn tendons is assessed by pulling on the stay sutures. To ensure a successful repair, the edges of the torn tendon should reach the anatomical neck of the humerus with the arm in a functional position of 10–15° of forward elevation and 10° of abduction.

There are several manoeuvres which can be performed if sufficient tendon cannot be mobilized to bring the leading edge of the cuff to the anatomical neck. The rotator interval and coracohumeral ligament should be released at the base of the coracoid (Figure 23.4). The coracohumeral ligament is often contracted, thus inhibiting the lateral and distal advancement of the supraspinatus tendon. This complete release of the rotator interval and coracohumeral ligament at the base of the coracoid is termed 'the interval slide', and will allow the supraspinatus to be mobilized up to 1.0–1.5 cm. We have avoided the need to transfer the upper portion of the subscapularis by using this manoeuvre. However, if the subscapularis transfer is performed, it is important not to transfer the underlying capsule as this may lead to instability.

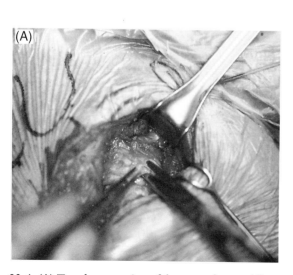

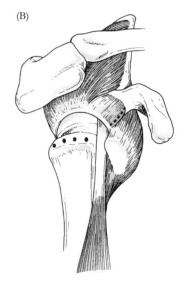

Fig. 23.4 (A) To release scarring of the coracohumeral ligament at the base of the coracoid, an interval release is sharply performed with scissors beginning laterally and incising directly to the coracoid base. (B) The complete release of the rotator interval and coracohumeral ligament is termed the interval slide as the tissues, once incised, are slid along the dotted line, thus mobilizing the retracted tissue in a lateral direction. Sliding the tissues in a lateral direction at the interval allows for 1.0–1.5 cm of new length for repair.

If more mobilization is required, further releases can be performed along the posterior and superior aspect of the cuff on the glenoid rim. Since we have been releasing the rotator interval, however, these manoeuvres have rarely been necessary. When required, capsular release along the glenoid rim should be performed bluntly or cautiously with scissors, spreading more than cutting. Sharp dissection in this area can injure the muscle belly of the infraspinatus and/or the suprascapular nerve and should be avoided. In the majority of cases, these manoeuvres will provide sufficient mobilization to allow the torn rotator cuff tendons to reach the anatomical neck with the shoulder in the desired position. Of note, we have not found the use of synthetic material or allografts to be helpful in our repairs. With mobilization complete, the next step becomes the actual repair of the rotator cuff to bone.

The greater tuberosity is prepared for tendon repair by 'scarifying' the anatomical neck area with a large curette. A deep trough is not used as it increases the amount of tendon mobilization required and has not been found necessary to promote tendon-to-bone healing. Multiple drill holes (four or five) are then placed into the greater tuberosity starting medially in the anatomical neck. Corresponding lateral tuberosity holes are made, leaving a 1.0–1.5 cm bridge of tuberosity bone between the holes and thereby creating a bony tunnel for suture repair to bone. Zero or no. 1 braided nylon sutures are then passed through the tunnels with a curved needle. Although suture anchors can be used in the greater tuberosity, the bone may be osteoporotic allowing for potential pull-out of the anchors.

During the repair, the arm is held in approximately 10–15° of flexion and 10° of abduction and the sutures are tied over the bony bridges. This allows excellent apposition of the bone and rotator cuff edge. If an interval slide has been performed, the rotator interval should be closed in such a way as to realign the mobilized supraspinatus edge further laterally than the corresponding subscapularis edge of the interval. If there is a split between the infraspinatus and teres minor (generally the 'apex' of the tear), this should also be closed. The side-to-side 'apex stitch' should be sutured before reapproximation of the distal edges of the tear to allow proper restoration of the intratendinous relationships of the posterior cuff.

If there is a large or massive cuff tear with deficiency of the superomedial aspect of the coracoacromial arch, the preserved coracoacromial ligament is now reattached medially, As mentioned, this provides a superomedial buttress which may provide restraint from superior migration of the humeral head. The deltoid is then meticulously repaired to the cuff of strong deltoid origin which was preserved, and the stay suture in the distal deltoid split is removed. If the cuff of the deltoid origin tissue is of poor quality, drill holes are placed in the acromion and the deltoid is repaired directly to bone. A few subcutaneous absorbable sutures are placed followed by a subcuticular skln closure with an absorbable suture. The arm is immobilized in a sling and swathe for approximately 24 h. We do not use abduction braces, as we feel this tends to put the arm in too much extension, increasing tension across the repair. The swathe is removed at 24 h and precise range of motion exercises are initiated.

Rehabilitation

In large and massive tears, the normal Neer Phase I Rehabilitation Program[38] is altered. In the first 6 weeks, only three exercises are performed. These include pendulum exercises, supine external rotation using a stick to 30°, and assisted passive forward elevation to 140°. We like to avoid extension and pulley exercises in the first 4–6 weeks, as this puts stress across the rotator cuff repair. Isometric and active assisted exercises are usually started at the 6–8-week period. These generally begin with active supine external rotation, theraband exercises and active supine forward elevation. Once these exercises are performed, erect forward elevation with the help of a stick is started. This is performed initially with a stick alone, then followed with weights of 1–5 lbs. A hand weight can then be used in the supine position to raise the arm. Weights can be increased to 3 lbs but should not increase past this weight to avoid placing undue stress on the cuff repair. Once these exercises can be performed without difficulty, more active strengthening exercises can then be added.

ISOLATED RUPTURE OF THE SUBSCAPULARIS TENDON

Tears of the most anterior portion of the rotator cuff, the subscapularis tendon, are uncommon and rarely occur in isolation.[47,48] The majority of these lesions have been reported in association with biceps tendon pathology, more extensive rotator cuff tears, fractures to the tuberosities, or as a part of an instability complex of the shoulder.[48] Gerber and Krushell[44] have reported the clinical features of 16 patients who had isolated rupture of the subscapularis tendon, all of which were associated with significant traumatic events. Patients complained of anterior shoulder pain as well as difficulties with activities both above and below shoulder level; however, none experienced recurrent anterior shoulder instability. Each patient exhibited a 'pathological lift–off test'[47] on physical examination. Arthrography can be misinterpreted in the anteroposterior view with subscapularis tears[47] and MRI has been shown to be diagnostic, not only of the tear but also of the status of the biceps tendon.

In patients with symptoms of pain and functional disability, an anterior deltopectoral incision identifies the subscapularis tear and enables adequate exposure for repair of the tendon with sutures through bone or with suture anchors. Chronic cases may necessitate anterior mobilization techniques as previously described. The long head of the biceps tendon should be carefully examined; if intact but medially dislocated, soft tissue reconstruction of the transverse humeral ligament should be performed. If the biceps tendon is significantly damaged or ruptured, a biceps tenodesis should be performed. It is important to limit external rotation after surgery to approximately 30°, or to a comfortable rotation as determined at the time of surgery for 6 weeks to allow time for tendon-to-bone healing. Although large series of results of isolated subscapularis repair are not yet currently available, reported

preliminary results have been favourable in both pain relief and functional improvement.[47]

MANAGEMENT OF ROTATOR CUFF DEFICIENCY IN ASSOCIATION WITH GLENOHUMERAL ARTHRITIS

In 1983, Neer et al[49] described the clinical and pathological findings of cuff tear arthropathy: degenerative arthritis of the shoulder secondary to massive rotator cuff deficiency. Superior migration of the humeral head causes subacromial impingement and eventual erosion of the anterior portion of the acromion and the acromioclavicular joint such that the humeral head articulates not only with the superior aspect of the glenoid but also the coracoacromial arch. Owing to the presence of concomitant arthritis, isolated rotator cuff repair does not provide adequate relief of symptoms. In an attempt to improve postoperative results, some authors have advocated a total shoulder arthroplasty using a semiconstrained glenoid component.[50] Others have advocated the fixed fulcrum prosthesis, subacromial spacers or a reverse ball-and-socket prosthesis. These interventions have had technical difficulties, including limitation of abduction, a higher rate of wear and mechanical failure and loss of external rotation.[51]

Unconstrained shoulder arthroplasty has also been recommended for patients with rotator cuff deficiency.[49,50] These arthroplasties, along with rotator cuff repair, are undertaken with the understanding that achievement of Neer's 'limited goals' should be the aim of surgery in this subgroup. However, at long-term follow-up, investigators have noted an association between glenoid loosening and irreparable rotator cuff deficiencies. They postulated that superior migration of the humeral component leads to eccentric loading of the glenoid, which has been termed the 'rocking-horse glenoid'.[52]

Humeral hemiarthroplasty with rotator cuff reconstruction emphasizing anteroposterior stability has evolved as the preferred alternative in this difficult patient population.[52,53] Although glenohumeral arthrodesis is an option in these rotator-cuff-deficient patients,[52] Arntz et al have reported that the results of humeral hemiarthroplasty are preferable.[53] The subacromial soft tissue buttress provided by the coracoacromial ligament is preserved superiorly, and the rotator cuff is repaired as best possible with local remaining cuff tissue. The prosthetic head is allowed to articulate with the coracoacromial arch, which allows a new stable fulcrum in the face of altered glenohumeral relationships and kinematics. Although functional improvements after this procedure are modest at best, pain relief can be achieved in a majority of patients.[54]

ARTHROSCOPIC MANAGEMENT OF THE ROTATOR CUFF

Overview

Although a thorough discussion of shoulder arthroscopy is beyond the scope of this chapter, some relevant aspects regarding the arthroscopic evaluation and management of rotator cuff disease are included. It must be emphasized that the rationale for arthroscopic intervention in rotator cuff disease should be based upon sound principles established in the open treatment of the rotator cuff.

Despite early beliefs that the arthroscope's major benefit would be in diagnosis, isolated diagnostic arthroscopy is rarely indicated. Its most frequent use is in 'overlap patients', especially throwing athletes, in whom the relative contributions of instability and impingement are unclear. Far more commonly, diagnostic arthroscopy is combined with an operative procedure, both to confirm preoperative assessment of the extent of the tendon damage (e.g. in deciding whether to convert to an open procedure) and to uncover associated pathology (e.g. glenohumeral arthrosis).

There has been controversy as to the importance of information gained in this way. Cofield noted that although adjunctive arthroscopy allowed the accurate assessment of the presence and size of rotator cuff tears, this was already

known from preoperative studies in all cases in his series, and did not reliably determine the quality or mobility of the tissue.[55] Grana and co-workers[56] found that treatment of glenohumeral pathology discovered at arthroscopy did not affect the results of the rotator cuff procedure, except to increase the cost. However, many investigators have found the additional information clinically useful.[33,52,57–59] An impending biceps rupture may suggest the need for tenodesis; an articular surface partial rotator cuff tear which is extensive may require mini-open excision and repair;[60–62] labral pathology may require treatment;[63] and early arthritic changes of the articular surfaces may allow the surgeon to counsel the patient about a less favourable prognosis.

Arthroscopic treatment of partial-thickness tears

Although young athletic patients with minor degrees of partial-thickness rotator cuff damage may benefit from debridement alone,[64] this procedure resulted in a 50% failure rate when applied to a series of older patients with chronic shoulder pain and partial-thickness tears. Snyder[65] reported good results following an algorithm by which decompression was added to debridement of partial-thickness tears only if there was visible damage to the bursal side of the tendon (Figure 23.5). However, most investigators have included an acromioplasty as a routine part of the procedure.[66–68] The major unanswered question in both open and arthroscopic management of partial-thickness rotator cuff tears is when is more than simple decompression and debridement indicated? Fukuda et al[69] recommended open excision of the involved tendon along with decompression, an approach also used by Neviaser and co-workers.[68] Ellman[60] noted that of 20 incomplete tears treated by arthroscopic subacromial decompression, five (25%) required reoperation and two were found to have progressed to full-thickness tears. Weber and Schaefer[62] reported a series of patients with partial tears involving 50% or more of the tendon thickness: 40 were treated arthroscopically, while 35 under-

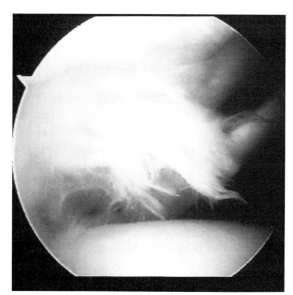

Fig. 23.5 Arthroscopic view of partial undersurface rotator cuff tear before debridement and arthroscopic subacromial decompression.[62]

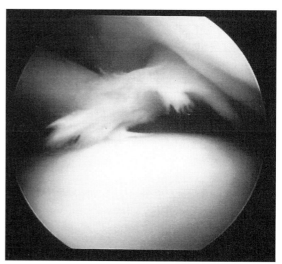

Fig. 23.6 Arthroscopic view of full-thickness rotator cuff tear before arthroscopic subacromial decompression combined with a mini-open tendon repair.

went mini-open repair. A higher percentage of the arthroscopic group had less than excellent results, and two patients developed complete tears. Healing of the partial tears was never seen at second-look arthroscopy. Open treatment with tendon repair has also been advised by others when more than half of the tendon is involved.[17,60,70] However, hard data to establish this criterion are not available. In the era before arthroscopy, excision and repair of significant partial tears seemed logical and added little morbidity to the already open procedure.[17] Currently, however, we generally treat patients with partial thickness tears with arthroscopic debridement and decompression, but warn them that their results may be less predictable, especially if a new trauma tears the weakened tendon. However, reoperation has in our experience been so rarely required that routine open treatment seems unnecessary.

Arthroscopic treatment of full-thickness tears

As previously outlined, open rotator cuff repair has been a reliable treatment for full-thickness tendon defects and remains the gold standard.

Options available for arthroscopic treatment of full-thickness tears include debridement without repair, arthroscopic subacromial decompression combined with a mini-open tendon repair and arthroscopic tendon repair (Figure 23.6).

Rockwood et al[71] have reported the results of subacromial decompression, debridement and rehabilitation for massive tears of the rotator cuff in 50 patients followed for an average of 6.5 years. Their results were satisfactory in 83% of shoulders which was attributed to a thorough decompression and intensive rehabilitation of the subscapularis, teres minor, deltoid and scapular stabilizers. However, in a prospective randomized study, Montgomery et al[72] compared 38 shoulders with chronic full-thickness tears of the rotator cuff treated with arthroscopic anterior acromioplasty and cuff debridement to 50 shoulders treated by open anterior acromioplasty and rotator cuff repair. They found that the open surgical repair group (78% satisfactory results) faired significantly better than the arthroscopic debridement group (39% satisfactory results) and they were unable to delineate any factors that would allow preoperative selection of patients who might do well after decompression alone. Five of their 38 patients treated by decompression and debridement developed cuff-tear arthropathy and the results from this procedure seemed to deteriorate with time. Apoil and co-workers[73] have abandoned debridement of massive tears, noting that more than a quarter of these patients developed arthropathy and superior subluxation with follow-up greater than 10 years. Harryman and colleagues[74] found that maintained integrity of the rotator cuff tendon at follow-up (as determined by ultrasonography) was the factor most significantly associated with a good functional result after repair. Although early arthroscopic experience with decompression without repair has been promising,[75,76] longer follow-up has documented results inferior to open repair in many independent series.[64,69,74–76] Burkhart[80–82] has proposed that better understanding of the pathomechanics will aid in patient selection for debridement, but further follow-up is needed to validate this approach.

Wiley[83] reported a serious complication of decompression and debridement without repair of large rotator cuff tears: superior humeral dislocation. As previously discussed, in patients with massive tears and associated superior migration of the humeral head, we have recently reported removal of the coracoacromial ligament, conservative anterior acromioplasty, and reinsertion of the coracoacromial ligament to the acromion in a more medial position in an attempt to prevent this complication.[40,41] In rare cases we have performed decompressions without repair, for example, an infirm elderly patient in severe pain who cannot comply with the protracted rehabilitation needed after tendon repair. We have not aggressively resected the coracoacromial arch but smoothed and contoured it, recognizing that it will continue to function as an articulating surface with the superiorly translating humeral head. Results from rotator cuff repair of large and massive tears[42,84] would suggest that this treatment offers reliable pain relief and provides a high percentage of satisfactory results which do not deteriorate with time. Until further compelling evidence is presented, subacromial decompression and rotator cuff repair, rather than decompression and debri-

dement, should be considered the standard for symptomatic tears of the rotator cuff.

The combination of arthroscopic subacromial decompression with an open tendon repair through a small deltoid split has become widely popular and increasingly accepted.[62,85–93] Arthroscopic localization of the tear allows precise incision placement, and newer suture-passing devices as well as implants have allowed the procedure to be performed through very small incisions. Reported results have been gratifying.[62,85–93] Perceived advantages over traditional open repair include deltoid preservation, quicker rehabilitation, shorter hospitalization, reduced early morbidity, a smaller scar and the addition of glenohumeral inspection to elucidate other pathology. Weber found similar long-term results but decreased early morbidity in patients undergoing arthroscopically assisted mini-open repair as compared with those undergoing traditional open cuff repair.[62]

Small easily mobilized tears are ideal for this approach, and tissue quality and elasticity are more important than exact tear size in determining repair potential.[94,95] Indeed, with a combination of arthroscopic and open releases, it is often surprising how large a tear may be repaired in this fashion. Tears involving multiple tendons with retraction, however, are preferably treated with the traditional open technique, as releases and tendon mobilization are facilitated, especially posteriorly. MRI can be extremely helpful in elucidating the size and morphology of the defect.

Despite the already low morbidity of mini-open repair, efforts have continued to find methods for entirely arthroscopic tendon repair. Transfixing implants, such as staples, have been used,[90] but problems with the metal staples have been worrisome.[90,95,96] Biodegradable tacks have also been employed.[90] However, primate studies have shown that cuff repairs take up to 2 years to regain full strength,[94,95] and are immediately stressed by early motion. Thus most investigators have preferred permanent fixation.

Suture anchors have been used in open rotator cuff surgery. Snyder & Bachner[97] have developed a technique of repair utilizing small screw suture anchors in arthroscopic surgery, and early results are encouraging. Nevertheless, the poor quality of greater tuberosity bone often seen in patients with cuff disease and osteoporosis has made this region seem less promising for implant technology than, say, the glenoid neck. At present, suture anchors are most helpful in the repair of subscapularis tears where the bone quality in the lesser tuberosity is better. This area is also more difficult to place bony tunnels because of the low profile of the lesser tuberosity. Continued experimental investigations into the possibility of suture repair to bone continues. Further advancements in this evolving area and analysis of long-term results will facilitate definition of the appropriate indications for arthroscopic rotator cuff repair.

RESULTS

Since Neer's report on the routine use of anterior acromioplasty in combination with rotator cuff mobilization and repair in 1972,[13] rotator cuff repair has been associated with improved results in many studies. In a review on rotator cuff tears, Cofield[25] found that an average of 85% of patients could be expected to achieve satisfactory results after repair, with a range from 65 to 100% reported in the literature. We have recently reported our results of rotator cuff repair on 481 patients and found 92% of patients had a satisfactory result, with pain relief reliably achieved in 96% of patients.[84] The fact that pain relief is predictable and nearly universally achieved reinforces the premise that pain remains the primary indication for rotator cuff repair.[13,25,84,97–99]

Functional results after rotator cuff repair, however, are more difficult to quantify and have been a topic of controversy. Walker et al[46] showed by isometric strength testing of 33 postoperative shoulders that external rotation strength reached 90% of normal by 1 year after surgery, which was an improvement over that measured at 6 months. They also showed no difference in external rotation strength when comparing small and large tears. Heikel,[100] on the other hand, demonstrated that 55% of patients had moderate or considerable weakness in shoulder abduction

and flexion at an average of 35 months after rotator cuff repair. Gore et al[101] objectively measured postoperative isokinetic strength in 63 shoulders at an average of 5.5 years after cuff repair and found abduction strength to be 78% of normal and flexion strength 90% of normal; abduction strength, however, significantly decreased as the size of the tear increased. They also found a positive correlation between the objective results of isometric shoulder strength and range of motion with their patient's subjective results after surgery. Although the degree of functional improvement reported in studies is difficult to compare, most reports indicate that approximately 75–95% of patients have significant improvement in shoulder function after rotator cuff repair.

A significant shortcoming in comparing these functional results is the lack of a standardized tool of measuring outcomes. Outcomes research is important to promote communication between investigators, permit and encourage multicentre trials, and to allow the exchange of useful and relevant outcome data to physicians, healthcare administrators and the general public. The membership of the American Shoulder and Elbow Surgeons have recently adopted a single standardized method of assessing shoulder function and have called for its universal adoption.[102] Although studies to test its applicability and validity across different patient populations have yet to be performed, it may serve as a useful means of facilitating accurate comparisons between studies.

Separating and categorizing potential clinical factors which may affect the result after rotator cuff surgery is extremely difficult, as they are frequently highly interdependent. The most commonly cited factor that affects surgical outcome is rotator cuff size. Owing to different shapes of tendon defects as well as varying degrees of cuff elasticity and mobility, the development of a consistent and accurate classification for reporting rotator cuff tear size has also been difficult. The most commonly used system is that proposed by Post and co-workers[19] who defined small tears as those less than 1 cm at greatest diameter, medium tears 1–3 cm, large tears 3–5 cm, and massive tears greater than 5 cm in diameter. In addition, Gerber et al[103] described a classification of rotator cuff size based on the size of the defect after mobilization as well as the ability of the surgeon to approximate the tear to a bony trough near the greater tuberosity.

Although McLaughlin et al and others have stated that the overall results of rotator cuff surgery were not significantly affected by cuff tear size, Cofield and co-workers[104] found that tear size is the single most important factor influencing long-term results. Also, several studies have found that results after rotator cuff repair are better and more predictable with smaller tears.[15,17,42–44,105] When results are unsatisfactory after rotator cuff repair, the majority are due to decreased strength and function which is attributable to the poor quality of existing rotator cuff tissue in patients with larger tears, rather than unsatisfactory pain relief. Bigliani et al[42] reported 92% satisfactory pain relief after repair of massive rotator cuff tears, which is in agreement with the observation of Hawkins et al[16] and others that the achievement of satisfactory pain relief after rotator cuff repair is independent of cuff tear size. Although it is now generally agreed that the best overall results are seen with repair of smaller rotator cuff tears, surgical repair of massive tears is worthwhile because of the high level of pain relief achievable in this difficult patient population. Bigliani et al[42] concluded that, although repair of a massive rotator cuff tear is a tedious, demanding procedure, the results are rewarding if technical principles are strictly followed.

The results of alternatives to repair of massive rotator cuff tears have been mixed. Decompression, debridement of the tendon edges and rehabilitation is advocated by some; however, as previously outlined, this procedure is not currently widely accepted because of concerns about function and deteriorating results with time. Cofield[106] has recommended transposition of the subscapularis tendon superiorly for repair of large cuff defects, particularly those involving the supraspinatus tendon. Gerber[107] has described transfer of the latissimus dorsi as a reconstructive procedure for a cuff-deficient shoulder, but warns that it should not be considered as an alternative to repair. Its use is primarily indicated for patients with loss of external rotation strength and irreparable defects of the posterior cuff, including the infraspinatus and teres minor. Gerber reported approximately 80% restoration of normal shoulder function when using the latissimus dorsi transfer, provided subscapularis function was intact. Other local tendon flaps, fascia lata grafts, freeze-dried rotator cuff and prosthetic grafts have all been described to repair massive cuff defects, with variable success. Experience with these different techniques is limited.

Another factor that may potentially affect surgical outcome is the timing of repair. Although some authors have recommended early repair after acute rotator cuff tears, many have reported that delaying repair does not negatively affect the outcome. The question is whether the acute tear is the endpoint of a degenerative process brought on by a trivial traumatic event, or whether it is an avulsion of an otherwise normal rotator cuff which occurs with forced contraction of an eccentrically loaded tendon. Many factors, such as age, previous symptoms, history of corticosteroid injections, degree of traumatic injury, are incorporated into this decision-making process. The assocation of rotator cuff disruption occurring in the setting of concomitant acute anterior shoulder dislocation has been well described, and unrecognized and untreated disruption of the rotator cuff tear in this patient population has a poor prognosis. Newer imaging technology, especially MRI, has helped in determining the size of the rotator cuff defect and amount of retraction of its tendons. Bassett and Cofield[108] show that in patients who have a significant acute injury and a full-thickness rotator cuff tear, repair carried out within 3 weeks of injury afforded the best surgical results. They recommended early surgical repair of acute rotator cuff tears in active patients who place high demands on their shoulders.

Rotator cuff injury in athletes often presents a more confusing clinical scenario than that of the non-athletic population. Sports requiring repetitive overhead movements cause injury to the rotator cuff as a result of creating large amounts of strain within the tendon during both the deceleration phase of throwing and from compression.[109] This overuse causes fatigue of the rotator cuff tendons which often leads to rotator cuff tendinitis and functional weakness, bursal scarring and coracoacromial ligament hypertrophy. Thus secondary subacromial impingement[33,109–111] and subsequent rotator cuff damage may ensue. Also, it is not uncommon to find the association of secondary subacromial impingement in the overhead athlete with primary subtle glenohumeral instability. When faced with this differential, it should be emphasized that all overhead athletes cannot be placed in a single treatment category. Efforts to try to determine the relative contributions of impingement or instability in these overlap patients is necessary before treatment can be rendered. This information should then be used to guide therapy.

Non-operative management of rotator cuff problems in the overhead athlete should be aggressively pursued initially, including stretching with rotator cuff and periscapular muscle strengthening. If non-operative treatment fails, rotator cuff surgery in this population can provide satisfactory relief of pain, although return to previous level of sporting activity has been inconsistent.[15,105,109,111] Controversies continue in regard to stabilization versus decompression, arthroscopic versus open procedures, and repair of partial-thickness rotator cuff tears versus debridement. It is generally agreed, however, that the principal underlying diagnosis based on the entire clinical picture should be used to dictate the appropriate surgical procedure for each individual athlete.

COMPLICATIONS

With recent technical advances, most symptomatic tears of the rotator cuff can be repaired successfully, with good relief of pain and improvement of function. However, operative repair is not always successful in these patients. Complications may occur and several factors have been associated with failure of repairs, including a large or massive tear, a rotator cuff tendon of poor quality, an inadequate repair due to technical problems, damage to the deltoid origin with or

without a lateral or radical acromionectomy at the time of the procedure, inadequate subacromial decompression,[18,43] insufficient postoperative external support and improper rehabilitation. By following technical considerations as previously outlined in this chapter, many complications and/or poor outcomes can be avoided.

The approach to a failed repair of a rotator cuff must be thoughtful and comprehensive. Potential concomitant diagnoses, such as cervical spine abnormalities, acromioclavicular arthritis, adhesive capsulitis and calcific tendinitis must all be thoroughly evaluated. Every attempt must be made to determine the cause of failure before reoperation. Previous operative notes should be reviewed to determine the exact procedure performed. The history and physical examination should focus not only on the shoulder, but the entire cervical spine and extremity. It is important to determine what the patient's symptoms were before the initial procedure and how he or she fared after the operation. What was the postoperative rehabilitation protocol? Was there ever pain relief and/or functional improvement? Was there additional trauma to explain the poor outcome? Differential injections can play an important role in working through the differential diagnosis. Plain radiographs should be repeated and examined for persistent acromial or acromioclavicular joint spurs. Electrodiagnostic studies may be indicated if significant weakness persists, to rule out suprascapular or axillary nerve damage. Although the role of MRI is controversial in this situation, it may be helpful in determining the size of the rotator cuff tear and/or the amount of retraction as well as potential humeral head and articular surface damage.

The primary indication for revision rotator cuff repair is pain relief. The ability to provide functional improvements has been shown to be much less reliable. Factors associated with unsatisfactory results from revision repair, which have ranged from 48–58%,[43,105,112] include a previous lateral acromionectomy, a detached deltoid origin and/or deltoid dysfunction, and the finding that the tissue of the rotator cuff that was available at the time of the repeat operation was of poor quality. If these findings are present, DeOrio and Cofield[43]

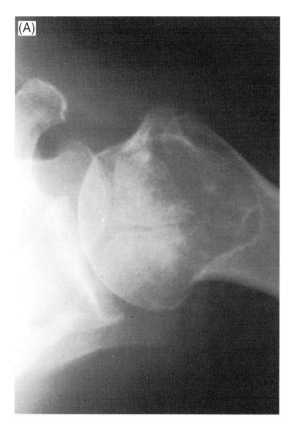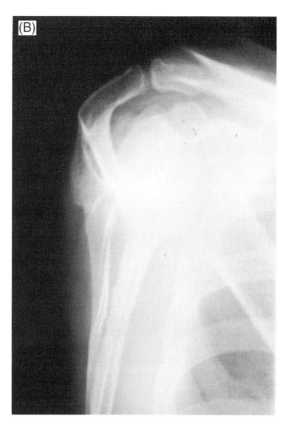

Fig. 23.7 Axillary (A) and supraspinatus outlet (B) radiographs of shoulder with os acromionale in a patient with subacromial impingement and a full-thickness rotator cuff tear.

have recommended consideration of immediate glenohumeral arthrodesis rather than revision repair.

An unrecognized unfused acromial epiphysis may occasionally cause persistent impingement and pain after rotator cuff repair (Figure 23.7). This can be a very difficult problem to correct. If there is no motion at the site of the non–union and there is a stable fibrous union, a routine anterior acromioplasty should be performed. If a small fragment is encountered, it can be excised without difficulty. Removal of a large anterior fragment of the epiphysis can lead to weakness and retraction of the deltoid. However, others have reported satisfactory results with excision. Furthermore, a repair of the acromion can be extremely difficult, with a high prevalence of failure of the hardware. We no longer use metal devices for internal fixation.[113] Instead, we split

the deltoid anterior to the acromion and remove the undersurface of the bone, leaving the superior cortex. Recently, several patients have had a satisfactory result after use of this technique.[113,114]

SUMMARY

Symptomatic tears of the rotator cuff can be successfully managed with operative repair. Performing an adequate subacromial decompression, maintaining the integrity of the deltoid, mobilizing and preserving the remaining rotator cuff tissue, and carefully staging and supervising the rehabilitation programme are factors that will lead to favourable results. Patient satisfaction and pain relief are reliably achieved in the majority of patients. By following the techniques of repair as presented, the presence of a large or massive tear does not preclude a satisfactory result and/or adequate pain relief.

Arthroscopy has improved our diagnostic assessment of rotator cuff disease, especially in understanding patterns of articular surface partial thickness tears. Despite continued controversy, most partial thickness rotator cuff tears may be satisfactorily treated by arthroscopic debridement and decompression. The role for debridement and decompression without repair for full-thickness rotator cuff tears seems less than initially suggested, as several recent independent studies have documented results inferior to open repair. Arthroscopically assisted mini-open repair of small full-thickness rotator cuff tears is a reliable procedure. Arthroscopic repair appears promising, but it is not yet well enough documented to be considered a standard of treatment.

REFERENCES

1. Smith, J.G. (1834) Pathological appearances of seven cases of injury of the shoulder joint with remarks. *London Med. Gaz.* **14:** 280.
2. Codman, E.A. (1911) Complete rupture of the supraspinatus tendon: Operative treatment with report of two successful cases. *Boston Med. Surg. J.* **164:** 708–710.
3. Codman, E.A. (1934) *The Shoulder, Rupture of the Supraspinatus Tendon and Other Lesions in or about the Subacromial Bursa.* Boston: Thomas Todd.
4. Wilson, P.D. (1931) Complete rupture of the supraspinatus tendon. *J. Am. Med. Assoc.* **96:** 433–438.
5. Bosworth, D.M. (1940) An analysis of twenty-eight consecutive cases of incapacitating shoulder lesions, radically explored and repaired. *J. Bone Joint Surg.* **22:** 369–392.
6. McLaughlin, H.L. (1944) Lesions of the musculotendinous cuff of the shoulder: 1. The exposure and treatment of tears with retraction. *J. Bone Joint Surg.* **26:** 31–51.
7. McLaughlin, H.L. (1963) Repair of major cuff ruptures. *Surg. Clin. North Am.* **43:** 1535–1540.
8. McLaughlin, H.L. & Asherman, E.G. (1951) Lesions of the musculotendinous cuff of the shoulder. IV: Some observations based upon the results of surgical repair. *J. Bone Joint Surg.* **33A:** 76–86.
9. Bartolozzi, A., Andreychik, D. & Ahmad, S. (1994) Determinants of outcome in the treatment of rotator cuff disease. *Clin. Orthop.* **308:** 90–97.
10. Watson, M. (1985) Major ruptures of the rotator cuff.

11. Wolfgang, G.L. (1974) Surgical repair of tears of the rotator cuff of the shoulder: factors influencing the result. *J. Bone Joint Surg.* **56A:** 14–26.
12. Codman, E.A. (1937) Rupture of the supraspinatus. *J. Bone Joint Surg.* **19:** 643–652.
13. Neer, C.S. II (1972) Anterior acromioplasty for the chronic impingement syndrome in the shoulder: a preliminary report. *J. Bone Joint Surg.* **54:** 41–50.
14. Cofield, R.H. (1985) Current concepts review: rotator cuff disease of the shoulder. *J. Bone Joint Surg.* **67A:** 974–979.
15. Ellman, H., Hanker, G. & Baer, M. (1986) Repair of the rotator cuff: end-result study of factors influencing reconstruction. *J. Bone Joint Surg.* **68A:** 1136–1144.
16. Hawkins, R.J., Missnore, G.W. & Hobecka, P.E. (1985) Surgery for full-thickness rotator cuff tears. *J. Bone Joint Surg.* **67A:** 1349–1355.
17. Neer, C.S. II, Flatow, E.L. & Lech, O. (1988) Tears of the rotator cuff. Long term results of anterior acromioplasty and repair. *Orthop. Trans.* **12:** 735.
18. Packer, N.P., Calvert, P.T., Bayley, J.I.L. & Kessel, L. (1983) Operative treatment of chronic ruptures of the rotator cuff of the shoulder. *J. Bone Joint Surg.* **65B:** 171–175.
19. Post, M., Silver, R. & Singh, M. (1983) Rotator cuff tear. Diagnosis and treatment. *Clin. Orthop.* **173:** 78–92.
20. Burns, T.P. & Turba, J.E. (1992) Arthroscopic treatment of shoulder impingement in athletes. *Am. J. Sports Med.* **20:** 13–16.
21. Ellman, H. & Kay, S.P. (1991) Arthoscopic subacromial decompression for chronic impingement: two- to five-year results. *J. Bone Joint Surg.* **73B:** 395–398.
22. Esch, J.C., Ozerkis, L.R., Helgager, J.A., Kane, N. & Lilliott, N. (1988) Arthroscopic subacromial decompression: results according to the degree of rotator cuff tear. *Arthroscopy* **4:** 241–249.
23. Miniaci, A., Dowdy, P.A., Willits, K.R. et al. (1995) Magnetic resonance imaging evaluation of the rotator cuff tendons in the asymptomatic shoulder. *Am. J. Sports Med.* **23:** 142–145.
24. Sher, Uribe, Posada, et al. (1995) Abnormal findings on magnetic resonance images of asyptomatic shoulders. *J. Bone Joint Surg.*
25. Cofield, R.H. (1985) Rotator cuff disease of the shoulder. *J. Bone Joint Surg.* **67A:** 974–979.
26. Neer, C.S. II (1983) Impingement lesions. *Clin. Orthop.* **173:** 70–77.
27. Bigliani, L.U., Morrison, D.S. & April, E.W. (1986) The morphology of the acromion and its relationship to rotator cuff tears. *Orthop. Trans.* **10:** 228.
28. Bigliani, L.U., Ticker, J.B., Flatow, E.L., Soslowsky, L.J. & Mow, V.C. (1991) The relationship of acromial architecture to rotator cuff disease. *Clin. Sports Med.* **10:** 823–838.

The results of surgical repair in 89 patients. *J. Bone Joint Surg.* **67B:** 618–624.

29. Soslowsky, L.J., An, C.H., Johnston, S.P. & Carpenter, J.E. (1994) Geometric and mechanical properties of the coraco-acromial ligament and their relationship to rotator cuff disease. *Clin. Orthop.* 10–17.

30. Zuckerman, J.D., Klummer, F.J., Cuomo, F., Simon, J. & Rosenblum, S. (1992) The influence of the coraco-acromial arch anatomy on rotator cuff tears. *J. Shoulder Elbow Surg.* **1:** 4–14.

31. Walch, G., Boileau, P., Noel, E. & Donell, S.T. (1992) Impingement of the deep surface of the supraspinatus tendon on the posterosuperior glenoid rim: an arthroscopic study. *J. Shoulder Elbow Surg.* **1:** 238–245.

32. Uhthoff, H.K., Hammond, D.I., Sarkar, K., Hooper, G.J. & Papoff, W.J. (1988) The role of the coracoacromial ligament in the impingement syndrome. A clinical, radiological and histological study. *Int. Orthop.* **12:** 97–104.

33. Jobe, F.W. & Bradley, J.P. (1988) Rotator cuff injuries in baseball: prevention and rehabilitation. *Sports Med.* **6:** 378–387.

34. Rathburn, J.B. & Macnab, I. (1970) The microvascular pattern of the rotator cuff. *J. Bone Joint Surg.* **52B:** 540–553.

35. Fukuda, H., Hamada, K., Nakajima, T. & Tomonaga, A. (1994) Pathology and pathogenesis of the intratendinous tearing of the rotator cuff viewed from en bloc histologic sections. *Clin. Orthop.* **11:** 60–67.

36. Nakajima, T., Rokuuma, N., Hamada, K., Tomatsu, T. & Fukuda, H. (1994) Histologic and biomechanical characteristics of the supraspinatus tendon: reference to rotator cuff tearing. *J. Shoulder Elbow Surg.* **3:** 79–87.

37. Nicholson, G.P., Goodman, D.A., Pollock, R.G., Flatow, E.L. & Bigliani, L.U. (1993) The acromion: morphology and age related changes. A study of 420 scapulae. *Orthop. Trans.* **17:** 976.

38. Flatow, E.L., Soslowsky, L.J., Ticker, J.B., Pawluk, R.J., Hepler, M., Ark, J., Mow, V.C. & Bigliani, L.U. (1994) Excursion of the rotator cuff under the acromion: patterns of subacromial contact. *Am. J. Sports Med.* **22:** 779–788.

39. Neer, C.S. II (1990) *Shoulder Reconstruction*, pp. 41–142. Philadelphia: W.B. Saunders.

40. Flatow, E.L., Weinstein, D.M., Duralde, X.A., Compito, C.A., Pollock, R.G. & Bigliani, L.U. (1994) Coracoacromial ligament preservation in rotator cuff surgery. *J. Shoulder Elbow Surg.* **3:** S73.

41. Weinstein, D.M., Bucchieri, J.S., Pollock, R.G., Flatow, E.L. & Bigliani, L.U. (1993) Arthroscopic debridement of the shoulder for osteoarthritis. *Arthroscopy* **9:** 366.

42. Bigliani, L.U., Cordasco, F.A., McIlveen, S.J. & Musso, E.S. (1992) Operative treatment of massive rotator cuff tears: long-term results. *J. Shoulder Elbow Surg.* **1:** 120–130.

43. DeOrio, J.K. & Cofield, R.H. (1984) Results of a second attempt at surgical repair of a failed initial rotator cuff repair. *J. Bone Joint Surg.* **66A:** 563–567.

44. Neer, C.S. II & Marberry, T.A. (1981) On the disadvantages of radical acromionectomy. *J. Bone Joint Surg.* **63A:** 416–419.

45. Swointkowsky, M.F., Iannotti, J.P., Boulas, H.J. et al. (1990) Intraoperative assessment of rotator cuff vascularity using laser doppler flowmetry. In Post, M., Morrey, B.F. & Hawkins, R.I. (eds) *Surgery of the Shoulder*, pp. 202–212. St. Louis: Mosby-Year Book.

46. Walker, S.W., Couch, W.H., Boester, G.A. et al. (1987) Isokinetic strength of the shoulder after repair of a torn rotator cuff. *J. Bone Joint Surg.* **69:** 1041–1044.

47. Gerber, C. & Krushell, R.J. (1991) Isolated rupture of the tendon of the subscapularis muscle. Clinical features in 16 cases. *J. Bone Joint Surg.* **73B:** 389–394.

48. Mendoza Lopez, M., Cardoner Parpal, J.C., Samso Bardes, F. et al. (1994) Lesions of the subscapular tendon regarding two cases in arthroscopic surgery. *Arthroscopy* **10:** 239.

49. Neer, C.S. II, Craig, E.V. & Fukuda, H. (1983) Cuff tear arthropathy. *J. Bone Joint Surg.* **65A:** 1232–1244.

50. Neer, C.S., Watson, K.C. & Stanton, F.J. (1982) Recent experience in total shoulder replacement. *J. Bone Joint Surg.* **64A:** 319–337.

51. Neer, C.S. (1985) Unconstrained shoulder arthroplasty. *Instr. Course Lect.* **34:** 278–286.

52. Franklin, J.L., Barrett, W.P., Jackins, S.E. & Matsen, F.A. (1988) Glenoid loosening in total shoulder arthroplasty. *J. Arthroplasty* **3:** 39–46.

53. Arntz, C.T., Jackins, S. & Matsen, F.A. III (1993) Prosthetic replacement of the shoulder for the treatment of defects in the rotator cuff and the surface of the glenohumeral joint. *J. Bone Joint Surg.* **75A:** 485–491.

54. Pollock, R.G., Deliz, E.D., McIlveen, S.J., Flatow, E.L. & Bigliani, L.U. (1992) Prosthetic replacement in rotator cuff deficient shoulders. *J. Shoulder Elbow Surg.* **1:** 173–186.

55. Cofield, R.H. (1984) The role of arthroscopy in surgery of the shoulder. In Bateman, J.E. & Welsh, R.P. (eds) *Surgery of the Shoulder*, pp. 45–50. Philadelphia: Decker.

56. Grana, W.A., Teague, B., King, M. & Reeves, R.B. (1994) An analysis of rotator cuff repair. *Am. J. Sports Med.* **22:** 585–588.

57. Jobe, F.W. & Kvitne, R.S. (1989) Shoulder pain in the overhand or throwing athlete. The relationship of anterior instability and rotator cuff impingement. *Orthop. Rev.* **18:** 963–975.

58. Miller, C. & Savoie, F.H. (1993) Glenohumeral abnormalities associated with full thickness rotator cuff tears. *Orthop. Trans.* **17:** 449.

59. Paulos, L.E. & Franklin, J.L. (1990) Arthroscopic shoulder decompression development and application. A five year experience. *Am. J. Sports Med.* **18:** 234–244.

60. Ellman, H. (1990) Diagnosis and treatment of incomplete rotator cuff tears. *Clin. Orthop.* **254:** 64–74.

61. Ogilvie-Harris, D.J., Wiley, A.M. & Sattarian, J. (1990)

Failed acromioplasty for impingement syndrome. *J. Bone Joint Surg.* **72B:** 1070–1072.

62. Weber, S.C. & Schaefer, R. (1993) 'Mini-open' versus traditional open repair in the management of small and moderate size tears of the rotator cuff. *Arthroscopy* **9:** 365–366.

63. Cordasco, F.A., Steinmann, S., Flatow, E.L. & Bigliani, L.U. (1993) Arthroscopic treatment of glenoid labral tears. *Am. J. Sports Med.* **21:** 425–431.

64. Andrews, J.R., Broussard, T.S. & Carson, W.G. (1985) Arthoscopy of the shoulder in the management of partial tears of the rotator cuff: a preliminary report. *Arthroscopy* **1:** 117–122.

65. Snyder, S.J. (1993) Evaluation and treatment of the rotator cuff. *Orthop. Clin. North Am.* **24:** 173–192.

66. Ellman, H. (1989) Arthroscopic treatment of impingement of the shoulder. *Instr. Course Lect.* **38:** 177–185.

67. Gartsman, G.M. (1990) Arthoscopic acromioplasty for lesions of the rotator cuff. *J. Bone Joint Surg.* **72A:** 169–180.

68. Neviaser, T.J., Neviaser, R.J. & Neviaser, J.S. (1994) Incomplete rotator cuff tears. A technique for diagnosis and treatment. *Clin. Orthop.* 12–16.

69. Fukuda, H., Craig, E.V. & Yamanaka, K. (1987) Surgical treatment of incomplete thickness tears of rotator cuff: long term follow-up. *Orthop. Trans.* **11:** 237–238.

70. Neviaser, T.J., Neviaser, R.J., Neviaser, J.S. & Neviaser, J.S. (1982) The four-in-one arthroplasty for the painful arc syndrome. *Clin. Orthop.* **163:** 107–112.

71. Rockwood, C.A., Williams, G.R. & Burkhead, W.Z. (1995) Debridement of degenerative, irreparable lesions of the rotator cuff. *J. Bone Joint Surg.* **77A:** 857–866.

72. Montgomery, T.J., Yerger, B. & Savoie, F.H. (1994) Management of rotator cuff tears: a comparison of arthroscopic debridement and surgical repair. *J. Shoulder Elbow Surg.* **3:** 70–78.

73. Apoil, A. & Augereau, B. (1990) Anterosuperior arthrolysis of the shoulder for rotator cuff degenerative lesions. In M. Post, B.F. Morrey & R.J. Hawkins (eds) *Surgery of the Shoulder*, pp. 257–260. St. Louis: Mosby Year Book.

74. Harryman, D.T., Mack, L.A., Wang, K.Y., Jackins, S.E., Richardson, M.L. & Matsen, F.A. III (1991) Repairs of the rotator cuff: correlation of functional results with integrity of the cuff. *J. Bone Joint Surg.* **73A:** 982–989.

75. Levy, H.J., Gardner, R.D. & Lemak, L.J. (1991) Arthroscopic subacromial decompression in the treatment of full-thickness rotator cuff tears. *Arthroscopy* **7:** 8–13.

76. Olsewski, J.M. & Depew, A.D. (1994) Arthroscopic subacromial decompression and rotator cuff debridement for stage II and stage III impingement. *Arthroscopy* **10:** 61–68.

77. Ogilvie-Harris, D.J. & Demaziere, A. (1993) Arthroscopic debridement versus open repair for rotator cuff tears: a prospective cohort study. *J. Bone Joint Surg.* **75B:** 416–420.

78. Seitz, W.H. Jr & Froimson, A.I. (1992) Comparison of arthroscopic subacromial decompression in partial and full thickness rotator cuff tears. *J. Bone Joint Surg.* **74B** (Suppl. III): 294.

79. Zvijac, J.E., Levy, H.J. & Lemak, L.L. (1994) Arthroscopic subacromial decompression in the treatment of full-thickness rotator cuff tears: a 3- to 6-year follow-up. *Arthroscopy* **10:** 518–523.

80. Burkhart, S.S. (1993) Arthroscopic debridement and decompression for selected rotator cuff tears: clinical results, pathomechanics, and patient selection based on biomechanical parameters. *Orthop. Clin. North Am.* **24:** 111–123.

81. Burkhart, S.S. (1994) Reconciling the paradox of rotator cuff repair versus debridement: a unified biomechanical rationale for the treatment of rotator cuff tears. *Arthroscopy* **10:** 4–19.

82. Burkhart, S.S., Nottage, W.M., Ogilvie-Harris, D.J., Kohn, H.S. & Pachelli, A. (1994) Partial repair of irreparable rotator cuff tears. *Arthroscopy* **10:** 363–370.

83. Wiley, A.M. (1991) Superior humeral dislocation: a complication following decompression and debridement for rotator cuff tears. *Clin. Orthop.* **263:** 135–141.

84. Black, A.D., Codd, T.D., Rodosky, M.W. et al. (1995) Surgical management of rotator cuff disease. Presented at the American Academy of Orthopaedic Surgeons 62nd Annual Meeting, February 16–21, Orlando, Florida.

85. Baker, C.L. & Liu, S.H. (1995) Comparison of open and arthroscopically assisted rotator cuff repairs. *Am. J. Sports Med.* **23:** 99–104.

86. Flynn, L.M., Flood, S.J., Clifford, S., Brown, T., Jongko, T., Brannan, J. & Sloan, K.W. (1991) Arthroscopically assisted rotator cuff repair with the Mitek anchor. *Am. J. Arthroscopy* **1:** 15–18.

87. Levy, H.J., Uribe, J.W. & Delaney, L.G. (1990) Arthroscopic assisted rotator cuff repair: preliminary results. *Arthroscopy* **6:** 55–60.

88. Liu, S.H. (1994) Arthroscopically-assisted rotator-cuff repair. *J. Bone Joint Surg.* **76B:** 592–595.

89. Liu, S.H. & Baker, C.L. (1994) Arthroscopically assisted rotator cuff repair: correlation of functional results with integrity of the cuff. *Arthroscopy* **10:** 54–60.

90. Paletta, G.A. Jr, Warner, J.J.P., Altchek, D.W., Wickiewicz, T.L., O'Brien, S.J. & Warren, R.F. (1993) Arthroscopic-assisted rotator cuff repair: evaluation of results and a comparison of techniques. *Orthop. Trans.* **17:** 139.

91. Paulos, L.E. & Kody, M.H. (1994) Arthroscopically enhanced mini approach to rotator cuff repair. *Am. J. Sports Med.* **22:** 19–25.

92. Seltzer, D.G. & Zvijac, J. (1994) The technique of

arthroscopy-assisted rotator cuff repair. *Tech. Orthop.* **8:** 212–224.

93. Warner, J.J.P., Altchek, D.W. & Warren, R.F. (1991) Arthroscopic management of rotator cuff tears with emphasis on the throwing athlete. *Op. Tech. Orthop.* **1:** 235–239.

94. Paulos, L.E., France, E.P., Boam, G.W., Tearse, D.S., Grauer, J.D., Stonebrook, S.N. & Healey, J.E. (1990) Augmentation of rotator cuff repair: *in vivo* evaluation in primates. *Orthop. Trans.* **14:** 404.

95. France, E.P., Paulos, L.E., Harner, C.D. & Straight, C.B. (1989) Biomechanical evaluation of rotator cuff fixation methods. *Am. J. Sports Med.* **17:** 176–181.

96. Flatow, E.L. & Bigliani, L.U. (1992) Complications of rotator cuff repair. Complications in Orthop. **8:** 298–303.

97. Snyder, S.J. & Bachner, E.J. (1993) Arthroscopic fixation of rotator cuff tears: a preliminary report. *Arthroscopy* **9:** 342.

98. Bigliani, L.U., Kimmel, J., McCann, P.D. & Wolfe, I. (1992) Repair of rotator cuff tears in tennis players. *Am. J. Sports Med.* **20:** 112–117.

99. Flatow, E.L., Fischer, R.A. & Bigliani, L.U. (1991) Results of surgery. In J.P. Ianotti (ed) *Rotator Cuff Disorders: Evaluation and Treatment,* pp. 53–63. American Academy of Orthopaedic Surgeons, Park Ridge, Illinois.

100. Heikel, H.V.A. (1968) Rupture of the rotator cuff of the shoulder: experience of surgical treatment. *Acta Orthop. Scand.* **39:** 477–492.

101. Gore, D.R., Murray, M.P., Sepic, S.B. et al. (1986) Shoulder muscle strength and range of motion following surgical repair of full-thickness rotator cuff tears. *J. Bone Joint Surg.* **68A:** 266–272.

102. Richards, R.R., An, K.N., Bigliani, L.U. et al. (1994) A standardized method for the assessment of shoulder function. *J. Shoulder Elbow Surg.* **3:** 347–352.

103. Gerber, C., Schneeberger, A.G., Beck, M. & Schlegel, U. (1994) Mechanical strength of repairs of the rotator cuff. *J. Bone Joint Surg.* **76B:** 371–380.

104. Cofield, R.H., Hoffmeyer, P. & Lanzar, W.H. (1990) Surgical repair of chronic rotator cuff tears. *Orthop. Trans.* **14:** 251–252.

105. Bigliani, L.U., Cordasco, F.A., McIlveen, S.J. & Musso, E.S. (1992) Operative treatment of failed repairs of the rotator cuff. *J. Bone Joint Surg.* **74A:** 1505–1515.

106. Cofield, R.H. (1982) Subscapular muscle transposition for repair of chronic rotator cuff tears. *Surg. Gynecol. Obstet.* **154:** 667–672.

107. Gerber, C. (1992) Latissimus dorsi transfer for the treatment of irreparable tears of the rotator cuff. *Clin. Orthop.* **275:** 152–160.

108. Bassett, R.W. & Cofield, R.H. (1983) Acute tears of the rotator cuff. The timing of surgical repairs. *Clin. Orthop.* **175:** 18–24.

109. Hawkins, R.J. & Kennedy, J.C. (1981) Impingement syndrome in athletes. *Am. J. Sports Med.* **6:** 151.

110. Jackson, D.W. (1976) Chronic rotator cuff impingement in the throwing athlete. *Am. J. Sports Med.* **4:** 231–240.

111. Tibone, J.E., Elrod, B. & Jobe, F.W. (1986) Shoulder impingement syndrome in athletes treated by an anterior acromioplasty. *J. Bone Joint Surg.* **68A:** 887–891.

112. Neviaser, R.J. & Neviaser, T.J. (1989) Reoperation for failed rotator cuff repair: analysis of forty-six cases. *Orthop. Trans.* **13:** 241.

113. Armengol, J., Brittis, D., Pollock, R.G., Flatow, E.L., Self, E.B. & Bigliani, L.U. (1994) The association of an unfused acromial epiphysis with tears of the rotator cuff: a review of 41 cases. *J. Shoulder Elbow Surg.* **3:** S14.

114. Hutchinson, M.R. & Veenstra, M.A. (1993) Arthoscopic decompression of shoulder impingement secondary to os acromiale. *Arthroscopy* **9:** 28–32.

24

The Biceps Tendon

SA Copeland

INTRODUCTION

The function of the biceps tendon at the shoulder has been surprisingly difficult to define. As the tendon anatomically crosses two joints, the shoulder and the elbow, it is difficult to consider its function of one joint without considering the other. Initially it was thought to be a primary head depressor acting in concert with the rotator cuff, but more recent work by Jobe and co-workers[1] indicates that the electrical activity in biceps is more associated with movement of the elbow than it is of the shoulder. However, Glousman and associates[2] report an increased activity in the biceps during throwing in patients with unstable shoulders. It seems therefore that the biceps may take on more importance as a primary stabilizer in the injured shoulder. Additional evidence for this view comes from the occasional finding in a massive rotator cuff tear of hypertrophy of the remaining biceps tendon. However, if the biceps is subluxed out of its groove, this does not occur. It therefore does appear to have some head depressor effect in the cuff-deficient shoulder. Berlemann & Bayley[3] have shown the long-term results of biceps tenodesis, and upward subluxation of the humeral head is noted, although this may be in part due to rotator cuff deterioration.

Warner and McMahon[4] have recently shown that the tendon of the long head of biceps acts as a stabilizer of the humeral head in the glenoid during abduction of the shoulder in the scapular plane.

It therefore appears to have a contributory role in many aspects of shoulder function, but little primary function that can be isolated. It is for this reason that there is no one clinical test that can reliably determine pain arising in the biceps tendon region. Many tests have been described, but the 'palm up' test appears to be the most reliable. The patient is asked to turn the palm upwards with elbow extended and elevate the straight arm against resistance. A positive test is denoted by pain in the region of the biceps groove. If this pain is abolished by localized injection into the biceps groove, this may confirm it as the site of pathology.

BICEPS TENDINITIS

In the majority of patients the tendinitis of the long head of biceps is part of an anterior rotator cuff impingement syndrome as the biceps passes through the 'impingement area'. In the majority, decompression alone by anterior acromioplasty can relieve symptoms. However, rarely, primary biceps tendinitis does occur. Berlemann & Bayley[3] carried out an interesting long-term study of patients who had had biceps tenodesis at an average follow-up of 7 years. In this series, approximately half of the patients had prior decompression, but with persistent symptoms relieved by eventual tenodesis.

If considering either repair or tenodesis of the biceps tendon, then decompression must also be part of the procedure.

Anterior acromioplasty and excision of the coracoacromial ligament are routinely performed at repair or fixation of the tendon. Injection of the biceps groove with a local anaesthetic has been shown to be a good predictive factor in isolating pain arising in the biceps tendon. Injection of the biceps groove is surprisingly difficult especially in the well-covered patient. If it is required, then it may have to be performed by screening X-ray control unless the groove can be easily palpated.

Bicipital tendinitis may be part of an overuse syndrome in the throwing athlete's shoulder. The biceps is a great decelerator. It can be shown that biceps may be avulsed from the supraglenoid tubercle by maximal stimulation of the biceps.[5] The so-called SLAP lesion described by Snyder[6] is discussed elsewhere in this book.

BICEPS TENODESIS

Isolated biceps tenodesis should be a relatively rarely performed procedure, but may be carried out at the time of rotator cuff repair if the biceps tendon is found to be badly eroded.

If more than 50% of the fibres are disrupted, then biceps tenodesis is a reasonable option. Occasionally, after a degenerative rupture of the long head of biceps in the middle aged and elderly, symptoms of aching in the muscle belly may remain and the patient may dislike the bunched 'popeye' appearance of the muscle in the upper arm. In this circumstance, tenodesis is indicated.

Technique

The first part of this procedure is to decompress the rotator cuff by performing an anterior acromioplasty and excision of the coracoacromial ligament. A strap incision is used and the deltoid is split to allow the cuff to be viewed.[7] The arm is internally rotated and the biceps groove palpated. A window is then made in the biceps sheath with a flap of bone so that this can be repaired at the end of the procedure. The biceps tendon is chased proximally and dis-inserted from the supraglenoid tubercle. A vertical split is made into the rotator interval to achieve this. Excision of this proximal fragment may also be achieved arthroscopically.

The distal groove is now explored to find the distal stump of the tendon. The elbow is flexed and the muscle 'milked' up to the proximal wound to retrieve the tendon. If the tendon is retracted more distally, a second small incision may be required to expose this just proximal to the bunched muscle. The long head of biceps is found and a suture passer is then passed from proximal to distal to emerge in the distal wound. A stay suture is passed through the distal stump of the biceps tendon and then passed through the eye of the passer and pulled proximally to deliver the tendon into the proximal wound.

There are two common methods for actually achieving the biceps tenodesis in the groove: (1) the keyhole method (Figure 24.1); (2) the suture method. (1) In the keyhole method a knot is tied in the proximal tendon itself and secured by a through-and-through absorbable suture. This knot is then grasped and pulled proximally to assess tension within the biceps muscle itself. It is checked that the elbow can fully extend whilst maintaining tension on the tendon. Once the position for tenodesis has been decided on, the distal end of the knot in the tendon is marked in the groove using a small osteotome. A keyhole-shaped hole is then made in the biceps groove with its distal extremity at the level of this mark. Using a burr and small osteotome the proximal

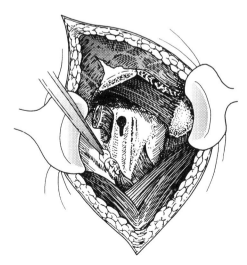

Fig. 24.1 Keyhole tenodesis.

part of this hole is made just wide enough to admit the knot into the tendon and the distal part of the hole just wide enough for the tendon itself. Once the knot in the tendon has been pushed into the hole, extension of the elbow and tension distally on the biceps will allow the tendon to be locked into the distal groove. This is a secure method of fixation and no other ancillary fixation is required.

(2) Sometimes knotting the biceps tendon leaves the knot rather too bulky to allow the keyhole method, so the suture method is used. The base of the groove is decorticated down to bleeding bone, and sutures are passed through drill holes in the bone and passed through and through the tendon. Again tension in the biceps muscle itself is judged to allow the elbow to extend fully, and then the sutures tied. The flap of the tendon sheath is then closed over this to allow additional security of the repair.

Postoperative management

The patient is treated in a sling with gentle passive mobilizing as far as pain allows; active movements are started at 3 weeks. Berlemann & Bayley[3] reviewed, at an average of 7 years, 15 shoulders in 14 patients treated by keyhole tenodesis of the long head of biceps. Eight of these patients had undergone rotator cuff decompression before the biceps tenodesis. Eight achieved an excellent result, one a good result, four fair results, and there were two failures. Seven shoulders had an improved result from short to long term and only two deteriorated. An upward migration of the humeral head on X-ray evaluation was noted, but was without clinical significance. Other authors have noted good shorter-term results.

RUPTURED LONG HEAD OF BICEPS

Spontaneous rupture of the long head of biceps is a relatively common occurrence in the middle aged and elderly. Its clinical effect may be surprisingly variable. In some, the spontaneous rupture is associated with great pain, swelling and extensive

bruising, but in the majority it is a relatively silent occurrence, sometimes the patient only noticing it as a chance finding of a bulge in the distal part of the arm. In the early stages of discomfort and bruising, the patient should be reassured that it will settle spontaneously and that surgical repair is not usually possible or wise. However, if symptoms persist for several months, then tenodesis may be considered to relieve the symptoms.

ACUTE TRAUMATIC RUPTURE OF THE BICEPS

This can occur usually in the younger patient associated with a sudden forced extension of the flexed elbow or during very heavy weight lifting. The diagnosis is easily made as it is associated with pain and distal migration of the muscle belly of the long head of biceps. In this rare circumstance in the young patient, it is worth while considering repair of the tendon within the groove. The earlier this is carried out, the better. However, if on exploration, the rupture is found to be associated with degenerative change, then tenodesis is the better option.

RUPTURE OF THE DISTAL BICEPS

This is a relatively infrequent occurrence, but may occur in the younger patient associated with a forced extension pronation of the semi-flexed elbow. The pain of this injury is usually more severe and more prolonged. The muscle with this injury is noted to migrate proximally and the bruising extends downwards into the antecubital fossa.

If this injury is seen early enough, then repair is very definitely worth while. An anterior lazy 'S' incision is made in the antecubital fossa and the proximal disrupted tendon found. It is usually a complete avulsion from the bone and the tendon has to be reimplanted directly into bone. This has been made a much easier procedure with the advent of suture anchors. Two suture anchors are drilled into the bone and then the sutures are used to reimplant the tendon distally. If no suture anchors are available, then a grasping suture is put into the tendon, drill holes are made in the bone and the suture is passed through and through and tied on the extensor surface of the radius via a second incision in the forearm.

BICEPS INSTABILITY

Subluxation of the long head of biceps may occur as an acute event in association with dislocation of the shoulder or more usually as a more degenerative process in association with cuff disease.

Acute biceps subluxation

Acute biceps subluxation is a relative rarity. It can be associated with acute anterior dislocation of the shoulder. The history usually indicates that the shoulder was reduced adequately, but the patient continues with symptoms of pain over the anterior aspect of the shoulder. There is acute tenderness over the long head of biceps and the patient may feel the tendon flicking in and out on rotation with the elbow flexed and abducted. In the acute situation, this is always associated with partial rupture of the subscapularis tendon. The tendon of the long head of biceps subluxes anteriorly out of the groove and disrupts the upper part of the insertion of the subscapularis. If the diagnosis is made, then acute repair is very worth while in association with repair of the subscapularis insertion. The main stabilizer of the biceps tendon is the musculocutaneous cuff and the coracohumeral ligament. These structures should be repaired. It is important to remember the diagnosis of a dislocated biceps tendon almost by definition means that there is a consequent rotator cuff tear also and this must be repaired.

Chronic subluxation of the biceps tendon

This is almost invariably associated with degenerative disease of the rotator cuff. Once the cuff has disrupted, there is direct impingement and wear of the musculotendinous cuff and the cor-

acohumeral ligament. Once the stabilizing structures are destroyed, the biceps flips over the anterior lip of the biceps groove. The diagnosis can be most easily made by using ultrasound. Stabilization of the biceps tendon is only part of the treatment. If indicated, the rotator cuff is repaired and adequate decompression acromioplasty performed. In younger patients if the long head of biceps is in reasonable condition, then this is stabilized within the groove. The groove may have to be deepened and a flap of tissue fashioned from the base of the groove to take over the top of the tendon to stabilize the tendon in the groove (Figure 24.2). In the older patient, if there is positive pre-existing attrition wear in the biceps tendon and rupture is imminent, then tenodesis is a better option to relieve pain.

In summary biceps tendon subluxation should

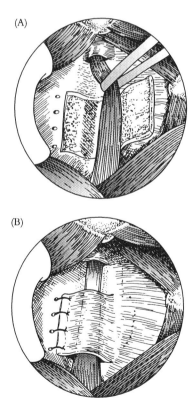

Fig. 24.2 Stabilization of the biceps tendon in the groove. An osteoperiosteal flap is raised from the base of the groove (A) and then sutured back over the top of the tendons with sutures passed through the bone after repair of the rotator cuff (B).

always be assumed to be associated with a tear of the rotator cuff whether this is acute or chronic. Treatment of the rotator cuff may take precedence over the long head of biceps itself.

REFERENCES

1. Jobe, F.W., Tibone, J.E., Perry, J. et al. (1983) An EMG analysis of the shoulder in throwing and pitching. A preliminary report. *Am. J. Sports Med.* **11**: 3–5.
2. Glousman, R., Jobe, F., Tibone, J. et al. (1988) Dynamic electromyographic analysis of the throwing shoulder with gleno-humeral instability. *J. Bone Joint Surg.* **70A**: 220–226.
3. Berlemann, U. & Bayley, I. (1995) Tenodesis of the long head of biceps brachii in the painful shoulder; improving results in the long term. *J. Shoulder Elbow Surg.* **4**: 429–435.
4. Warner, J.P. & McMahon, P.J. (1995) The role of the long head of biceps brachii in superior stability of the glenohumeral joint. *J. Bone Joint Surg.* **77A**: 336–372.
5. Andrews, J., Carson, W. & McCleod, W. (1985) Glenoid labrum tears related to the long head of biceps. *Am. J. Sports Med.* **13**: 337–341.
6. Synder, S.J., Karzel, R.P., Delpizzo, W., Ferkel, R.D. & Friedman, M.J. (1990) Slap lesions of the shoulder. *Arthroscopy* **6**: 274–279.
7. Copeland, S.A. (1995) *Biceps Tendon Repair and Tenodesis in Operative Shoulder Surgery*. Edinburgh: Churchill-Livingstone.

25

Total Shoulder Replacement

PM Connor and LU Bigliani

INTRODUCTION

The French surgeon Pean performed the first reported prosthetic arthroplasty of the shoulder in 1893 for tuberculosis.[1] Although this platinum and rubber prosthesis was removed 2 years later for uncontrolled infection, the initial postoperative result was excellent. The modem era of shoulder arthroplasty was pioneered by Neer, who used his first prosthesis for the treatment of severe proximal humeral fractures in 1951.[2] In his 1955 report of 12 patients who were treated by prosthetic replacement of the humeral head, Neer noted that the procedure was followed by a 'remarkable painfree convalescence'.[3] Since that time, unconstrained shoulder arthroplasty has become a commonly performed procedure for many acute and chronic disease processes which afflict the shoulder, and its success has been well established. Several recent series of unconstrained total shoulder replacements with an average follow-up of 46 months have reported only a 8.2% overall revision rate.[4] This is quite favourable since these series represent first-generation total shoulder replacements and included more complex reconstructive problems as well as primary degenerative disease. The indications and techniques for total shoulder replacement have evolved dramatically so that glenohumeral resection or arthrodesis is now rarely required.[4,5]

Over the last decade, there has been a proliferation of new designs for shoulder arthroplasty intended to improve clinical results and longevity of the prosthesis. Although many of these recent designs offer novel features, the major causes of imperfect results after shoulder arthroplasty are inadequacies of the soft tissues of the disease process (as in rheumatoid arthritis or post-traumatic arthritis) as well as improper patient selection, operative technique and postoperative rehabilitation. Just as design and technique modifications of total hip arthroplasty should provide improvements in the long-term results of Charnley's design before being universally advocated, the same can be said of Neer's total shoulder design. In his personal series of 408 total shoulder replacements, of which more than half of the patients were under 60 years of age, only a 3.6% revision rate was reported with follow-up ranging from 2 to 15 years.[6] These results provide a basis for the comparison of improvements in outcome and durability that may be achieved with newer designs and techniques of total shoulder arthroplasty.

CLINICAL EVALUATION

History

A thorough history is essential to gather as much information as possible for evaluation of the arthritic shoulder. It is best obtained in a systematic fashion to avoid overlooking factors which the patient may think unimportant but which may nevertheless be quite relevant in evaluating the shoulder problem at issue. Hand dominance, occupation and athletic activities should all be recorded in an effort to understand functional demands and future expectations.

The precise nature of the patient's chief complaint, usually pain, stiffness and/or loss of function, should be well understood and kept in mind when considering treatment. For example, if a patient with rotator cuff deficiency and arthritis is most concerned with pain relief, then shoulder arthroplasty is a reasonable intervention. If loss of strength and overhead function is the chief complaint, then surgery is less likely to meet the goals of this same patient. Pain is usually deep inside the arthritic shoulder, but may radiate down the arm or up into the neck. The patient with severe glenohumeral arthritis will complain of constant pain and the inability to perform even simple activities of hygiene and dressing. Less extreme cases will often present with muscle fatigue while lifting and carrying, and difficulty with functions at the limits of motion such as fastening a bra strap or reaching for shelves.

It is important to document the duration, provocation, severity, and timing of symptoms, especially pain. Rest pain and night pain are especially common in patients with shoulder arthritis and are not necessarily indicative of infection or tumour, although these possibilities must always be considered. The mechanism of any injury, as well as the nature of exacerbating activities, should be noted.

It may be difficult to separate complaints emanating from the shoulder from those due to adjacent regions such as the neck, chest, heart, upper back and arm. Cervical disease can be especially difficult to differentiate from intrinsic mechanical shoulder disorders, and the two frequently coexist. Nevertheless pain from a cervical source is often referred to the posterior shoulder and trapezius, and may radiate down the arm into the hand. Shoulder disorders more frequently hurt deep inside the shoulder or down the front of the upper arm, not usually extending beyond the elbow. Furthermore, neck pain is often related to the position of the cervical spine, and becomes more severe after driving or long periods of sitting. Numbness or tingling in the hand may be indicative of cervical disc disease or peripheral nerve entrapment. A general medical history should be obtained, with special care to elicit any symptoms suggestive of a systemic or rheumatological disorder. In addition, conditions such as diabetes mellitus and metastatic cancer can be associated with a painful stiff shoulder.

The history should also be specifically directed to the most common aetiologies of shoulder arthritis. Questions pertaining to other joint involvement, arthritis of the spine and/or other physical limitations is important in patients with osteoarthritis, rheumatoid arthritis or arthritis due to seronegative spondyloarthropathies. A history of corticosteroid use or excessive alcoholism may suggest avascular necrosis of the humeral head. In patients with a history of trauma, all details pertaining to the timing of the event, mechanism, instability, fractures and treatment must be addressed. For patients who have had previous shoulder surgery a thorough review of the indications is required, including surgical technique and operative report(s), convalescence and subsequent injuries, which all combined enable the most appropriate treatment plan to be rendered. Although infrequent, the possibilities of infection and neoplasm must be examined and questions regarding previous injections, procedures with a history of wound healing problems, coexistent immunosuppressive disorders, systemic symptoms, night pain and a history of primary neoplasm should all be addressed.

Physical examination

The patient should be examined with both shoulders fully exposed: men disrobe above the waist and women are given gowns that are tied under the shoulder in the axilla so that they are 'strapless'. Inspection is performed both from in front and behind the patient. Careful note is made of muscle atrophy and contour, bone prominences and deformity. Patients with rheumatoid arthritis often have 'medialization' of the humerus due to loss of glenoid bone, and the shoulder may lose its normally round contour.[6] Asymmetry in the shoulder with wasting of the supraspinatus and infraspinatus is often a sign of either rotator cuff disease in association with rheumatoid arthritis or cuff tear arthropathy or suprascapular nerve entrapment or injury. Sometimes the subdeltoid bursa may be palpably distended ('fluid sign'), often seen in cuff tear arthropathy. Rheumatoid bursitis without a cuff defect is less common but can also result in a distended bursa on examination.

With the examiner standing behind the patient, palpation is performed, checking for areas of localized tenderness. The acromioclavicular joint should always be carefully palpated, as it is a frequently overlooked source of symptoms. Posterior glenohumeral joint line tenderness is commonly noted in arthritis, as is crepitus with range of motion. A thorough examination of the cervical spine should be performed and, if the patient's 'shoulder' pain is reproduced by cervical manipulation or Spurling's sign, strong consideration should be given to a cervical aetiology.

Range of motion is evaluated and recorded. Forward elevation is measured in the scapular plane. Passive elevation is more acurately measured in the supine position as substitution through lumbar lordosis is minimized. No effort is made to 'isolate' glenohumeral motion: total elevation, consisting of both glenohumeral and scapulothoracic motion, is more reproducibly measured and more functionally relevant. Active elevation is measured erect. External rotation, with the arm at the side, is also measured supine, to eliminate trunk rotation. Internal rotation is measured erect, by recording the highest vertebral level to which the thumb may be brought up the patient's back. When arthritis progresses and capsular tightness and glenohumeral incongruity become severe, shoulder motion gradually becomes restricted to scapulothoracic motion. Since scapular movement does not contribute significantly to rotation, limitation of external rotation is a much more sensitive physical finding of glenohumeral arthritis than limitation of forward elevation (which can be performed well with scapulothoracic motion).[6]

Manual strength testing is usually difficult in the arthritic shoulder because pain precludes quantitative assessment. External rotation weakness can be present in long-standing rotator cuff tears, but may be secondary to pain, cervical radiculopathy or suprascapular nerve palsy. It is best to test external rotation power with the elbow flexed and the arm at the side, to avoid a contribution from the deltoid muscle. A careful neurological assessment is necessary to rule out cervical spine disease and electromyography may occasionally be indicated when weakness is severe.

Specific provocative tests or signs such as the impingement sign for rotator cuff tendinitis, anterior apprehension for glenohumeral instability and cross-body adduction for acromioclavicular joint arthritis are generally not useful in the presence of significant glenohumeral arthritis since all motions are painful. Differential anaesthetic injections of the acromioclavicular joint, the glenohumeral joint and the subacromial space have been reported to be of value in sorting out the source of pain in rheumatoid shoulders,[7] especially when the glenohumeral joint is not felt to be the major source of pain and an arthroplasty may be avoided. However, by the time surgical treatment is considered, the glenohumeral joint is usually obviously symptomatic and arthritic, and deep injections are neither needed nor indicated, because of the risk of introducing infection.

Imaging studies

Plain radiographs are generally all that is needed to diagnose and assess the clinically significant arthritic shoulder. The classic radiographic changes of glenohumeral arthritis present in the later reactive stages of the disease process. Thus it is important to emphasize that glenohumeral arthritis is often clinically underappreciated because of the inability to radiographically demonstrate early cartilage pathology. A standard series includes anteroposterior and lateral views in the plane of the scapula and an axillary view. The true anteroposterior view of the scapula will show the glenohumeral joint space far better than an 'AP view of the shoulder', which in most cases provides an anteroposterior view in the plane of the thorax and an oblique view of the glenohumeral joint.

The hallmark of glenohumeral arthritis is loss of joint space and irregular articular contours. The axillary view is often the most sensitive indicator of loss of glenohumeral joint space. Osteoarthritic shoulders will generally show subchondral sclerosis and cysts, flattening of the humeral and glenoid surfaces, and a ring of osteophytes around the

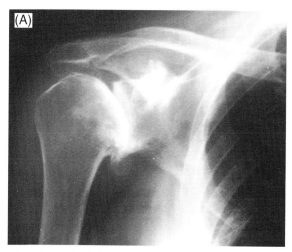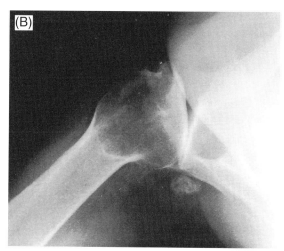

Fig. 25.1 (A), (B) Characteristic deformity of late glenohumeral osteoarthritis, with subchondral sclerosis of the humeral head, inferior humeral head osteophytes, asymmetric loss of joint space, eccentric posterior glenoid wear and loose bodies.

humeral anatomical neck (often projecting as an inferior humeral osteophyte on the anteroposterior view as the inferior portion of the ring is in profile). A characteristic deformity in late glenohumeral osteoarthritis is posterior humeral subluxation with eccentric wear of the posterior glenoid (Figure 25.1). This is usually well seen on axillary radiographs, and computed tomography (CT), which will show glenoid bone loss most accurately, is generally not required.

Osteopenia, juxta-articular erosions and cystic changes are common in the rheumatoid shoulder. Glenoid erosion is more irregular than in osteoarthritis and is often central. As the glenoid bone resorbs, the humerus 'medializes' in a protrusio fashion. A common error is to assume that, as in a non-arthritic shoulder, superior humeral translation indicates a large or massive tear of the rotator cuff. The rheumatoid shoulder loses its glenohumeral fulcrum as the joint surfaces are destroyed, and the head often ascends before a large cuff tear is present.[6] However, the pattern of end-stage rheumatoid arthritis, with severe erosion of the upper glenoid, coracoid base and acromioclavicular joint, is often associated with a massive rotator cuff defect.

Plain radiographs can differentiate other causes of glenohumeral arthritis. In cuff tear arthropathy, sclerosis and rounding of the greater tuberosity are seen, along with humeral ascent, acromial spurs, head collapse and superior glenoid wear.[6,8] Shoulders with post-traumatic arthritis will have joint loss in association with the deformities resulting from trauma and/or any associated surgery. Patients who develop arthritis after instability surgery have a pattern similar to osteoarthritis except that the posterior humeral subluxation and posterior glenoid wear are very pronounced (due to anterior soft-tissue tightening), inferior glenoid osteophytes may be especially large and hardware may be present. The radiographic appearance of avascular necrosis parallels that of the femoral head as described by Ficat.[6,9]

More specialized studies, such as CT, magnetic resonance imaging (MRI), arthrography and bone scans can provide additional information when evaluating the causes of arthritic shoulder pain, especially when planning operative intervention. CT is very useful in the preoperative evaluation of severe glenohumeral arthritis as it can accurately assess the degree of posterior glenoid deficiency and bone stock available for reconstruction. It can also be useful in evaluating post-traumatic deformities of the humeral head before humeral head replacement. Three-dimensional reconstruction of CT scans has been helpful in understanding acute fractures, but is not necessary for assessing arthritis of the shoulder. MRI is useful for the diagnosis of rotator cuff tears and is currently favoured over arthrography as it is non-invasive, accurate and able to assess the size of rotator cuff defect. It may also demonstrate intra-articular pathology in rheumatoid arthritis more effectively than plain films, but whether this is of clinical benefit has yet to be demonstrated. However, the cost of MRI has limited its use to the rare case where a potential change in the treatment plan is dependent upon the results. A technetium bone scan or an indium-labelled white blood cell scan may be useful in the diagnosis of infection, or in assessing patients with arthritis after deep infections or persistent infection.

Laboratory tests

In general, laboratory tests for specific arthrides of the shoulder (e.g. rheumatoid disease, ankylosing spondylitis, systemic lupus erythematosus) will be performed in conjunction with a rheumatologist or internist and are beyond the scope of this chapter. However, a basic screening set of blood tests are generally obtained: electrolytes, erythrocyte sedimentation rate, white blood cell count with differential. These are useful in assessing general health and candidacy for surgery, activity of any underlying inflammatory arthritis and the possibility of active infection (especially in the post-traumatic, postoperative or multiply injected shoulder).

Ancillary studies

Electromyograms (EMG) and nerve conduction studies (NCS) are useful in the evaluation of peripheral nerve injuries and entrapments, brachial plexus disorders and cervical radiculopathies, but are rarely needed in the routine arthritic shoulder. However, in a shoulder where a nerve lesion is suspected, especially those after trauma or prior surgery, electrical studies may be helpful in avoiding a futile reconstruction of denervated muscles (which may be difficult to assess clinically due to severe pain and stiffness). Cervical CT or MRI may also be needed in conjunction with an EMG if a cervical aetiology is strongly suspected. Somatosensory evoked potential testing may also

occasionally be useful, especially when the predominant symptoms are sensory. Cybex muscle testing can document functional deficits and serve as a baseline for the evaluation of rehabilitation protocols, but is rarely used in the arthritic shoulder since pain and stiffness usually have an unpredictable effect on effort.

INDICATIONS

The primary indication for shoulder arthroplasty is pain which has persisted despite non-operative management. Although stiffness and functional difficulties with activities of daily living are also important, they are secondary indications for surgery. Shoulder arthroplasty is rarely performed to improve range of motion and/or function without concomitant pain. The health, activity and motivation of the patient are also important factors to consider before surgical intervention; some patients clearly are not good surgical candidates for various reasons. In addition, the patient must be ready and able to play an essential role in his or her own rehabilitation. As noted by Neer,[6] total shoulder arthroplasty merely sets the stage for the patient to actively participate in the rehabilitative process so his or her result can be maximized.

While most patients with arthritis of the shoulder are encouraged to delay reconstructive surgery as long as possible, the timing of surgery is not always quite this simple. The rheumatoid shoulder, for example, presents a special problem because delay in reconstruction can allow further loss of bone stock and rotator cuff. Early replacement arthroplasty of a rheumatoid shoulder can result in excellent function, while surgery on an end-stage rheumatoid shoulder with a massive rotator cuff tear and severe bone loss may achieve gratifying pain relief but disappointing function. Also, some authors have advocated that total shoulder arthroplasty for osteoarthritis be considered once cartilage damage is irreversible and stiffness and functional limitations ensue before the patient develops end-stage soft tissue contractures and/or posterior glenoid bone loss which would make reconstructive efforts less reliable.[10]

It can be considered more conservative, in fact, to advise patients to undergo shoulder arthroplasty rather than continuing potentially harmful medications and allowing the further destruction of the rotator cuff and glenoid bone.[6] The ultimate decision regarding the timing of surgery, however, should be based on all factors pertaining to the patient, the disease process and the expected outcome.

Absolute contraindications to shoulder arthroplasty are active infection and/or extensive paralysis with complete functional loss of both rotator cuff and deltoid function. Neither bone loss nor a deficient rotator cuff is considered a contraindication to shoulder replacement surgery.[6]

ALTERNATIVES TO ARTHROPLASTY

The original prosthesis was designed for the treatment of acute fractures and fracture/dislocations of the proximal humerus because the alternatives to treatment, namely resection arthroplasty and fusion, were found to be unsatisfactory.[2] However, other alternative treatments have evolved and all should be included in the surgeon's armamentarium for the care of patients with glenohumeral arthritis. It is important to be familiar with these available options and to know their indications and limitations.

Debridement, soft tissue balancing

Although Neer[11] reported uniformly poor results after open release, debridement, removal of osteophytes and soft tissue balancing for osteoarthritis, MacDonald et al[12] reported favourable early results after open release of soft tissue contractures with concomitant arthritis after instability repair. The goals of this treatment are to normalize the biomechanics of the shoulder joint through soft tissue balancing so that the articular congruity of the humeral head and the glenoid will be restored and the joint forces will be more evenly distributed throughout the glenoid surface. Although the indications for this procedure are narrow, it may prove to be useful in young patients with mild or moderate arthritis after instability repair with a concomitant internal rotation contracture.

The use of arthroscopy for glenohumeral irrigation and debridement, combined with capsular release and bursal surgery, may have a role in patients who are poor candidates for joint replacement, especially those unwilling or unable to modify their activities to protect the implant.[13] In addition, coexisting pathological conditions that contribute to symptoms may be addressed.[13,14] In the study of Weinstein et al,[13] arthroscopy for glenohumeral arthritis provided significant pain relief and increased motion in 78% of patients at an average of 2.5 years follow-up. This procedure is contraindicated if there is complete loss of joint space, large osteophytes or posterior humeral subluxation.

Certainly the arthritis is not arrested by arthroscopy, but early failures are uncommon. Furthermore, complications are rare. Patients with glenohumeral arthritis may be advised that arthroscopy is not a cure but an attempt to delay the need for joint replacement. However, the long-term value of arthroscopic management of shoulder arthritis is as yet undocumented and economic considerations are sure to play a role in the decision-making process in the future.

Synovectomy and bursectomy

Isolated glenohumeral synovectomy is rarely indicated. There may be a very small group of patients with rheumatoid arthritis who present with signs of intra-articular inflammation and synovitis but still have a congruent joint with no evidence of cyst formation or joint degeneration who will benefit from this procedure. Simpson and Kelly[15] recently reported promising early results using bursectomy, acromioplasty and distal clavicle excisions as determined by selective preoperative xylocaine injections in patients with rheumatoid arthritis. The long-term results of this approach are not available. It appears, however, that the majority of patients with rheumatoid inflammation have significant cartilage involvement and would not be candidates for this more limited surgical approach.

Core decompression

The idea of drilling the medullary bone in early avascular necrosis to stimulate revascularization has been popularized in the hip literature. This has been somewhat successful in the early stages of avascular necrosis of the proximal femur where collapse of the articular surface has not occurred. There is little in the shoulder literature regarding decompression for avascular necrosis of the proximal humerus, perhaps because the majority of cases do not present until the articular surface and head are more severely involved.[18,19]

With the increasing use of MRI, it is likely that avascular necrosis may be detected earlier. Preliminary studies[20] have shown promising early results with this technique, which involves placement of a small reamer into the necrotic segment of the humeral head under fluoroscopic guidance using a deltoid-splitting approach. Again, long-term results are needed in order to recommend this procedure and, at present, its role is controversial.

Humeral head resection

Humeral head resection has been used as a reconstructive and salvage procedure for a variety of shoulder disorders. This procedure is used today only in the presence of resistant infections (e.g. Gram-negative osteomyelitis of the humeral head) or failed arthroplasties with extensive bone loss in which reimplantation is contraindicated.[5] Although Neer et al[2] reported satisfactory overall results in 14 of 19 patients after resection arthroplasty, glenohumeral motion and function were severely limited. In a review of the indications and results of humeral head excision, Cofield[5] stated that only approximately one-half to two-thirds of patients will achieve satisfactory pain relief, and range of motion is limited on the average to 40–90° of active forward elevation, no active external rotation and minimal active internal rotation.

When humeral head resection is indicated, a standard deltopectoral incision is used. Special care is taken not to injure the deltoid or pectoralis major insertion. The joint is opened and the humeral head is resected at the level of the anatomical neck. The humerus is then smoothed with a rasp or burr to round the edges. A synovectomy and thorough debridement of the joint is then performed. The tendons of the rotator cuff can be reattached to the neck of the humerus through drill holes for soft tissue coverage and interposition; however, it has been shown that function is not enhanced with this rotator cuff 'repair'.[5] The patient is placed in a sling for 6–8 weeks and only allowed to perform pendulum range of motion exercises. The aim is to allow a certain degree of stiffening and scar formation to establish stability. This scarring suspends the humerus to some degree to prevent traction on the brachial plexus and also minimizes grating of the resected humerus on the glenoid and other adjacent structures. Often, in cases of infection, the possibility of later conversion to a prosthetic implant is considered after the infection has been eradicated.[21] However, patients may decline further surgery if the resection alone has provided adequate pain relief.

Shoulder arthrodesis

The indications for shoulder fusion have markedly diminished since the introduction of shoulder replacement in 1953.[3] These are paralysis of both the rotator cuff and deltoid muscles (as are commonly seen in upper brachial plexus injuries), active septic arthritis and/or osteomyelitis, severe degenerative joint disease in combination with a massive rotator cuff tear and anterosuperior instability for which previous attempts at repair and stabilization have failed, and occasionally severe bone and soft tissue loss which occurs after radical excision of the shoulder girdle after tumour surgery.

The results after glenohumeral fusion have been variable. Hawkins and Neer[22] reviewed 17 patients at an average of 4 years after the operation and found that none could use their extremity in an overhead position and most had difficulties with personal hygiene. In addition, nearly 50% complained of either moderate or severe shoulder and/or periscapular pain. The pain and functional limitations combined with the risk of non-union (reported as high as 42%) led these authors to recommend careful consideration before fusion is advised. Even if the ideal position of fusion is achieved (25–40° abduction, 20–30° flexion, 25–30° internal rotation), arthrodesis produced significant limitations in function.[5,22] Other studies[5,23,24] have led to the agreement that, because of unreliable pain relief, variable functional results and the risk of complications, shoulder fusion should be confined to the indications as listed above and be considered a salvage procedure.

DESIGN CONSIDERATIONS

Anatomical design

Neer's approach[6] to the design of his initial humeral head replacement in 1951 was based on components of normal anatomy. In addition, his principles emphasized minimal removal of bone, the avoidance of mechanical blocking of prosthetic motion which might lead to mechanical failure, and soft-tissue balancing and reconstruction to maximize rehabilitation potential.[25] This approach has been widely accepted. Most attempts to improve on this design (e.g. hooded components to resist superior humeral subluxation) have been abandoned. Indeed, recent controversies in design have centred on the degree of precision with which prosthetic components should replicate anatomy. For this reason, the various non-anatomical replacements (e.g. ball-on-the-glenoid/socket-on-the-humerus designs, constrained designs, bipolar arthroplasties, etc.) which have been largely unsuccessful[6,25–32] will not be discussed. Rather, the issues involved in the design of anatomical shoulder arthroplasties will be explored.

Bone anatomy

The proximal humerus has a flared metaphyseal shape. Many humeral component designs use a relatively straight stem, often with added fins to provide rotational control of the component by either cancellous bone or cement. Recently, designs with wedge-shaped proximal geometry have been used to achieve proximal endosteal fit.

Yet, intraoperative humeral fractures have been reported to occur during implantation of humeral components caused by the thin cortex of osteoporotic bone in the proximal humerus.[4,33,34] It is unclear, however, whether these bulky metal components increase the risk of this complication. Nevertheless, humeral loosening is extremely uncommon, and the value of proximal fit has yet to be established.

The humeral head is inclined relative to the shaft at an angle of 130–150°, and its centre is offset about 6 mm medially and 3–5 mm posteriorly from the axis of the shaft.[33] Most systems use a standard head inclination, but components are available in which a modular assembly allows adjustment of the neck-shaft angle. For posterior offset to be reliably reproduced, either left and right components must be designed, or the (modular) head component must have a peg system so that it can affix to the stem only in right or left offset orientations. However, this type of complexity increases the possibility of surgeon error and of component fretting at the modular interfaces. Because total shoulder replacements are generally performed not in normal shoulders but in grossly arthritic shoulders with extensive anatomical distortions, it is unclear whether such precise adjustments are clinically justified.

Humeral retroversion has been extensively studied. Since the proximal humerus lacks a structure analogous to the femoral neck (the axis of which is reliably measured to assess hip version), determination of humeral version requires definition of the edges of the proximal humeral articular surface. However, the articular margin is irregular, and varies from the top of the head to the bottom. Because of this and the various radiographic techniques and choices for the distal axis (especially given a 6° difference between the transepicondylar axis and the distal humeral articular surface), estimates of normal humeral retroversion have varied. While most studies have reported average humeral retroversion to be from 26° to 31°, average values as low as 18° and as high as 40° have also been found.[33] More importantly perhaps is the finding that there is a wide range of retroversion in shoulders of patients free of known shoulder disorders and even between the two shoulders in one individual. This has led to a shift in emphasis from putting the humeral component in the 'correct' degree of retroversion to adjusting the version to that particular shoulder, being guided more by the local anatomy such as the cuff insertion and biceps groove than by an exact predetermined number.[35]

The bony architecture and density of the native glenoid have been investigated, and most glenoid components use either pegs or a short keel for fixation in the limited amount of available bone. There is often significant glenoid bone loss at the time of shoulder arthroplasty, especially posteriorly. While reaming or sculpting the surface may to some degree correct this problem, it has been recommended that in some instances it is better to accept slightly altered glenoid version (more retroversion) and compensate by reducing humeral retroversion.[6] Canal-filling deep glenoid component keels makes it difficult to adjust version; shorter-finned or pegged components may facilitate more precise titration of component version.

Articular geometry

Modern stereophotogrammetry has been used to show that the articular geometry of the glenohumeral joint surfaces are very closely approximated by spheres.[36] As such, the majority of glenohumeral replacements are spherical in design. However, some have recommended elliptical designs based on studies that showed deviations from sphericity in normal shoulders.[37]

A significant controversy concerns the optimum degree of glenohumeral conformity desirable in a total shoulder system. Neer[6,11,25] originally obtained good pain relief after uncemented humeral head replacement for osteoarthritis, but found that heads could sublux on the flat arthritic glenoids. He introduced glenoid resurfacing to provide a stable fulcrum for the muscles,[25] and used a glenoid that conformed to the curvature of the prosthetic humeral head. Many authors, studying bone shape, have shown that the normal glenoid is generally less curved

than that of the corresponding humeral subchondral bone. However, on examination of the cartilage articular surfaces, the glenohumeral joint has been found to be highly conforming, with the average difference between the radius of curvature of the humeral head and that of the glenoid being less than 0.1 mm.[36] Because articular cartilage is more compliant than a polyethylene prosthetic surface, however, the issue still remains as to whether it is better to model the prosthetic surfaces closer to the radii-mismatched subchondral bone or to the conforming articular surfaces.

Proponents for a mismatch in curvature of the prosthetic components argue that any translations that occur in a conforming total shoulder replacement will cause eccentric loading of the humeral head on the rim of the glenoid component. This may lead to potential polyethylene deformation and wear. In addition, a rocking moment of the glenoid component may be introduced since the contact force is at the periphery and thus has a longer moment arm. Opponents of mismatch designs, however, argue that, when the prosthetic humeral head is centred on the glenoid, the articulating portion of the less curved glenoid is over a smaller area, potentially leading to increased contact stresses and linear polyethylene wear.

Severt and co-workers[38] differentiated between constraint (the relative surface area of the glenoid, e.g. increased with superiorly hooded components) and conformity (the relative curvature). Constraint will improve resistance to subluxation, which may be an asset if stability is otherwise compromised. However, the force that resists this subluxation is transmitted to the interface between the component and bone, which leads to rocking of the component and mechanical loosening. An example of this effect is in total shoulder arthroplasty with concomitant rotator cuff deficiency. The tendency of the superiorly subluxing humerus to load the superior rim of the glenoid, transmitting a bending moment, has been suggested by clinical studies of glenoid loosening and by finite element modelling.[30] Increased conformity also increases stability; however, once again, rim loading can cause both material failure of the polyethylene and rocking of the glenoid component.[39] Severt et al[38] concluded that the use of less conforming and less constrained designs may reduce the potential for mechanical loosening of the glenoid component.

On the other hand, Buechel et al[40] and others[41] have suggested that curvature mismatch in total shoulder replacement would increase contact stresses, leading to debris and resultant inflammation. This also parallels the experience with total knee arthroplasties, as less conforming tibial components have led to increased linear polyethylene wear. One solution has been to search for materials that can withstand higher stresses. However, stronger polyethylenes may also be stiffer, such that there is less deformation under load, and thus a smaller contact area when a more curved head contacts the glenoid.

It has been anecdotally noted that rim wear is often seen at the time of glenoid component revision.[31] Although there is no denying that this may occur, rim wear is usually in the setting of gross instability, malpositioned components, or when an adequate release of a tight anterior capsule was not performed at the time of initial arthroplasty.[42] Adequate release and soft-tissue balancing needs to be performed at the time of total shoulder replacement. It remains to be seen whether a curvature mismatch in the prosthetic component surfaces will increase or decrease polyethylene wear in an adequately released properly rehabilitated shoulder.

It has been shown that passive manipulation causes glenohumeral translations at the extremes of motion.[43] However, it is unclear if this translation is relevant to the active use of the arm in activities of daily living as reports regarding this issue have provided conflicting opinions.[33,43,44] Nevertheless, given that glenohumeral joint forces are highest during muscle loading in the midrange of motion, especially when raising a weight in the arm, it is certainly possible that the risk of polyethylene wear from increased stresses caused by curvature mismatch is greater than the risk of wear from edge-loading caused by subluxations in a conforming design. It is clear that long-term follow-up studies are needed before definitive clinically based recommendations can be made.

Component sizing

Several studies have been performed on the range of normal glenohumeral sizes and dimensions.[37,45] Parameters include the curvature and thickness of the head component, and the thickness and shape of the glenoid component. Whereas it is generally believed that replacements should be modelled on normal anatomy, the bone and soft-tissue distortions seen in shoulders requiring arthroplasty may require components beyond the normal range of sizes (e.g. a small head may be needed if the soft-tissue envelope is too tight despite soft-tissue releases). Thus it may be desirable to have a range of sizes available. Modularity in shoulder arthroplasty components allows a larger range of choices without a similar increase in inventory storage requirements.

The glenoid has been found to average 3–4 cm in height and 2–3.5 cm in width.[45] The arthritic glenoid is often larger, especially if there are large marginal osteophytes. Occasionally it can be smaller, as in juvenile rheumatoid arthritis. Although the normal glenoid is shaped like a teardrop or comma, most glenoid components are symmetrical and either oval or rectangular with rounded edges.

The humeral head has a radius of curvature from 20 to 30 mm, usually about 25–26 mm.[36,45] The thickness of the humeral head is generally from 15 to 25 mm.[45] There tends to be an association in normal shoulders between humeral head thickness and radius of curvature.[45] Even if a conforming total shoulder system is used, the choice of radius is important. Contracture release at the time of surgery creates a soft-tissue space or effective joint space. By varying the radius of curvature of the head for a fixed head thickness, the use of this effective joint space can be maximized and the location of the joint centre of rotation restored. Thus total shoulder systems that offer a wide range of humeral head thicknesses and curvatures are used to accommodate these parameters thereby recreating anatomical relationships and biomechanics.

Inserting oversized components can make rotator cuff repair difficult and can markedly restrict motion,[31] while the use of components that are too small can lead to instability. A larger humeral head component theoretically increases the moment arm of the shoulder and also offers an increased articular arc for motion. This would argue for a relatively thin glenoid component, to leave room for an appropriately sized head in the limited soft-tissue space that exists to accommodate both components. Metal backing, for example, tends to increase glenoid component thickness with no documented benefit in stress transmission.[27,33] Whether or not its role in uncemented implantation for bone ingrowth is of value is as yet unclear. In addition, the bulk of the metal backing necessitates a concomitant decrease in the thickness of the polyethylene component for a given amount of space. Experience in metal-backed patellar components of total knee arthroplasties reminds us of the potential problems with this design. Also, the optimum polyethylene thickness of the glenoid component has yet to be determined. Despite a great deal of discussion about glenohumeral offset and soft-tissue space during total shoulder replacement, clinical experience has suggested that intraoperative releases and assessment of soft-tissue tension are more important than any preoperative radiographic measurements or templating. Nevertheless, investigations continue in this area.

Materials

There is little data specific to the shoulder on the optimum choice of materials, and these considerations generally draw on hip and knee implant experience. Given the poor track record of titanium as a bearing surface, most humeral head components are cobalt–chrome. Polyethylene glenoids have performed well, but improved polyethylene has been suggested as a way of coping with the increased contact stresses that may result from designs with a mismatch between the curvature of the humeral and glenoid surfaces. However, as previously noted, the increased stiffness of this material also decreases contact area since it deforms less when loaded by the humeral surface, thus increasing stresses and partially reducing the benefit of the increased strength.

Porous surfaces for bone ingrowth have unproved value in the humerus, and may be deleterious. Since aseptic humeral loosening is infrequent,[6,46] strategies to avoid loosening are less important than in the glenoid or other joints. Furthermore, revision of humeral components is more commonly performed for instability, component malposition or infection.[25,34] One concern prompting the use of a tissue ingrowth humeral component is that revision of cemented humeral components may be nearly impossible to perform without destroying the upper end of the humerus.[46] In our experience, removing a well-fixed porous-coated stem is equally difficult with a high risk of humeral fracture or perforation. Thus the advantage of simplifying revision surgery seems unjustified. There is no current information as to whether other strategies derived from lower-extremity implants, such as precoating, hydroxyapatite or polished tapered stems, will be of value in the shoulder.

Modularity

Modular humeral head replacements allow a larger selection of sizes for a given inventory, provide the ability to adjust soft-tissue tension after stem implantation, and facilitate glenoid implantation or revision without removing the humeral stem. Reverse Morse taper designs in which the socket is on the stem allows easy access to the glenoid after the modular head has been removed. Potential disadvantages include the risk of fretting products from the Morse taper interface, taper disassembly[47,48] and decreased head size (and thus the angular arc of the head segment to allow range of motion) for a given soft-tissue space.[39]

Blevins et al[48] reported that from 1988 to 1992, 13 clinical dissociations of the Morse taper were known to have occurred with one design of a modular humeral head replacement. Retrieval analysis failed to document wear or defects at the metal surfaces. Laboratory studies were performed suggesting that allowing fluid or blood into the socket may be a causative factor in these dissociations.[47] This particular design is a reverse-Morse taper, and because the socket sits on the stem, it may be more prone to filling with fluid. If modular designs are used, care must be taken to dry the Morse taper interface completely before engagement.

Another concern with these designs is that they use an average-sized baseplate on the stem below the Morse taper. If a large head is used, a portion of its thickness will project beyond this baseplate. This may increase the risk of dissociation if any mechanical impingement occurs on the undersurface of the head, for example by displaced tuberosities with a fracture or by the glenoid rim with a dislocation. Nevertheless, taper junction dissociation is uncommon and modularity is beneficial in many situations. It will probably always be preferable, however, to have available one-piece components for cases in which modular components are either at increased risk of dissociation or represent an unnecessary expense.

Bone interface

Aseptic loosening of cemented humeral components is rare. Although glenoid loosening has been more of a clinical problem, it still remains uncommon. In a recent review of over 1400 glenoid components reported in the literature, the revision rate was 2.9%.[27] Furthermore, classic aseptic loosening is even more rare. The majority of revisions of glenoid failure have been due to technical errors, especially failure to support the glenoid component with bone, component malposition and failure to properly release and balance the soft tissues.[42] Thus implantation technique is probably more important to glenoid component survival in the long run than design features. Still, several design issues have been investigated.

Fully constrained replacements transmitted applied loads to the bone and failed catastrophically.[6,25–32] Early partially constrained designs had superior hoods or overhangs to provide superior constraint in rotator-cuff-deficient shoulders. This has fallen out of favour for two reasons. First, the superior overhang cannot reproduce the active rotational torque of an intact rotator cuff, and thus the patient cannot externally rotate the arm to allow full elevation.[6] Second, the superior

hold is subjected to asymmetric vertical forces which potentially 'rock' the glenoid, increasing the risk of mechanical loosening.[6,30] Thus efforts to improve glenohumeral stability and mechanics have centred on soft-tissue balancing, rotator cuff repair and rehabilitation in unconstrained arthroplasties.

Finite element modelling and photoelastic models have been used to investigate stresses in the scapula resulting from glenoid implantation.[49] One problem with modelling is that it is unclear what the desirable endpoint should be. Would the best design transfer the load to the cortex, reduce peak stress magnitude or reproduce normal glenoid stress patterns? Clearly more work needs to be done before definitive conclusions may be drawn. Nevertheless, Friedman[44] found that the all-polyethylene component provides the most physiological and natural stress distributions in the glenoid, that subchondral bone should be preserved and that newer keel designs may better approximate normal physiological glenoid stresses.[44]

Bone density studies have been performed to identify the best bone for implant fixation. The normal glenoid vault is deepest and has the best bone anterosuperiorly, at the coracoid base, and inferiorly, along the axillary 'lateral mass' of the scapula.[6] However, the arthritic glenoid may have an extremely variable pattern, and implantation techniques are often individualized.

Uncemented glenoid designs have been advocated to maximize bony ingrowth and minimize the incidence of lucent lines about the glenoid and glenoid loosening.[46] Although early results have reported a decrease in the incidence of lucent lines, this design has three substantial drawbacks: it is thicker (because of metal backing), it is stiffer (also because of metal backing) and thus may be more prone to rock under an off-centre load, and it usually uses screws for initial fixation, thus providing a conduit (screw holes) for polyethylene wear particles. In addition, dissociation of the metal-backed and polyethylene components has been reported.[50] The potential advantages of uncemented glenoid components await confirmation by long-term clinical studies.

Studies of glenoid component failure have

identified lack of adequate bone support of the component as a factor in component loosening or fracture.[42] Collins et al,[51] in a laboratory study, showed less glenoid component deformation attributable to an applied off-centre load when the bone was mechanically sculpted to conform exactly to the back of the glenoid component. Although asymmetric components have been considered to allow bone support in cases of uneven glenoid wear, usually sculpting the existing bone, adjusting component version as necessary, is preferred. The need to graft a glenoid deficiency is rare.

Cost

Technical improvements in shoulder replacement technology can increase cost, and the burden will be on innovators to prove the value of these changes. For example, data collection has shown that despite the wide variety of head sizes available in many modular systems, only a few common sizes are used for the vast majority of cases.[33] Furthermore, strategies to improve implant longevity can rarely be validated until 10 or more years of follow-up has been obtained. The cost to study these systems over time is significant. These economic issues will continue to play an ever bigger role in future discussions of arthroplasty design.

Summary

The Neer design of shoulder arthroplasty has been remarkably effective and durable in the treatment of glenohumeral arthritis.[33] The achievement of the proper balance between innovation and conservatism in arthroplasty design is always difficult. Because the major causes of imperfect results are inadequacies of the soft tissues of the disease process, improper patient selection, technical considerations and/or postoperative rehabilitation, attention should not deviate from these issues when attempting to affect outcome. Nevertheless, there are many promising and exciting areas in implant design that may ultimately improve the care of the patient with an arthritic shoulder.

TECHNIQUE

Within each diagnostic category of shoulder arthritis, there is too much variability in the condition of the soft tissues and bone to permit one comprehensive discussion of surgical technique.[53] Thus the surgeon must tailor the operative procedure to the specific pathology at hand. Nevertheless, an overview of the general technique of humeral head replacement and glenoid resurfacing is provided. Special circumstances relevant to each diagnostic category are then presented.

Humeral head replacement

The operative technique is based on that described by Neer.[6,25] Either general anaesthesia or regional interscalene brachial plexus anaesthesia may be used. We prefer the interscalene block technique as many of the unpleasant side effects associated with general anaesthesia are avoided and pain control in the perioperative period is improved. Appropriate perioperative antibiotics are administered. The patient is placed in a semi-sitting or beach chair position and the head is secured to a padded head rest, avoiding hyperextension of the neck. The patient is placed high on the table, with the affected shoulder over the corner of the table. It is important to be able to fully extend the humerus over the side of the table to facilitate adequate exposure. Towels are placed under the medial border of the scapula, and a small arm board is placed on the surgical side. The shoulder girdle is then shaved, prepped with an antimicrobial scrub solution and betadine, and draped in the standard fashion.

An extended deltopectoral approach is employed to preserve the deltoid origin and insertion. A 15–17 cm incision is made inferior to the clavicle and proceeding over the coracoid and obliquely toward the deltoid insertion. The interval between the deltoid and the pectoralis major is identified and developed, retracting the cephalic vein either medially or laterally. At this point, slight abduction of the arm will release tension on the deltoid and facilitate this dissection.

In patients with a significant joint contracture, there may be medialization of the deltopectoral interval and therefore it is important not to inadvertently dissect medial to the coracoid. The clavipectoral fascia is then incised, starting lateral to the coracoid and conjoined tendon. The coracoid is not osteotomized, and retraction of the conjoined tendon is performed gently to avoid injuring the musculocutaneous nerve and brachial plexus. The subacromial space is freed of bursal adhesions or scar. Care must be taken in clearing the subacromial space, especially in cuff arthropathy and advanced rheumatoid arthritis, as the torn edge of the rotator cuff may be adherent to the undersurface of the acromion. The coracoacromial ligament is preserved in cases with massive rotator cuff tears to preserve a buffer against anterosuperior humeral ascent. If the cuff is intact but there is evidence of impingement, an acromioplasty and coracoacromial ligament resection may be performed at the time of shoulder arthroplasty. However, this is rarely needed. The tendon of the long head of the biceps functions as a humeral depressor and superior stabilizer of the humerus and should also be preserved if intact. Inferiorly, the leading edge of the pectoralis major insertion may be released for enhanced exposure and tagged for later repair. Care must be taken during this manoeuvre to protect the underlying biceps tendon.

The axillary nerve is identified by gentle palpation at the inferiomedial border of the subscapularis. Care must be taken to identify and protect this nerve during the subscapularis dissection as it may be adherent to the underlying capsule. The subscapularis and capsule are then released together at their humeral insertion to maintain maximum length. Traction sutures are placed in the cut edge of the subscapularis and used to allow gentle mobilization, while minimizing tissue trauma. Most arthritic shoulders have some degree of anterior soft-tissue contracture and loss of external rotation. Release of the anterior capsule along its glenoid insertion along with circumferential release of the subscapularis insertion are extremely important steps in enabling full postoperative external rotation as well as avoiding posterior humeral subluxation. The coracohum-

eral ligament should be released if it is contracted and thus hindering external rotation. Sharp dissection of the rotator interval between the supraspinatus and the subscapularis tendons to the area of the coracoid base is also helpful. Repairing the subscapularis, which was removed from the lesser tuberosity, to the articular edge more medially at the end of the procedure effectively lengthens this tendon. In addition, removing bulky osteophytes will also maximize the length of the subscapularis (Figure 25.2). Formal coronal step-lengthening of this tendon is usually only used if the patient has had a prior subscapularis shortening procedure (e.g. in a patient with glenohumeral arthritis after a Putti–Platt repair).

The humeral head is next dislocated by gently externally rotating the shoulder and extending the humerus off the side of the table. Dislocation is facilitated by an adequate release of the inferior and posteroinferior capsule from the humeral neck. If the biceps tendon is intact, care is taken to preserve it. At this point, it is helpful to visualize fully the posterior cuff insertion on the greater tuberosity in order to avoid damage during humeral head resection. In addition, osteophytes can be removed, especially inferiorly along the calcar, with a rongeur or osteotome to better delineate more clearly the true articular surface of the humerus (Figure 25.3). Osteophytes are often found to be more impressive in size and amount than preoperative radiographs would suggest.[11] The excision of these humeral osteophytes helps with exposure if there is difficulty in dislocating the humeral head, is necessary to prevent impingement of the humerus on the glenoid, and is used to allow maximal subscapularis and capsular mobility. A cutting guide template or the trial humeral component is used to mark the planned osteotomy. A blunt retractor is placed under the calcar of the humerus to protect the axillary nerve, and the humeral head is then resected with an oscillating saw, removing minimal bone (Figure 25.4).

As has been previously outlined, there has been a shift in emphasis from placing the humeral component in the 'correct' degree of retroversion to adjusting the version to the specific pathology present. Preliminary version in resecting the head

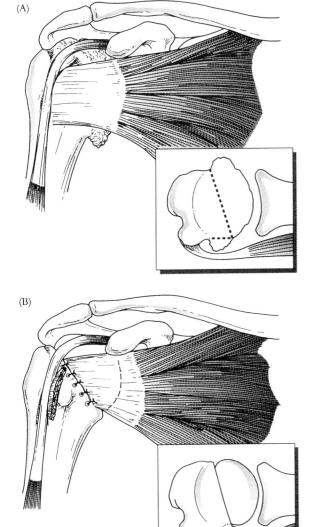

Fig. 25.2 (A) Resecting anterior osteophyte (inset) effectively lengthens anterior soft tissues. (B) Repairing subscapularis to anatomical neck medial to its original insertion also functionally lengthens the anterior soft tissue.

can be guided in several ways. In general the humeral cut is made orthogonal to the humeral shaft by externally rotating the humerus 30–35° and cutting directly parallel or judging from the humeral epicondyles and making the cut approximately 30–35° retroverted to these. Tillet et al[35] have shown that the central axis of the humeral

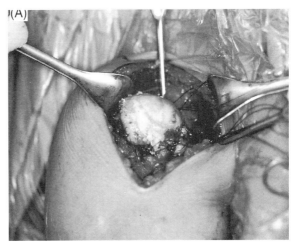

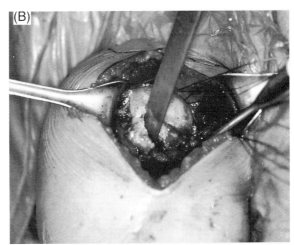

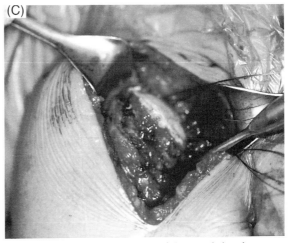

Fig. 25.3 (A)–(C) Removal of humeral head osteophytes more clearly delineates the true articular surface of the humerus.

(A)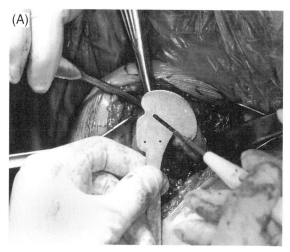

(B)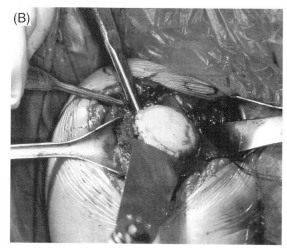

Fig. 25.4 A cutting guide template is used to mark the planned humeral head osteotomy (A), which is performed with an oscillating saw (B).

head is symmetrical to the position of the bicipital groove; thus the proper amount of retroversion can be accomplished by making the cut to allow the lateral fin of the prosthesis to be approximately 9 mm posterior to the posterior margin of the bicipital groove. The superior aspect of the osteotomy should exit just at the insertion of the posterior cuff and should not violate the infraspinatus and teres minor tendons. The rotator cuff insertion is never detached posteriorly, as this can lead to significant weakness of external rotation.

The medullary canal of the humerus is then prepared with progressive manual reaming. A slot is then made for the lateral fin of the prosthesis, just posterior to the bicipital groove. This can be done with a small rongeur or curette. Care should be taken during this process as the humerus is often soft and, especially in rheumatoid disease, can be fractured during reaming. A trial implant is then placed in the humeral canal in the appropriate amount of retroversion and the shoulder is then reduced. Humeral head height is checked to avoid excessive prominence of the tuberosity and possible impingement which occurs if the prosthetic head is below the level of the greater tuberosity. Preliminary version and soft tissue laxity are also assessed. The humeral head should be directed toward the glenoid with the arm in the anatomical position of neutral rotation.

Regarding the appropriate head size for implantation, the goal is to use a prosthetic humeral component approximately the same size as the head that was removed. The goals for shoulder motion with the prosthesis in place and the subscapularis reduced are to have 50% posterior and inferior translation, as well as external rotation to 45°. If a modular prosthesis is used, it is advisable to try several different sizes of head components to appreciate the different degrees of soft tissue laxity that each provides.

Once appropriate humeral sizing is obtained, the humeral trial is removed. If the glenoid articular surface is worn and there is adequate bone stock and either an intact cuff or functioning rotator cuff muscle–tendon unit that will centre the head on the resurfaced glenoid which can be restored by cuff repair, consideration is given to implanting a glenoid component (see next section). Otherwise, glenoid resurfacing is avoided and a humeral hemiarthroplasty is performed.[54,55]

Using bony drill holes, no. 2 non-absorbable braided sutures are placed through the anterior humeral neck region for later reattachment of the subscapularis (Figure 25.5). The humeral component is either press-fit or cemented, depending on the quality of bone. Cement is used routinely in rheumatoid arthritis, acute fractures and osteoporotic humeri with broad intramedullary canals

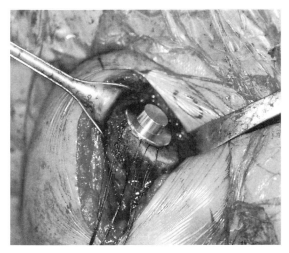

Fig. 25.5 Modular humeral component in place, with non-absorbable braided sutures placed through the surgical neck for subscapularis repair.

and thin cortical bone. A bone or synthetic cement plug is recommended in patients for whom elbow reconstruction may be a later consideration. After implantation, the subscapularis is then repaired using the bone sutures that had been placed before implanting the prosthesis.

In patients with preoperative acromioclavicular joint tenderness, an arthroplasty of this joint is performed by a technique derived from arthroscopic procedures. The joint is palpated through the deltoid muscle, and a small, 1–2 cm vertical split in the deltoid is made to allow access to it. An incision is made in the anterior and inferior acromioclavicular joint capulse, and a power burr is used from below to resect the distal clavicle. This technique preserves the superior and posterior capsule. Manual rhinoplasty rasps are used to ensure that the resection is even and that the edges are smooth. Generally, 6–8 mm of bone resection from the distal clavicle is sufficient. This approach spares the deltoid muscle, as no deltoid origin is removed, and the coracoacromial arch is preserved as well.

The wound is thoroughly irrigated. Suction drains may be used and are placed between the deltoid and rotator cuff and are brought through the deltoid and the skin through separate stab incisions. The deltopectoral interval is closed, and

finally the skin is closed with a subcuticular suture. The patient's arm is placed in a well-padded sling and swathe in neutral rotation in the operating room. It is important to avoid excessive internal rotation in the immediate perioperative period as this may lead to posterior dislocation, especially as the patient's extremity remains paralysed from a long-acting regional block.

On the first postoperative day, the swathe is removed and the arm is maintained in a sling. Suction drains are likewise removed. Administration of perioperative antibiotics is continued for 24–48 h. Passive range of motion exercises begin on the first postoperative day, consisting of pendulums, elevation in the scapular plane and external rotation exercises. The limitations of postoperative physical therapy are established by the surgeon and are based upon the specific diagnosis, integrity of the soft tissues and motion achieved at the time of surgery. These exercises are performed with a physical therapist, under the surgeon's supervision, to maintain motion and prevent the formation of adhesions in the perioperative period.[6,56] When the patient is familiar with the exercises and has achieved a sufficient passive range of motion (usually approximately 130–140° of forward elevation and 30–40° of external rotation), the patient may be discharged from the hospital to a supervised, home therapy programme.

Glenoid resurfacing

The decision on whether or not to resurface the glenoid is made during the operation based on the amount of glenoid arthritis along with the adequacy of soft tissue and bone stock available for reconstruction. Once the decision to resurface the glenoid is made, technique is important in obtaining an excellent result as the majority of glenoid revisions are for technical errors.[42] The choice of the component itself can be dictated by surgeon preference. Certain components have had a high failure rate and have been abandoned. These include oversized 200%, 600% and semiconstrained glenoid components. As previously outlined, the indications, if any, for a metal-backed glenoid are unclear. The metal-backed glenoid is particularly contraindicated, however, in the presence of significant glenoid bone loss and/or glenoid bony erosions (e.g. in rheumatoid arthritis) which would preclude initial stable fixation. The polyethylene glenoid component implanted with cement fixation has been used the most extensively and can be considered the gold standard.[25,27]

Glenoid loosening has been remarkably rare, even in active patients. Over 800 glenoid components have been implanted at our centre over 23 years, and we have revised only 12 for all causes, only four of which were due to aseptic mechanical loosening.[42] Nevertheless, loosening can occur, and in young active patients, especially those who are unwilling to limit their activities, humeral head replacement without glenoid resurfacing has been employed. The soft-tissue releases combined with humeral replacement can result in gratifying improvements in motion and pain. Neer[6] noted that he personally had not revised any humeral head replacements due to deterioration of the glenoid. However, he noted that postoperative stiffness will predispose the glenoid cartilage to damage and may necessitate conversion to a total shoulder arthroplasty, Thus the importance of adequate soft-tissue balancing and rehabilitation are emphasized. However, when the glenoid is diseased, it does seem that glenoid resurfacing offers quicker and more reliable pain relief than humeral head replacement alone.[25,57] The rate of acetabular cartilage degeneration has been shown to be greater than normal in response to articulation with a metallic hemiarthroplasty component in the hip.[58] Although destruction of the glenoid surface from the articulation of a metal humeral head is rare, it can occur. Furthermore, it has not been proven that hemiarthroplasty is a better long-term option overall than total shoulder replacement, even given the risks of glenoid loosening.

After the humerus has been prepared for prosthetic implantation, attention is turned to the glenoid for resurfacing. A Fukuda or other humeral head retractor is placed along the posterior glenoid neck and the humerus is retracted posteriorly (Figure 25.6A). A small arm board at the side of the table combined with a bolster of sterile towels will elevate the distal humerus and facilitate posterior retraction of the proximal humerus. Care is taken not to crush the exposed humeral bone; if the humerus is soft and osteopenic, the trial modular humeral component can occasionally be maintained in position to protect the proximal humerus. However, this technique may limit exposure if visualization is restricted. The anterior capsule and subscapularis are completely freed and mobilized at this time, if not done previously. A blunt retractor is placed along the anterior neck of the glenoid. Any remaining labrum is sharply resected to view the entire glenoid so accurate keel placement can be achieved. Care is taken at the inferior aspect of the glenoid during labral and capsular debridement to avoid injuring the axillary nerve. Because glenoid resurfacing is technically demanding and requires precision, it is important to maximize glenoid exposure during this aspect of the procedure.

A power burr or drill is used to penetrate the glenoid face in a vertical orientation corresponding to keel placement (Figure 25.6A). Several commercial guides are available, but the landmarks to be used to ensure adequate orientation of the keel are the coracoid base and the anterior surface of the glenoid neck. These landmarks should help to achieve the goal of placing the keel into the glenoid neck and vault of the coracoid. The use of a small curette will often aid in spatial orientation of the glenoid vault and allows the surgeon to orient the axis of further reaming to avoid penetration of the anterior or posterior glenoid neck. A common error is to orient the slot with respect to the face of the remaining glenoid rather than with its bony vault. If the slot is created 90° to the face before correcting for asymmetric posterior wear (and resulting retroversion), anterior perforation can easily occur. Also, if inadequate exposure is achieved, the surgeon's hand will be directed posteriorly during glenoid preparation and posterior perforation will occur. A power burr is then used to progressively deepen and widen the slot so that it is approximately 2–3 mm larger than the keel of the glenoid in all directions (Figure 25.6B).

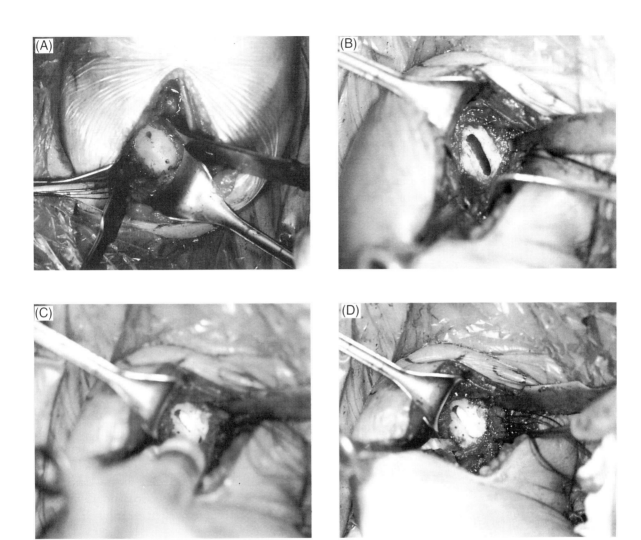

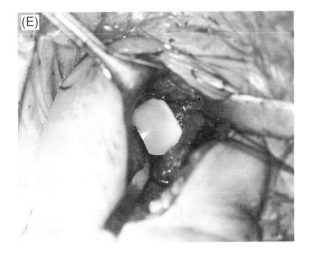

Fig. 25.6 (A) Glenoid exposure with ring humeral head retractor posteriorly and glenoid neck retractor anteriorly; drill holes placed corresponding to proper keel position. (B) Glenoid keel slot fashioned with power burr, approximately 2–3 mm larger than prosthetic keel in all directions. (C), (D) Cement placement in dry keel slot. (E) Position of all-polyethylene glenoid component.

A trial glenoid is now implanted and proper seating of the component is assessed. If the glenoid component does not rest on bone circumferentially, it will rock. To avoid this, the glenoid is contoured with the burr to allow complete seating. Collins et al[51] have emphasized the importance of preparing the bony glenoid so that it matches the contour of the back of the polyethylene. This stabilizes the component against eccentric loads which are encountered over the life of the prosthesis. The most common occurrence of glenoid asymmetry is posterior wear; when this occurs, the high anterior side of the glenoid is lowered to allow complete seating of the component.[6] If necessary, some altered glenoid version (more retroversion) is accepted and compensated for by reducing humeral retroversion.[6] In extremely rare instances, focal glenoid deficiency will be large enough that lowering the glenoid will create insufficient bone for glenoid seating. In these cases, bone grafting with the previously removed humeral head can be performed.[52] A portion of the bone from the excised humeral head is shaped using hand and power tools into a defect-filling wedge. This bony wedge is then placed posteriorly and fixed in place with small AO screws.[52] However, the need for a bone graft to support a glenoid component is rare. Use of cement to build up the defect is not recommended as the cement wedge can extrude, leading to glenoid component breakage or loosening.[42]

After the glenoid face has been adequately sculpted to allow stable seating of the glenoid trial, preparation is made for implantation. Haemostasis is obtained with a variety of techniques, as bleeding in the glenoid vault has been implicated as one cause of glenoid lucent lines. First, pulsatile lavage is used. Then a combination of thrombin-soaked gauze, peroxide, use of the electrocautery, and/or pressure can in most cases create a dry keel slot. The technique of 'double cementing' can be useful: a small amount of liquid cement is inserted and pressurized by packing the corner of a sponge into the slot. After a dry keel slot is ensured, a second infusion of cement is inserted and the prosthetic glenoid is implanted and held firmly in place to allow solid

fixation (Figure 25.6C and D). Any excess cement must be carefully removed at this time. After the component is solidly fixed and the cement cured (Figure 25.6E), the humeral component can then be sized and inserted by the techniques outlined in the preceding section on humeral replacement.

SPECIAL CONSIDERATIONS

Osteoarthritis

The surgical techniques for humeral head replacement and glenoid resurfacing as outlined above are most applicable to patients with primary osteoarthritis. It is important to differentiate this diagnosis from isolated rotator cuff disease as well as those conditions that lead to secondary osteoarthritis (post-traumatic arthritis, avascular necrosis, cuff tear arthropathy, septic arthritis, etc.).[59] Patients with primary osteoarthritis may have a positive family history of arthritis, as well as multiple joint involvement. The affected shoulder will often have decreased range of motion in all planes, with external rotation being relatively the most limited.[6] In most cases, standard plain radiographs are all that is needed for the diagnosis. However, it is felt that because standard shoulder radiographs are not weight-bearing films, the incidence of mild or moderate osteoarthritis is underestimated.[60] In fact, with the advent of arthroscopy, many patients with presumed impingement and/or rotator cuff disease have been found to have underlying osteoarthritis as their primary diagnosis.[13,14]

Neer[6] has stated that the rotator cuff probably plays some role in the aetiology of primary osteoarthritis by providing compressive joint forces required to produce this disease process in shoulders subjected to ordinary activities. This theory is supported by the fact that the incidence of full-thickness rotator cuff tears in shoulders with primary osteoarthritis which are treated with shoulder arthroplasty is exceedingly low. In fact, only four of a combined 110 shoulder arthroplasties performed for primary osteoarthritis had full-thickness rotator cuff tears.[11,20] The average age of these patients was nearly 60 years. Given our current knowledge of the incidence of rotator cuff tears in the general population, one would expect anywhere from 30 to 50% of this particular patient population to have rotator cuff tears. Thus, although the aetiology of primary osteoarthritis is probably multifactorial with genetic, biochemical, biomechanical and environmental causes, the integrity of the rotator cuff may play a significant role in its clinical expression.

Intraoperative findings in patients with primary osteoarthritis include varying degrees of anterior soft-tissue contractures, marginal osteophytes on the humeral head as well as the glenoid, loose bodies which often migrate to the subcoracoid recess and need to be removed to allow maximal excursion of the subscapularis, and posterior glenoid wear. Concomitant acromioclavicular arthritis is uncommon, but the acromioclavicular joint should be carefully evaluated before surgery, as persistent pain in this joint can lead to an unsuccessful outcome.

Recent reports have shown that total shoulder arthroplasty for primary osteoarthritis reliably provides excellent pain relief and nearly normal motion and function. In a recent review[61] of 59 patients (68 shoulders) who underwent total shoulder arthroplasty for primary osteoarthritis, 91% achieved excellent results, near-total pain relief was consistently achieved, average active forward elevation was 163°, active external rotation was 63°, and functional improvements were excellent. A properly performed arthroplasty in a patient with primary glenohumeral osteoarthritis can be a very gratifying procedure, both for the patient and the surgeon (Figure 25.7).

Rheumatoid arthritis

Although rheumatoid arthritis rarely presents initially with shoulder pain, the majority of patients with established rheumatoid arthritis have been shown to have significant shoulder problems.[6,16,17,62] In fact, in a review of over 100 patients with rheumatoid arthritis, 91% reported shoulder pain or functional limitations referable to the shoulder, with approximately 33% of the

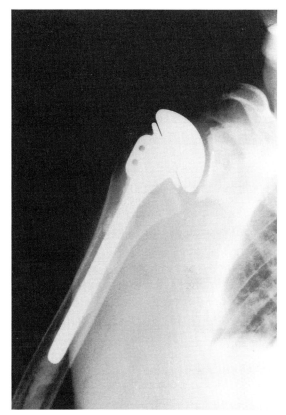

Fig. 25.7 Postoperative anteroposterior radiograph of total shoulder arthroplasty for glenohumeral osteoarthritis.

patients having severe complaints.[17] This same report concluded that once the destructive process of the rheumatoid shoulder is initiated, an inexorable downhill course ensues which inevitably provides painful restriction of shoulder motion and worsening of the patient's general functional ability.[17] This clinical course has been noted and emphasized by other authors as well.[6,7,16,25,62,63]

Patients with rheumatoid arthritis who present with shoulder pain are difficult to assess because of the systemic multiple joint involvement of their disease process.[6,62] These patients often have associated cervical spine disease with radiculopathy or myelopathy, may have referred pain from the acromioclavicular joint, subacromial bursa, rotator cuff, glenohumeral synovium, as well as pain emanating from the shoulder or hand, and are usually frail and have difficulties with manual muscle testing. Differential injections with xylocaine has been shown to be beneficial in evaluating these patients with shoulder girdle pain.[7,15]

Some patients with rheumatoid arthritis may benefit from isolated acromioclavicular arthroplasty, subacromial bursectomy, acromioplasty or rotator cuff repair if they present with these isolated findings. The more common scenario, however, is of a patient presenting with shoulder pain, weakness and radiographic evidence of humeral ascent with a narrowed joint space. Although it has been stated that conservative treatment of the rheumatoid shoulder should be carried out as long as possible,[64] most authors believe that once rheumatoid arthritis is clinically expressed as shoulder pain or functional loss, little can be done conservatively, including intra-articular steroid injections, to considerably influence the destructive course of the disease process.[6,16,17] The rate of progression, however, varies with the patient and the activity of the disease.[16,62]

Although many believe that a high-riding humerus in a patient with rheumatoid arthritis and glenohumeral joint destruction is a sign of a concomitant rotator cuff tear, most shoulder arthroplasties performed on patients with rheumatoid arthritis have an intact rotator cuff. In fact, the incidence of full-thickness rotator cuff tears has varied from 10 to 40% in patients undergoing shoulder arthroplasty.[6,62] The initial cause of the humeral ascent is thought to be loss of the superomedial aspect of the articular surface.[6] With this, the glenohumeral fulcrum is lost causing an imbalance of the force couple between a strong deltoid and a weak poorly rehabilitated rotator cuff which is no longer able to function as a humeral head depressor. Once the articular surface becomes more involved, the disease progresses. Superior translocation of the humerus eventually causes impingement erosion of the rotator cuff. In addition, severe bone loss from pannus erosion and disuse osteopenia occur. This cascade of events has led authors to recommend early shoulder arthroplasty before irreparable bone damage and cuff degeneration. As functional results from shoulder arthroplasty in patients with rheumatoid arthritis parallel the status of the bone and soft tissues, this approach is certainly reasonable. As stated by Neer,[6] the answer to an easier and more successful arthroplasty on a rheumatoid shoulder has become clear. The operation should be performed prior to the development of severe bone loss and rotator cuff damage. Thus, although clinical studies with long-term follow-up have yet to resolve this issue, the most conservative initial recommendation to the patient with rheumatoid arthritis and shoulder disability may very well be operative.[6,17,62]

In the rheumatoid patient with upper extremity involvement in multiple joints, the issue regarding the appropriate sequence of surgery is controversial. Although some have suggested that shoulder arthroplasty should take precedence over elbow arthroplasty and hand surgery,[6] others have found that elbow arthroplasty provides greater functional improvement of the upper limb if performed before shoulder arthroplasty.[63] Most agree, however, that the first surgical priority should be the joint(s) which causes the most pain and disability for the patient. Fortunately, the majority of rheumatoid patients present with a chief complaint referrable to a single joint. However, if one joint is not any more or less disabling than the others in a single extremity, surgical priority must be determined. Because the function of the shoulder and elbow are to position the hand in space for function, it seems reasonable to maximize hand and wrist function by an operation before shoulder or elbow surgery. Next, if both the elbow and shoulder appear to be equally involved, an informed and active patient can assist the surgeon in selecting which area first requires surgical attention.

The pathological findings at the time of surgery in patients with rheumatoid arthritis are variable. The humeral bone is often osteoporotic, predisposing to intraoperative fracture as well as humeral prosthetic loosening if a press-fit component is used. For this reason, cement is routinely used for humeral fixation in patients with rheumatoid arthritis. In addition, a long-stem humeral prosthesis should be available to bypass a humeral shaft fracture should it occur. The tendon of the long head of the biceps is commonly torn, and if the rotator cuff does have a full-thickness tear, it is often small and easily repaired. The glenoid bone is commonly deficient with a protrusio pattern of destruction. This often leaves the inferior glenoid pole intact, giving the face of the glenoid a cephalic tilt.[62] A burr is used to contour the inferior glenoid bone and readjust the orientation of the glenoid face before placement of the glenoid component. If there is excessive bony glenoid erosion or a massive rotator cuff tear, a glenoid component is not used. Glenoid replacement is also omitted if, despite extensive soft tissue releases, the tissues are excessively tight making it impossible to accommodate the humeral head and glenoid component while allowing a functional amount of soft-tissue laxity.[62] Involvement of the acromioclavicular joint is common, and an acromioclavicular arthroplasty is frequently required. The coracoacromial ligament, however, is maintained to provide a buttress to superior humeral migration.

The results of unconstrained total shoulder arthroplasty for rheumatoid arthritis are very much dependent on the functional integrity of the soft tissues. Although pain relief is reliably achieved, functional improvements have been less dependable. In a long-term (mean follow-up, 9.5 years) study of Neer total shoulder arthroplasties in 36 patients with rheumatoid arthritis, pain relief was excellent and 80% of shoulders could function at shoulder level at the time of final review. However, improvement in range of motion was moderate and component loosening as defined by progressive radiolucencies was present in nine humeral components and nine glenoid components. Three patients required revision for loose components.[62] Although some authors report equal pain relief and functional results in rheumatoid patients who undergo proximal humeral hemiarthroplasty,[64] most indicate that results of total shoulder arthroplasty, if indicated, are superior to those of humeral head replacement alone, both in pain relief and function.[57,62,65]

Post-traumatic arthritis

The difficulties in treating post-traumatic arthritis with shoulder arthroplasty lie not only in the abnormal bony anatomy afforded by non-unions, malunions, articular collapse and avascular necrosis, but also the significant soft-tissue contractures and scarring associated with the injury as well as any previous surgical procedures. The surgical management of post-traumatic arthritis is associated with a significant rate of complications.[66–68] Before embarking on this operative endeavour therefore a complete and detailed history, physical examination and radiographic evaluation should be performed.

The specific nature of the injury or injuries should be determined, as they will help to provide insight into the degree of soft-tissue damage that occurred. The patient's treatment, rehabilitation and convalescent course should also be determined. If previous surgery was performed, a history of infection or even a protracted healing course of the wound is important to establish. Any previous operative notes should be reviewed to help determine the pathology present at the time of surgery, pertaining especially to the management of the soft tissues. On physical examination, specific attention should be given to both active and passive glenohumeral motion in all planes, glenohumeral stability, muscle strength and a detailed neurological examination. Plain radiographs should include an anteroposterior view of the glenohumeral joint in the plane of the scapula with the humerus in neutral, internal and external rotation, a scapular lateral view, and an axillary view. It is not uncommon for malunions or nonunions to necessitate a preoperative CT to help determine the position and integrity of the tuberosities. MRI may be used to evaluate the extent of humeral head osteonecrosis or the status of the rotator cuff if clinically applicable. An EMG may also be needed to distinguish between weakness secondary to nerve injury from that associated with pain and joint incongruity. A complete blood count with white blood cell differential and an erythrocyte sedimentation rate should be obtained to rule out infection. The indication for shoulder arthroplasty in the post-traumatic setting is persistent pain and disability in a healthy well-motivated patient who has not been helped by conservative treatment.[6]

Because post-traumatic arthritis is such a broad category which encompasses many different pathological situations, there is no specific operative technique which would apply to all cases. Nevertheless, some more common intraoperative findings are worth mentioning. Soft-tissue contractures, usually in the form of internal rotation contractures, are universally present and necessitate mobilization techniques, including coracohumeral ligament and rotator interval releases, as previously described. The rare chronic locked anterior or posterior dislocation of the shoulder requires care in identification and protection of the axillary nerve, aggressive soft-tissue releases, modification of the humeral version approximately 30° away from the direction of dislocation, and glenoid sculpting or bone grafting for management of glenoid deficiency.[6,67,69–71] Tuberosity malunion may require tuberosity osteotomy before humeral head replacement if displacement is more than 1 cm in a superior direction, causing subacromial impingement, or more than 1 cm of anterior or posterolateral displacement, causing instability or coracoid impingement.[66] As outlined by Dines et al,[66] tuberosity osteotomy is performed with care to create a large osteotomy fragment which is subsequently trimmed to contour around the prosthetic head. The bicipital groove can be a helpful landmark for orientation of the osteotomy. In addition, a small modular prosthetic head is often necessary because soft-tissue contractures preclude the use of a full-sized head component.[66] Regardless of the aetiology, the importance of establishing the correct height of the humeral component has been emphasized by many authors[6,66–68] to restore the proper myofascial tension in the deltoid and rotator cuff and to prevent postoperative inferior instability. Gentle inferior traction is placed on the humerus at the time of humeral prosthetic insertion, maintaining the head adjacent to the glenoid fossa. Also, no more than approximately 50% of inferior translation should be possible with the prosthesis in place. The use of modular components is well suited in this setting.[66] Peri-operative protection and long-term rehabilitation are necessary to maximize results.

The results after shoulder arthroplasty for post-traumatic arthritis are also variable and reflective of the status of the soft tissues at the time of surgery.[6,25,68] Dines et al[66] reported a series of 20

shoulder arthroplasties performed for chronic post-traumatic arthritis with a modular prosthesis. The procedure addressed malunion or non-union in 14 patients, osteonecrosis in three and chronic fracture-dislocations in three. Hemiarthroplasty was performed in 14 patients and total shoulder arthroplasty in six who had significant glenoid changes. Excellent or good results were achieved in 14 patients; those who were older than 70 years of age and who required tuberosity osteotomy had less satisfactory results.[68] Tanner & Cofield[68] reported that better preoperative function and motion reflects a less severe insult to the cuff and tuberosity mechanisms at the original injury; thus patients with reasonable substance of the rotator cuff without scarring, or tuberosities in an anatomical position, had better results after arthroplasty. Given their experience, these authors recommended surgery be performed early to avoid the scarring and inelasticity that engender complications and limit functional recovery in shoulders with chronic fracture.

Avascular necrosis (AVN)

The natural history and management of AVN of the humeral head has received little attention in the literature.[6,18,19,72] In a review of 95 patients with AVN of bone treated by one surgeon, 18 had AVN of the humeral head and only five of these required shoulder arthroplasty due to persistent symptoms recalcitrant to non-operative treatments.[18] Patients may have a history of corticosteroid use, sickle cell disease, Gaucher's disease or previous irradiation after breast surgery or for other neoplasms.[6,18] The clinical manifestations are not unlike osteoarthritis; however, range of motion is usually maintained until late in the disease process. The radiological features parallel that of the femoral head as outlined by Ficat.[9] There is a characteristic location of articular surface collapse, corresponding to the area of contact between the humeral head and the glenoid from approximately 60° to 90° of abduction. Biomechanical studies have shown that the greatest force is exerted across the joint in this position, and it is probable that this mechanical stress determines the site of articular collapse.[18,19]

A series of 66 shoulders with atraumatic AVN of the proximal humerus has recently been reported.[72] Overall, 77% of the shoulders had clinical progression of the disease requiring surgery or resulting in severe pain and disability; 90% of these shoulders had articular incongruity of 2 mm or greater. Humeral head drilling was unsuccessful in preventing progression of the disease if articular collapse had occurred. They summarized that AVN of the proximal humerus had a relatively poor prognosis, especially with radiographic evidence of articular incongruity.[72]

Thus the management of AVN of the proximal humerus is based on articular congruity and the status of the glenoid articular surface. As mentioned by Cruess,[19] there are no prophylactic measures that can arrest the course of the disease process once it has begun. The investigational role of humeral head core decompression has previously been outlined. If a patient has disabling symptoms unresponsive to non-operative treatment, humeral hemiarthroplasty is indicated. The glenoid surface is rarely affected to the degree that glenoid resurfacing is required. Because of the lack of previous trauma, significant joint contractures or rotator cuff disease, results of shoulder arthroplasty for AVN are generally excellent.[6,18,19]

Cuff tear arthropathy[8]

Concomitant rotator cuff deficiency in patients with glenohumeral arthritis poses a formidable challenge in shoulder arthroplasty. Franklin et al[30] identified an association between loosening of the glenoid component and deficiency of the rotator cuff. In their series, six of seven cases of glenoid loosening occurred in patients with incompletely reconstructed rotator cuff tears. They found that the amount of superior migration of the humeral component correlated with the degree of glenoid loosening. The high-riding humeral prosthesis causes eccentric loading of the glenoid and results in upward tipping of the glenoid, which they refer to as a 'rocking horse glenoid'[30] (Figure 25.8). Hawkins et al,[73] in reviewing their series of 18 patients with glenohumeral arthritis and tears of the rotator cuff who underwent unconstrained total shoulder arthro-

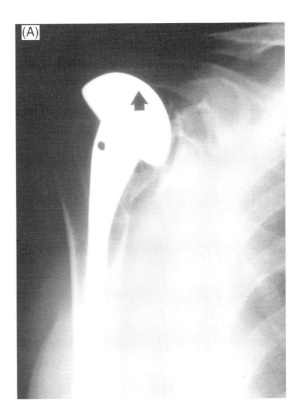

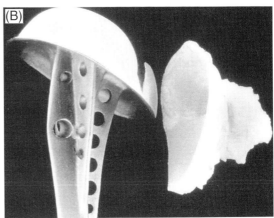

Fig. 25.8 (A) Cuff tear arthropathy with a high-riding humeral prosthesis causing eccentric superior loading of the glenoid, and subsequent glenoid component failure. (B) Components showing focal superior polyethylene wear of glenoid component.

plasty, found a similar association between rotator cuff deficiency and glenoid component loosening. Both revisions for glenoid loosening in this series were in patients who had rotator cuff deficiency and rheumatoid arthritis.

A number of treatment alternatives for this difficult problem have been reported. The use of different designs of constrained prostheses as a salvage procedure in this group of patients has led to higher rates of loosening and mechanical failure than are seen with unconstrained prosthesis; this has resulted in limited enthusiasm for constrained arthroplasty.[55] Neer et al[6,25] reported on the use of oversized glenoid prostheses in 12 patients who had massive rotator cuff tears. Two different oversized glenoids were used experimentally – ten that were 200% larger and two that were 600% larger – in an effort to provide some additional superior constraint. The 600% glenoid component did not allow the remaining rotator cuff to be closed and was therefore abandoned. Neer et al[25] noted a higher prevalence of radiolucent lines around the 200% glenoids, and at present prefer a standard-sized glenoid component for cuff tear arthropathy.[6,25] Amstutz et al[26] have also reported the use of a semiconstrained or hooded glenoid component in patients who have irreparable rotator cuff deficiency. Although postoperative pain and function were improved, range of motion was not significantly altered. Other authors have advocated standard unconstrained total shoulder arthroplasty for the treatment of cuff tear arthropathy.

Humeral hemiarthroplasty has been advocated independently[54,55] or in combination with a subacromial spacer[28,64] in patients with rheumatoid arthritis who have an irreparable rotator cuff. Marked relief of pain and improved function are achieved in most patients, and results are similar to those achieved with total shoulder arthroplasty in this subgroup of patients. Arntz et al[54] have reported satisfactory results from both glenohumeral arthrodesis and hemiarthroplasty. However, they prefer hemiarthroplasty because better motion and function is achieved. Pollock et al[54] reviewed a series of 30 shoulders in 25 patients with cuff tear arthropathy; 19 shoulders underwent humeral head replacement, and 11 had total shoulder arthroplasty. Total shoulder arthroplasty and humeral hemiarthroplasty were found to provide similar results with respect to pain relief, functional improvement and patient satisfaction. However, shoulders with hemiarthroplasty gained

significantly better range of motion, cuff repair was easier when a glenoid component was not used, and operative time, anaesthesia time and blood loss were all decreased with hemiarthroplasty alone. Because the lack of glenoid resurfacing did not adversely affect pain relief or function and avoided the potential problem of glenoid loosening, they recommend humeral hemiarthroplasty as the treatment of choice for glenohumeral arthritis in the rotator-cuff-deficient shoulder.[55]

The operative technique is basically the same as previously outlined, with some modifications.[55] Care is taken to maintain the coracoacromial ligamentous arch because this provides a superior stabilizer in these rotator-cuff-deficient shoulders. The subscapularis tendon is usually inferiorly retracted, and the head protrudes superiorly, creating a boutonniere type of deformity. The subscapularis can usually be mobilized so that there is sufficient tendon for superior transposition. It is important to examine the undersurface of the acromion because the leading edge of the posterior aspect of the rotator cuff may be adherent to this undersurface. The remaining rotator cuff tissue that composes the posterior aspect of the boutonniere deformity is freed superomedially and posteroinferiorly and is mobilized with the use of non-absorbable sutures. However, to avoid weakness of external rotation the remaining insertion of the posterior cuff is never detached. Several no. 2 non-absorbable sutures are placed through the greater tuberosity for reattachment of the posterior and superior cuff, as well as through the lesser tuberosity for reattachent of the subscapularis before implantation of the prosthesis. With the trial humeral component in place, the rotator cuff tissues are then pulled into proposed alignment, and the stability of the construct is assessed. The ability to repair the rotator cuff with the trial in situ is also judged. Because many of these glenoid surfaces are eroded (especially in patients with rheumatoid disease) and medialized, the aim is to implant as large a modular head as possible to fill the tuberosity–glenoid space. The head must still allow rotator cuff repair, however, and provide some anatomical laxity.

After the humeral head prosthesis is implanted, the rotator cuff defect is repaired and the other soft tissues are closed. The size of the tear and the quality of the remaining tendons determine the type of repair. Complete superior coverage may be obtained by transposing the subscapularis superiorly and by repairing the remnants of the posterior cuff and supraspinatus. When tissue is too deficient or is unable to hold sutures, attention is focused on achieving stable anterior and posterior buttresses to maximize postoperative stability.

The mechanical goal of total shoulder arthroplasty in the presence of an intact or reparable rotator cuff is to re-establish a painless fulcrum for the muscles. In the rotator-cuff-deficient shoulder, however, the humeral head has created a 'new fulcrum' under the coracoacromial arch.[55] The mechanics in this situation may be better than they appear. If a stable bony fulcrum has been created in the coracoacromial space, the major preoperative limitations may be due to pain secondary to joint incongruity (Figure 25.9). Humeral head replacement will relieve pain and

preserve this new fulcrum, thus allowing surprising functional gains. Attempts to relocate the fulcrum for the humerus down to the glenoid in the face of severe rotator cuff deficiency can be futile, resulting in a superiorly migrated humeral component that does not contact the resurfaced glenoid. Although it has been recognized that patients with massive tears of the rotator cuff with associated glenohumeral arthritis should expect more 'limited goals' from surgery than patients from other diagnostic categories,[6,25] patient satisfaction is high and complications are minimized with the use of humeral head replacement alone.

Arthritis after instability repair

Few reports have addressed the management of failed repairs for glenohumeral instability, and even fewer reports have evaluated the use of glenohumeral arthroplasty in the treatment of arthritis after surgery for instability repair.[6,25,74–76]

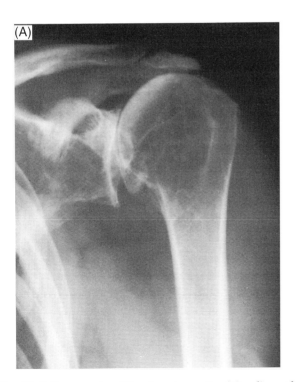 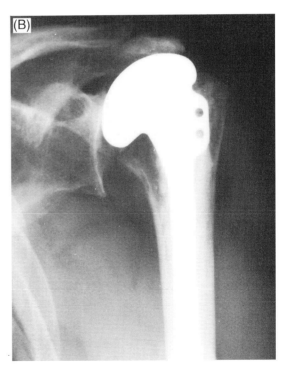

Fig. 25.9 Preoperative (A) and postoperative (B) radiographs of shoulder with cuff tear arthropathy that has undergone prosthetic replacement with humeral head component alone. The prosthesis rides high and articulates with both glenoid and acromion. The shoulder has satisfactory overall results; it is free of pain and can be used for most activities of daily living.

Arthritis is a devastating complication, because these patients are often young and athletically active. In a study of patients with arthritis after surgery for glenohumeral instability who underwent prosthetic replacement, Bigliani et al[74] reported the distorted anatomy found at the time of surgery, described special techniques to correct anterior soft-tissue contracture and to compensate for posterior glenoid bone loss, and provided results of 12 total shoulder replacements and five humeral head replacements in this subgroup of patients. At an average follow-up of 3 years, 13 (77%) patients achieved satisfactory results and four (23%) unsatisfactory results. Pain was relieved in 16 (94%) and range of motion improved by an average of 37° of elevation and 60° of external rotation

In this study,[74] the majority of patients were younger than 45 years of age and were severely limited in function by their arthritis. The operative treatment was complex as previous procedures had distorted anatomy, resulting in significant soft-tissue loss and bone deformities. Abundant scarring was encountered, making differentiation of tissue planes difficult. Most cases required lengthening of anterior joint structures. Uneven wear of the glenoid was also frequently encountered and was associated with posterior subluxation of the humeral head. It was often necessary to slightly alter the version of the glenoid component and to compensate by placing the humeral component in less than the usual 30–40° of retroversion to obtain stability.

The exact mechanism of development of the degenerative changes in the glenohumeral joint is unknown but is probably multifactorial.[36,41] Hawkins and Angelo[77] speculated that an excessively tight Putti–Platt capsulorrhaphy repair could lead to limitation of external rotation. Once the limit of external rotation is reached, any additional attempts at external rotation of the shoulder cause the humeral head to compress the surface of the glenoid, leading to deterioration of the joint.

Furthermore, if at the time of instability surgery excessive tightness is created on one side of the joint, a fixed subluxation or dislocation of the humeral head can occur in the opposite direc-

tion.[6] The subluxated head then wears unevenly on the glenoid, leading to articular damage and arthritis.[41] Posterior humeral subluxation is often seen in patients in this subgroup, indicative of overtightening of anterior structures. This problem requires anterior soft-tissue release and lengthening of the subscapularis tendon at the time of arthroplasty. Fenlin et al[78] emphasize that rim loading can occur in the anteroposterior plane after total shoulder arthroplasty in this patient population just as it can in the superior direction in rotator-cuff-deficient shoulders, predisposing to glenoid loosening. They recommend diligence in obtaining soft-tissue balance in the form of extensive anterior releases and occasional posterior capsular reefing to prevent eccentric loading of the glenoid component.

MacDonald et al[12] reported on ten patients who had an internal rotation contracture and pain after an anterior repair for recurrent dislocation. Six also had severe arthritic changes. All were treated with an anterior soft-tissue release and subscapularis lengthening and all had less pain and more external rotation at follow-up evaluation. However, the six patients with severe arthritis averaged only 15° of external rotation at follow-up evaluation (range 10–35°), whereas the four with mild to moderate arthritis averaged 51° of external rotation (range 25–70°). Although an isolated open soft-tissue balancing procedure may be an option in the patient with less severe arthritis, we prefer to combine replacement arthroplasty with soft-tissue balancing for shoulders with severe arthritis to achieve adequate pain relief and external rotation for function.[74] In the series of Bigliani et al,[74] the average preoperative external rotation was −2°. With the combination of soft-tissue releases and arthroplasty, the average external rotation after the operation improved to 58°.

Thus, glenohumeral replacement arthroplasty provides a satisfactory treatment for arthritis that develops after instability surgery.[6,25,74,76] Glenohumeral arthroplasty can be a rewarding procedure in a high percentage of these patients, leading to decreased pain and increased range of motion and thus greatly improved function. However, arthroplasty in this setting is a challenging task.

Soft-tissue contractures and asymmetric posterior glenoid wear make establishment and maintenance of component stability and restoration of motion more difficult than in, for example, primary glenohumeral arthritis.

Infection

Infection is a rare complication after prosthetic replacement of the glenohumeral joint. Several reviews have shown infection rates at or below 0.5%, suggesting lower occurrence than has been reported for other joints.[4,5,25] However, it is still a catastrophic complication causing pain, stiffness and loss of function.[5] Furthermore, there are very few reports in the literature on which to base clinical management decisions regarding the treatment of this problem. Reports on infections after knee and hip arthroplasty have suggested several treatment options, including irrigation and debridement, immediate exchange arthroplasty, staged reimplantation and resection arthroplasty. Historically, the recommended treatment for this complication of the glenohumeral joint has been resection arthroplasty.[5,25] In addition, previous deep infection has been generally regarded as a contraindication to implant arthroplasty.[6,25] Considering the recent literature on other major joint arthroplasties, these recommendations would appear to be quite conservative with regard to the management of infected shoulder arthroplasties.

The preoperative evaluation of patients with suspected infected arthroplasties can be quite difficult. The presentation of an aseptic failed shoulder arthroplasty can be similar to a septic one. In the series of Codd et al,[21] no single preoperative study was found to be 100% accurate. There was a 20% rate of false negative aspirations, a 40% rate of false negative bone scans and a 13% rate of false negative intraoperative cultures. In addition, white blood cell counts were usually within normal limits. While only 13% of sedimentation rates were normal before the operation only two were very high with values of 80 and 126 respectively. These results are comparable with literature on hip and knee operations which reports accuracy rates of approximately 80% for aspiration, 45% for bone scan and 70–75% for sedimentation rates. One difference in the preoperative presentation of shoulder infections, as opposed to that of hip and knee infections, is the relative lack of systemic findings; only two of the 16 patients in the study of Codd et al[21] had generalized malaise, and none were systemically ill. It is not uncommon, however, for these patients to be immunocompromised secondary to systemic disease and/or corticosteroid treatments.

Without a perfectly reliable test for infection, clinical judgment in interpreting preoperative studies becomes paramount. All issues such as a history of trauma, medical risk factors, concomitant illnesses, an immunocompromised host, history of wound healing problems, radiographs, sedimentation rates, aspirations, bone scans, intraoperative cultures and microscopic pathology can be used in combination to assist in clinical decision making. Because shoulder arthroplasty infection is such a rare entity, an exact algorithm has yet to be established for the clinical work-up of these patients. Microscopic pathology seems to be the most accurate 'study', however, correlating 100% with either operative cultures or the surgeon's clinical diagnosis in one study.[21] It should be emphasized that prosthetic arthroplasty for fractures may face a higher risk of infection, due to local tissue damage and haematoma that accompany acute fractures. In several series of arthroplasties for acute fractures, the reported incidence of infection has been from 3.1 to 4.8%, significantly higher rates than those encountered after prosthetic replacement.[6,21]

In a report of 16 patients in which infection was considered with prosthetic shoulder arthroplasty, Codd et al[21] concluded that reimplantation of another prosthesis after treatment of the deep prosthetic infection is a reasonable option. All of the patients in this category had no recurrence of infection at an average follow-up of 47 months. These patients were treated with resection arthroplasty, placement of an antibiotic-impregnated cement hemiarthroplasty spacer which provides local antibiotic delivery as well as maintaining normal soft-tissue relationships, and staged prosthetic reimplantation after an appropriate course of intravenous antibiotics. Similarly, prosthetic arthroplasty was found to be a safe alternative after primary glenohumeral joint infection if the infection had been treated and eradicated.[21]

Given the poor functional results for activities performed at or above shoulder level seen historically with resection arthroplasty,[2,5] reimplantation can generally be regarded as the treatment of choice.[21] The relative attributes of two- versus one-stage reimplantation are difficult to address due to the relative infrequency of this complication. Two-stage reimplantation has generally shown advantages in infection control, yet some studies have suggested that single-stage implantation is adequate when Gram-positive organisms are involved and antibiotic cement is used. The concerns with staging involve balancing the reduced infection risk against problems of scarring and joint contractures seen with two-stage procedures. Scarring and contractures have especially adverse implications in the shoulder, where functional mobility is easily lost. Some of these contractures can be reduced with the placement of an antibiotic cement hemiarthroplasty spacer which will maintain the soft-tissue relationships and minimize scarring. The decision on staging should be based on the relative virulence of the organism, the chronicity of the infection and the overall health of the patient.

Treatment of patients with infected shoulder arthroplasties should follow guidelines established for infected hip and knee arthroplasties, which are generally not treated with resection. It is not surprising that the shoulder can be treated similarly. With an infection rate less than 0.5% for all arthroplasties, including several large series reporting no infections, the shoulder appears to be well protected against postoperative infection. Its soft tissue coverage, excellent blood supply and excellent drainage properties perhaps make the shoulder better anatomically suited to fight infection than the hip or knee. It appears that arthroplasty can often be successfully performed in the shoulder once the infection has been eradicated.

Revision shoulder arthroplasty

Reconstruction after a failed shoulder arthroplasty is especially challenging. The problem differs from that of revision hip and knee arthroplasties because of the unique feature of the rotator cuff. The soft tissue around a 'failed' and immobile shoulder prosthesis soon becomes scarred and frozen, making revision arthroplasty one of the most difficult of all shoulder procedures.[25] Furthermore, the situation may be complicated by significant bone loss or muscle paralysis. The literature reflects revision rates from 0 to 17% after primary shoulder arthroplasty, but publications that specifically address revision shoulder surgery are rare.[25,34] In a prospective study of 40 consecutive humeral head and total shoulder arthroplasties, Neer and Kirby[25] outlined the various causes of failure and provided recommendations for treatment. More than one factor involved in failure was present in almost every case. These causes of failure included deltoid scarring and detachment, contractures of the subscapularis muscle and anterior capsule, adhesions and impingement of the rotator cuff, prominent or retracted tuberosities, loss of humeral length and uneven wear on the glenoid and/or 'centralization'. A universal problem present in all failed arthroplasties was scarring of the subacromial space and rotator cuff beneath the deltoid that had occurred as the result of immobilization. In many cases, it was found that the major cause of failure appeared to be an inadequate rehabilitation regime after the operation. These authors emphasize a surgeon-directed aggressive approach to rehabilitation in all primary arthroplasties.

Wirth & Rockwood[34] reviewed 38 consecutive unconstrained shoulder arthroplasty revisions performed from 1977 to 1983. The initial indication for arthroplasty was acute trauma in 19 shoulders, osteoarthritis in 12 shoulders, arthritis after instability repair in five shoulders and rheumatoid arthritis in two shoulders. Five patients had undergone eight prior attempts at revision arthroplasty. Revision surgery consisted of 19 total shoulder replacements, 11 hemiarthroplasties and eight resection arthroplasties. These authors also found causes of failure to be multifactorial; however, 43% were revised because of symptomatic instability which was correlated with inadequate humeral length, poor soft-tissue balancing and component malposition.

The indications for revision arthroplasty of the shoulder are the same as in the primary setting: pain and loss of function. Before embarking on surgery, however, every effort should be made to determine the exact aetiology of failure. As with any revision procedure, a thorough understanding of the indications, operative procedure and initial results from the primary surgery must be obtained. The history and physical examination should focus on the potential causes of failure as outlined above by Neer and Kirby, as well as infection, missed diagnosis (e.g. acromioclavicular arthritis, cervical disc disease), deltoid denervation, technical failure(s) and aseptic loosening of the humeral or glenoid component. Radiographs, laboratory tests and other special studies (EMG, CT, MRI, etc.) are used as needed to complete the necessary preoperative evaluation. Also, the patient must understand that he or she must play an active and integral part in the rehabilitation process, which is often prolonged in this setting, and that results after revision procedures are inferior when compared with other diagnostic categories.[25,34]

Regarding the technical aspects of revision shoulder arthroplasty, generalizations are difficult as each case must be approached individually according to the pathology. Previous surgical incisions should be incorporated into the approach, if possible, to avoid skin necrosis. Also, unnecessary skin flaps should be avoided as vascularity may be precarious. Intraoperative Gram stain and cultures should be taken and specimens sent for microscopic pathology to rule out infection. Prophylactic antibiotics are routinely administered, but not until all cultures have been obtained. Soft-tissue mobilization, as previously outlined, is universally necessary. Importantly, the subacromial space usually contains adhesions that must be fully lysed as they are a significant cause of loss of glenohumeral motion. Bone preservation should always be emphasized, especially when components require removal due to wear, malposition or infection or to gain proper access for glenoid revision.

In non-infected cases, the revision proceeds with dislocation of the humeral head replacement via external rotation and extension. The version of the humeral head replacement is measured and the component is also assessed for signs of loosening or damage. To gain proper access to the glenoid, the humeral head replacement must be removed. In cases in which the humeral component has the proper version and is well fixed with cement, this step is facilitated by a modular system as the modular head can be simply removed. However, well-fixed modular humeral stems can be extremely difficult to remove if necessary. The broad collar of a modular design often extends beyond the cortical edge of the humeral metaphysis, precluding the use of flexible osteotomes to help release the component. In contrast, a well-fixed Neer II humeral component with a smooth stem is less difficult to remove because the proximal geometry of this prosthesis permits the successful use of thin flexible osteotomes. In addition, the fixed humeral head is easily gripped and hammered out of the humeral canal. In some cases, small amounts of abnormal humeral version in well-fixed modular components can be overcome by upgrading the size of the humeral head, avoiding the potential damage that could occur to the proximal humeral bone stock. If the version is too excessive, however, the humeral component must be removed and replaced. In this instance, planned cortical windows or linear cortical cuts can help prevent excessive bone damage. Cerclage wires can be utilized later in the procedure to reconstruct these cortical defects. With the help of cement-removal tools, high-speed drills and ultrasonographic equipment, every effort is made to remove remaining humeral cement without damage to the native humeral bone stock. A long-stem prosthesis, allograft bone and cerclage wires should be available if an intraoperative humeral shaft fracture should occur, especially in patients with rheumatoid arthritis.

With the humerus retracted posteriorly with a Fukuda retractor, the glenoid can be adequately visualized. The failed glenoid component, if applicable, is removed. With loose glenoids, the component and its associated cement can often be easily removed. However, in broken or damaged glenoids with well-fixed stems, this step can be very difficult. Again, every effort should be made to preserve glenoid bone stock while removing all cement. A small thin osteotome is used to help release the glenoid platform. The component is then levered out of the glenoid. If a damaged or broken polyethylene component is encountered and is difficult to remove because of maintenance of fixation at the stem, the component can be fragmented and removed in a piecemeal fashion. A high-speed drill is often helpful in breaking up the cement and polyethylene.

The remaining glenoid bone stock is then surveyed. In cases where the bone stock is adequate and the articular surface worn, the native glenoid is contoured with a high-speed burr to allow for a concentric matched fit of a new glenoid component. If focal posterior or anterior bone loss is evident, the glenoid is contoured in the opposite direction to normalize the version of the glenoid. In many cases, much of the glenoid bone stock is lost. This can result in a native glenoid with massive central bone deficiency. The little remaining bone is often incapable of supporting a glenoid component. In these cases, it is preferred to remove the glenoid component and simply replace the humeral head component. The remaining rim of peripheral cortical glenoid bone allows for a concentric fit of the humeral head replacement. The head can be increased in size to allow for proper tensioning of the soft tissues.

The remainder of the operative procedure in revision arthroplasties differs little from that of primary surgery, as previously outlined.

The overall results of revision shoulder arthroplasty are not as reliable as in the primary setting. Neer et al reported seven excellent, three satisfactory and five unsatisfactory results after revision arthroplasty, with six additional patients achieving successful results with limited-goals rehabilitation.[25] Of 16 shoulders treated by revision shoulder arthroplasty and followed for at least 2 years, Wirth & Rockwood[34] reported five excellent, seven satisfactory, and four unsatisfactory results. All of the unsatisfactory results demonstrated marked anterior deltoid weakness and dysfunction before attempted revision.[34] Results can be maximized, however, by performing a thorough preoperative evaluation to determine the exact cause or causes of failure before revision shoulder arthroplasty.

POSTOPERATIVE MANAGEMENT

Postoperative rehabilitation after shoulder arthroplasty is the most underemphasized aspect of the procedure, although arguably the most important. Because of the unique anatomical arrangement and function of the rotator cuff, rehabilitation of the shoulder after surgery is also more difficult than that of any other joint. In many of these patients, muscles involved in the complex synchronous movements of the scapula and humerus have been atrophied from months or years of disuse. Also, the disease process itself may cause direct bone and soft-tissue damage. Nevertheless, because a good rehabilitation programme is necessary in restoring optimum function, the shoulder surgeon must not only understand this type of rehabilitation but also remain actively involved with the patient and therapist to make it successful. As emphasized by Neer, only the surgeon knows the intraoperative pathology and the stability of the soft-tissue repair and only the surgeon can use this knowledge to direct the therapist to achieve the maximum recovery of function.[25,28,79]

An important aspect of the comprehensive evaluation and management of a patient with shoulder pathology is for the surgeon to assess the patient's general health status and motivation for improvement. Patients must be very actively involved in their own rehabilitation process and this must be emphasized preoperatively. It is also helpful for the patient to meet his or her physical therapist before surgery to review the planned postoperative protocol. In addition, all arrangements necessary for immediate physical therapy after hospital discharge should be made before the operation.

Neer's[25] three-phase shoulder rehabilitation programme is based on a logical progression of joint mobilization, allowing tissue healing, followed by muscle strengthening. Phase I emphasizes local modalities (warm applications in preparation for shoulder exercises, ultrasound, etc.) to help achieve passive assisted motion in forward elevation and external rotation, with limitations set by the surgeon at the time of the procedure. Phase II progresses to active-assisted and active exercises of the shoulder when allowed by healing and continuity of the repaired tissues (usually between 4 and 8 weeks, depending on the pathology). Phase III advanced muscle stretching and progressive resistive strengthening exercises usually start approximately 3 months after surgery and continue indefinitely. Again, the patient's specific pathology, quality of soft tissue and motivation are all used by the surgeon to modify the timing of this programme appropriately.

A manual technique for early passive motion starting within the first 48 h of shoulder surgery has been outlined by Neer,[6,56] and remains the preferred technique of physical therapy during the perioperative phase of rehabilitation. Prerequisites for early passive motion include complete operative release of adhesions and short tendons to allow a full range of forward elevation and external rotation, a stable implant, sufficiently strong soft-tissue repair to enable passive motion without disruption, a knowledgeable person raising the arm (e.g. surgeon, physical therapist, trained family member) and complete relaxation of the arm. Premedication with oral narcotics is used to assist relaxation during the first several postoperative days. Pendulum exercises, passive motion in forward elevation in the scapular plane and external rotation are performed two to three times daily. Usually by the third or fourth postoperative day, the regular self-assisted progamme of exercises are started (e.g. pulley, external rotation with a stick, internal rotation, etc.) and advanced as tolerated. The success of this technique in shoulder arthroplasty has been reported by Neer.[6] Of 98 shoulders, 85% achieved over 140° of passive elevation by the sixth postoperative day, with 100% of patients with primary osteoarthritis achieving this motion. The exceptions were three of 16 patients with rheumatoid arthritis, two of seven with arthritis after instability repair, two of ten acute fractures, four of 14 post-traumatic arthritis, and three of five revision procedures. Hospital discharge occurred earlier in these patients, motion was maintained after discharge with self-assisted exercises and long-term follow-up showed no complications or detrimental effects of this early passive motion programme.[6]

Some patients with extensive loss of bone and/or soft tissue whose indication for arthroplasty is pain relief can achieve satisfactory results and function with the arm at the side through a limited-goals rehabilitation programme.[6,8,25] This programme was initiated to maintain glenohumeral rotation in patients treated with shoulder arthroplasty for a resected proximal tumour, cuff tear arthropathy or long-standing rheumatoid arthritis, rather than performing an arthrodesis. Limited-goals rehabilitation avoids overhead exercises and exercises extending into the extremes of rotation that make the glenohumeral joint unstable, as the muscles and/or bone are inadequate to move and stabilize the shoulder into these positions. During the first 3 months after surgery, passive elevation to 100° and external rotation to 20° with the arm at the side are maintained with pendulum exercises. Thereafter, the soft tissue usually permits isometric exercises to be performed in this functional range. After 6 months the patient progresses to activities as tolerated, and some patients may eventually become strong enough to be advanced to various aspects of the full rehabilitation programme.[6]

Potential rehabilitation problems not infrequently seen after humeral head replacement and total shoulder arthroplasty can occur with respect to each diagnostic category.[6] In osteoarthritis, posterior glenoid wear with a loose posterior capsule may predispose to postoperative posterior instability. Precautions should be taken to avoid early elevation in forward flexion (as opposed to forward elevation in the scapular plane) and adduction in patients with osteoarthritis. In patients with shoulder arthroplasty for rheumatoid arthritis, coexistent arthritis in the cervical spine, ipsilateral elbow and hand, contralateral upper extremity and/or both lower extremities may require improvisation with physical therapy. If significant rotator cuff defects were repaired at the time of surgery, strengthening rehabilitation should be delayed until healing. Also, the overall rehabilitation process in patients with rheumatoid arthritis is prolonged; the patient should be encouraged to persevere. In arthroplasties for post-traumatic arthritis, the potential for postoperative instability may be an issue due to long-standing soft-tissue contractures or failure to achieve proper humeral height, and rehabilitation should be tailored to the pathology present. In addition, nerve injuries, bone loss, cuff defects, deltoid muscle defects, and dense scar make rehabilitation especially challenging in this patient population. In arthroplasty for cuff tear arthropathy, limited-goals rehabilitation is advocated. In arthroplasties for arthritis after instability repair, decisions regarding postoperative positioning in a sling or brace as well as range limitations with physical therapy should be dictated by the degree and direction of preoperative instability. Rehabilitation after revision arthroplasty is of crucial importance in preventing postoperative adhesions, as scarring of the subacromial space and rotator cuff after immobilization after the primary procedure is a universal problem.[25]

COMPLICATIONS

The incidence of complications after shoulder arthroplasty has been less than for other major joint reconstructions.[4] However, when they occur, the sequel can be profound. Although many complications can be potentially avoided by proper indications, technique and rehabilitation of primary arthroplasty, some are unavoidable. They encompass a wide range and can be specific to certain diagnoses. It is important for the reconstructive shoulder surgeon to be aware of the potential complications of glenohumeral arthroplasty and be prepared to address them as needed.

Evaluation

The evaluation of complications following a total shoulder replacement should be as thorough as the initial work-up for a primary replacement. A complete history, including previous operative notes and physical examination, is essential. Pain, tenderness and loss of function must be determined. The presence of deformity, neurological injury, infection, instability and loss of motion must be clearly outlined. If infection is considered,

diagnostic laboratory tests, including a complete blood count and erythrocyte sedimentation rate as well as an aspiration, should be considered.

A complete shoulder series is needed, including an anteroposterior view in the plane of the scapula in internal rotation, neutral and external rotation, a scapular lateral or outlet view and an axillary view. The anteroposterior views help delineate the relationship of the humeral head prosthesis to the shaft and tuberosities as well as the superior and inferior position in reference to the glenoid. Also, glenoid loosening can be evaluated on these views. Rotational views are helpful to outline tuberosity displacement or ectopic bone formation. The axillary view will detect anterior or posterior instability of the humeral head as well as displacement of the glenoid prosthesis. The supraspinatus outlet view, a lateral in the scapular plane with 10° caudal angulation, will reveal subacromial impingement lesions.

An arthrogram is useful to evaluate the rotator cuff for complete-thickness rotator cuff tears. Also, loosening may be appreciated if the dye leaks between the cement–bone interface. A CT scan may be helpful to evaluate bone stock and component loosening, but special techniques must be used to decrease metal scatter. Bone scanning is useful to differentiate between aseptic loosening and infection. At present, standard MRI is not as useful as these other diagnostic procedures in the postoperative evaluation of total shoulder replacements. Arthroscopy may prove useful, especially in determining glenoid component loosening,[80] but this is still developmental.

Types of complications

Nerve injuries

Nerve injury during total shoulder arthroplasty is uncommon. Fortunately, these injuries most often represent neuropraxia, which can be treated expectantly. EMG and NCS can be useful in documenting the extent of injury as well as any serial improvement in nerve function. The axillary nerve is the most likely to be injured as it runs on the inferior aspect of the capsule curving posteriorly on the undersurface of the deltoid muscle. If there is a suspicion that the axillary nerve was lacerated at surgery and the EMG at 6 weeks reveals a complete lesion with no improvement at 3 months, early exploration and repair are suggested. If the initial lesion is partial and improving, observation is indicated.

Careful localization or palpation of the axillary nerve, particularly in revision or post-traumatic surgeries, is essential. If an intraoperative injury is identified, microsurgical repair should be performed at that time. Unfortunately, the muscle transfers presently available for deltoid paralysis are not satisfactory.

Fractures

Intraoperative fractures are uncommon but may occur, especially in osteoporotic or rheumatoid bone. The bone is extremely soft and the cortices are thin. Fracture commonly occurs with reaming, dislocation of the humeral head or reduction of the prosthesis. It is important while reaming the shaft to keep the reamers in the longitudinal direction of the humeral shaft. If there has been a previous prosthesis, the track of the previous stem may guide the reamers out of the cortex. Therefore it is important to break through the most inferior part of the previous stem track with a small drill. If a perforation occurs in the humeral shaft near the tip of the prosthesis, a long-stemmed prosthesis may be required to bridge the gap. A barrier should be used on the outside surface of the humeral shaft to avoid extravasation of cement into the soft tissues and possible radial nerve injury. Oblique fractures of the humeral shaft are treated in a similar fashion. However, sometimes the prosthesis will not allow for a secure stable fit. In this instance, the rehabilitation should be modified in the postoperative period to avoid active exercises for an 8–12-week period of time to allow sufficient fracture healing.

Postoperative fractures can be treated conservatively if the fracture is stable. However, if the fracture is unstable, further surgery is required.[81,82] Internal fixation may be extremely difficult, requiring special plates which incorporate cerclage wires as well as screws, autograft bone graft, allograft cortical struts or long-stemmed prostheses. Bonutti and Hawkins[81] have emphasized that periprosthetic fractures of the proximal humerus have a higher incidence of non-union, and aggressive treatment should be considered.

Tuberosity fractures can also occur in soft osteoporotic bone. Fortunately, these can be managed in the same fashion as four-part fractures with fixation via non-absorbable nylon sutures through the tuberosities. These should be attached to both the fin of the prosthesis and the proximal shaft.

Loosening

As mentioned, revision surgery for component loosening after shoulder arthroplasty is rare.[25,42,73] Very few cases of humeral component loosening have been reported. Neer[25] reported no significant loosening in the humeral component in his personal series of 776 cases. However, some cases of humeral head subsidence do occur, especially if there is osteoporotic bone. In this instance, cement should be used to avoid this problem. A press-fit technique is indicated only when there is sufficient bone stock to support the prosthesis, like that found in the younger patient.

Although radiolucent lines around the glenoid are common (30–83%), there has not been a direct correlation between radiolucent lines and clinical loosening.[42,73,83] A radiographic follow-up study of 69 total shoulder replacements found that 48 patients had glenoid lucent lines present before hospital discharge.[83] However, only six of these progressed, and one was symptomatic after an average follow-up of 5 years. Another series of 70 total shoulder replacements followed for 5–11 years noted a complete lucent line of 1.5 mm or more around one-third of glenoids, yet only three revisions were necessary for glenoid loosening.[73] And as previously reviewed, only 12 glenoid revisions have been necessary from over 800 total shoulder arthroplasties performed at our shoulder centre over the past two decades.[42]

The clinical relevance of radiolucent zones at the glenoid–bone interface is difficult to interpret. Since these lucent lines are frequently noted in the immediate postoperative period, they may reflect cementing technique or the poor quality of glenoid bone stock. Neer[6,25] attributed these radiolucent lines to a variety of factors, including inconsistent radiographic technique, variable density and strength of bone, stress shielding by the glenoid component and disuse osteoporosis.

Neer & Kirby[25] and Brems et al[83] both reported a higher incidence of complete lucent lines in the earlier cases in their series performed during the learning curve. Careful preparation of the glenoid slot with thorough lavage and adequate haemostasis will decrease the incidence of lucent lines. Also, the amount of cement used in the glenoid should be minimal: basically, only enough to fill the slot should be used. We have found that pressure lavage has been extremely helpful in removing debris and achieving haemostasis in the glenoid vault.

Instability

Fortunately, postoperative subluxation or dislocation has been reported to occur in only 1–2% of cases. Stability of an unconstrained implant depends on preservation of humeral length, proper version of the components and balancing of the soft tissues. Also, an intact rotator cuff is essential for superior stability. Careful attention to the maintenance of humeral length will help to prevent inferior subluxation, as it is important to maintain the proper myofascial sleeve tension. Neer[6] reported on 194 total shoulder replacements with an average of 37 months follow-up. There were four dislocations: two anterior and two posterior. All occurred within 3 weeks of surgery and all were reduced, immobilized for 3–6 weeks and then rehabilitated. None required further surgery, although one had recurrent subluxations.[6] Moeckel et al[84] reported on ten patients who had instability of the shoulder after arthroplasty. Anterior instability, which occurred in seven patients, was caused by a rupture of the repaired subscapularis tendon in each instance. The aetiology of posterior instability in three patients was multifactorial. Treatment was operative in each case: anterior instability was addressed by mobilization and repair of the subscapularis, and posterior instability was addressed by soft-

tissue balancing and revision of the prosthetic components as necessary. Three patients with recurrent anterior instability required Achilles allograft reconstruction of a deficient subscapularis tendon. Eventual stability was achieved in nine of ten patients.

The humeral component should be inserted in 30–40° of retroversion unless there is uneven glenoid wear. As previously mentioned, if there is significant posterior glenoid wear that cannot be addressed by sculpting the anterior glenoid, then less retroversion is needed. However, the decrease in retroversion should not be excessive, as anterior dislocation may occur. Revision of a dislocated prosthesis generally entails a correction of prosthesis malposition as well as soft-tissue procedures of both the capsule and the muscles about the shoulder to achieve soft-tissue equilibrium.[4,84]

Heterotopic bone

Clinically significant formation of heterotopic bone after total shoulder replacement is uncommon. However, a series from Denmark reported that 10% of their cases had ossifications bridging the glenohumeral and/or glenoacromial space and were associated with limited range of motion.[85] These authors reported no correlation between shoulder pain and the development of ossification. However, ectopic bone has not been clinically significant in most series.[6]

Rotator cuff tears

Postoperative tearing of the rotator cuff is one of the more frequent complications after total shoulder arthroplasty, with an incidence of 3–4%. Neer & Kirby[25] reported five traumatic cuff tears in a report on 194 total shoulder replacements. Two underwent surgical repair, two remained weak but without symptoms and one had intermittent pain but refused further surgery. Although patients with rotator cuff tears show some functional limitation, significant pain has not been an associated problem in the majority of reports. While further repair is not always required, the report by Franklin et al[30] concerning glenoid loosening and large cuff tears may support the repair of large postoperative rotator cuff tears.

CONCLUSIONS

As shoulder arthroplasty enters into the new era of implant design and materials research, modularity, tissue ingrowth and heretofore unknown advancements, the cornerstone of successful results has alway depended on proper patient selection, operative techniques and postoperative rehabilitation, and will probably continue to do so. Although promising and exciting research continues in this field, the basic principles and techniques of shoulder arthroplasty as outlined by Neer remain the standard. Hopefully, the maintenance of these principles will combine with the aforementioned advancements in shoulder arthroplasty, leading to improved patient care and ultimate outcomes.

REFERENCES

1. Lugli, T. (1978) Artificial shoulder joint by Pean (1893). *Clin. Orthop.* **133:** 215.
2. Neer, C.S., Brown, T.H. & McLaughlin, H.L. (1953) Fracture of the neck of the humerus with dislocation of the head fragment. *Am. J. Surg.* **85:** 252.
3. Neer, C.S. (1955) Articular replacement of the humeral head. *J. Bone Joint Surg.* **37A:** 215.
4. Miller, S.R. & Bigliani, L.U. (1993) Complications of total shoulder replacement. In Bigliani, L.U. (ed.) *Complications in Shoulder Surgery*, pp. 59–72. Williams & Wilkins.
5. Cofield, R.H. (1985) Shoulder arthrodesis and resection arthroplasty. *Instr. Course Lect.* **34:** 268–277.
6. Neer, C.S. II (1990) Glenohumeral instability. In *Shoulder Reconstruction*, pp. 143–271. Philadelphia: W.B. Saunders.
7. Kelly, I.G. (1994) The source of shoulder pain in rheumatoid arthritis: usefulness of local anesthetic injections. *J. Shoulder Elbow Surg.* **62:** 3–4.
8. Neer, C.S., Craig, E.V. & Fukuda, H. (1983) Cuff-tear arthropathy. *J. Bone Joint Surg.* **65A:** 1232–1244.
9. Ficat, R.P. (1985) Idiopathic bone necrosis of the femoral head. Early diagnosis and treatment. *J. Bone Joint Surg.* **67B:** 3–9.
10. Boyd, A.D., Aliabadi, P. & Thornhill, T.S. (1991) Postoperative proximal migration in total shoulder arthroplasty. Incidence and significance. *J. Arthroplasty* **6:** 31–37.
11. Neer, C.S. (1974) Replacement arthroplasty for glenohumeral arthritis. *J. Bone Joint Surg.* **56A:** 1.
12. MacDonald, P.B., Hawkins, R.J., Fowler, P.J. & Miniaci, A. (1992) Release of the subscapularis for internal rotation contracture and pain after anterior repair for recurrent anterior dislocation of the shoulder. *J. Bone Joint Surg.* **74A:** 734–737.
13. Weinstein, D.M., Bucchieri, J.S., Pollock, R.G., Flatow, E.L. & Bigliani, L.U. (1993) Arthroscopic debridement of the shoulder for osteoarthritis. *Arthroscopy* **9:** 366.
14. Ellman, H.A., Harris, E. & Kay, S. (1992) Early degenerative joint disease simulating impingement syndrome: arthroscopic findings. *Arthroscopy* **8:** 482–487.
15. Simpson, N.S. & Kelly, J.G. (1994) Extra-glenohumeral joint shoulder surgery in rheumatoid arthritis: the role of bursectomy, acromioplasty, and distal clavicle excision. *JSES* **66:** 3–4.
16. Crossan, J.F. & Vallance, R. (1982) The shoulder joint in rheumatoid arthritis. In I. Bayley and L. Kessel (eds), *Shoulder Surgery*, pp. 131–143. New York: Springer-Verlag.
17. Petersson, C.J. (1986) Painful shoulders in patients with rheumatoid arthritis. *Scand. J. Rheum.* **15:** 275–279.
18. Cruess, R.L. (1976) Steroid induced avascular necrosis of the head of the humerus. *J. Bone Joint Surg.* **58B:** 313.
19. Cruess, R.L. (1985) Corticosteroid-induced osteonecrosis of the humeral head. *Orthop. Clin. North Am.* **16:** 789–796.
20. Urquhart, M.W., Mont, M.A., Maar, D.C., Lennox, D.W., Krackow, K.A. & Hungerford, D.S. (1992–93) Results of core decompression for avascular necrosis of the humeral head. *Orthop. Trans.* **16:** 780.
21. Codd, T.P., Yamaguchi, K. & Flatow, E.L. (1995) Infected shoulder arthroplasties: treatment with staged reimplantation versus resection arthroplasty. Presented at the American Shoulder & Elbow Surgeons 11th Annual Open Meeting, Orlando, FL, February.
22. Hawkins, R.J. & Neer, C.S. (1987) Functional analysis of shoulder arthrodesis. *Clin. Orthop.* **233:** 65–76.
23. Harryman, D.T., Walker, Harris, S.L., Sidles, J.A., Jackins, S. & Matsen, F.A. (1993) Residual motion and function after glenohumeral or scapulothoracic arthrodesis. *J. Shoulder Elbow Surg.*
24. Richards, R.R. & Beaton, Hudson (1993) Shoulder arthrodesis with plate fixation: functional outcome analysis. *J. Shoulder Elbow Surg.* **225:** 9–10.
25. Neer, C.S. & Kirby, R.M. (1982) Revision of humeral head and total shoulder arthroplasties. *Clin. Orthop.* **170:** 189.
26. Amstutz, H.C., Thomas, B.J., Kabo, J.M. et al (1988) The Dana total shoulder arthroplasty. *J. Bone Joint Surg.* **70A:** 1174–1182.
27. Brems, J.J. (1993) The glenoid component in total shoulder arthroplasty. *J. Shoulder Elbow Surg.* **47:** 1–2.

28. Clayton, M.L., Ferlic, D.C. & Jeffers, P.D. (1982) Prosthetic arthroplasties of the shoulder. *Clin. Orthop.* **164:** 184.

29. Cockx, E., Claes, T., Hoogmartens, M. & Mulier, J.C. (1983) The isoelastic prosthesis for the shoulder joint. *Acta. Orthop. Belg.* **49:** 275–285.

30. Franklin, J.L., Barrett, W.P., Jackins, S.E. & Matsen, F.A. (1988) Glenoid loosening in total shoulder arthroplasty. *J. Arthroplasty* **3:** 39–46.

31. Harryman, D.T., Sidles, J.A., Harris, S.L., Lippitt, S.B. & Matsen, F.A. (1995) The effect of articular conformity and the size of the humeral head component on laxity and motion after glenohumeral arthroplasty. A study in cadavera. *J. Bone Joint Surg.* **77A:** 555–63.

32. McElwain, J.P. & English, E. The early results of porous-coated total shoulder arthroplasty. *Clin. Orthop.* **218:** 217–224.

33. Flatow, E.L. (1995) Prosthetic design considerations in total shoulder arthroplasty. *Semin. Arthroplasty* **6:** 1–12.

34. Wirth, M.A. & Rockwood, C.A. (1994) Complications of shoulder arthroplasty. *Clin. Orthop.* **307:** 47–69.

35. Tillett, E., Smith, M., Fulcer, M. & Shanklin, J. (1993) Anatomic determination of humeral head retroversion: the relationship of the central axis of the humeral head to the bicipital groove. *J. Shoulder Elbow Surg.* **255:** 9–10.

36. Soslowsky, L.J., Flatow, E.L., Bigliani, L.U. et al. (1992) Articular geometry of the glenohumeral joint. *Clin. Orthop.* **285:** 181–190.

37. Maki, S. & Gruen, T. (1976) Anthropometric study of the glenohumeral joint. *Trans. Orthop. Res.* **1:** 173.

38. Severt, R., Thomas, B.J., Tsenter, M.J., Amstutz, H.C. & Kabo, J.M. (1993) The influence of conformity and constraint on translational forces and frictional torque in total shoulder arthroplasty. *Clin. Orthop.* **292:** 151–158.

39. Ballmer, F.T., Lippitt, S.B., Romeo, A.A. & Matsen, F.A. (1994) Total shoulder arthroplasty: some considerations related to glenoid surface contact. *J. Shoulder Elbow Surg.* **3:** 299–306.

40. Buechel, F.F., Pappas, M.J. & DePalma, A.F. (1978) 'Floating-socket' total shoulder replacement: anatomical, biomechanical, and surgical rationale. *J. Biomech. Materials Res.* **12:** 89–114.

41. Flatow, E.L., Ateshian, G.A., Soslowsky, L.J. et al. (1994) Computer simulation of glenohumeral and patellofemoral subluxation: estimating pathologic articular contact. *Clin. Orthop.* **306:** 28–33.

42. Rodosky, M.W. & Bigliani, L.U. (1994) Surgical treatment of nonconstrained glenoid component failure. *Oper. Tech. Orthop.* **4:** 226–236.

43. Harryman, D.T., Sidles, J.A., Clark, J.M. et al. (1990) Translation of the humeral head on the glenoid with passive glenohumeral motion. *J. Bone Joint Surg.* **72A:** 1334–1343.

44. Friedman, (1992) Glenohumeral translation after total shoulder arthroplasty. *J. Shoulder Elbow Surg.* **312:** 11–12.

45. Iannotti, J.P., Gabriel, J.P., Schneck, S.L., Evans, B.G. & Misra, S. (1992) The normal glenohumeral relationships. An anatomical study of one hundred and forty shoulders. *J. Bone Joint Surg.* **74A:** 491.

46. Cofield, R.H. (1994) Uncemented total shoulder arthroplasty. A review. *Clin. Orthop.* **307:** 86–93.

47. Cooper, R.A. & Brems, J.J. (1991) Recurrent disassembly of a modular humeral prosthesis. A case report. *J. Arthroplasty* **6:** 375–377.

48. Blevins, F.T., Deng, X., Torzilli, P.A. et al. (1994) Dissociation of modular shoulder arthroplasty components. *Trans Orthop. Res. Soc.* **19:** 827.

49. Friedman, LaBerge, Dooley, O'Hara. (1992) Finite element modeling of the glenoid component: effect of design parameters on stress distribution. *J. Shoulder Elbow Surg.* **261:** 9–10.

50. Cofield, Daly (1992) Total shoulder arthroplasty with a tissue-ingrowth glenoid component. *J. Shoulder Elbow Surg.* **77:** 3–4.

51. Collins, D., Tencer, A., Sidles, J. & Matsen, F.A. (1992) Edge displacement and deformation of glenoid components in response to eccentric loading. The effect of preparation of the glenoid bone. *J. Bone Joint Surg.* **74A:** 501–7.

52. Neer, C.S. & Morrison, D. (1988) Glenoid bone grafting in total shoulder arthroplasty. *J. Bone Joint Surg.* **70A:** 1154.

53. Neer, C.S., Watson, K.C. & Stanton, F.J. (1982) Recent experience in total shoulder replacement. *J. Bone Joint Surg.* **64A:** 319.

54. Arntz, C.T., Jackins, S. & Matsen, F.A. (1993) Prosthetic replacement of the shoulder for the treatment of defects in the rotator cuff and the surface of the glenohumeral joint. *J. Bone Joint Surg.* **75A:** 485–491.

55. Pollock, R.G., Deliz, E.D., McIlveen, S.J., Flatow, E.L. & Bigliani, L.U. (1992) Prosthetic replacement in rotator cuff deficient shoulders. *J. Shoulder Elbow Surg.* **1:** 173–186.

56. Neer, C.S., McCann, P.D., Macfarlane, E.A. & Padilla, N. (1987) Earlier passive motion following shoulder arthroplasty and rotator cuff repair. A prospective study. *Orthop. Trans.* **2:** 231.

57. Boyd, A.D., Thomas, W.H., Scott, R.D., Sledge, C.B. & Thornhill, T.S. (1990) Total shoulder arthroplasty versus hemiarthroplasty. *J. Arthroplasty* **5:** 329–336.

58. Dalldorf, Banas, Hicks, Pellegrini. (1995) Rate of degeneration of human acetabular cartilage after hemiarthroplasty. *J. Bone Joint Surg.* **77A:** 877–882.

59. Neer, C.S. (1961) Degenerative lesions of the proximal humeral articular surface. *Clin. Orthop.* **20:** 116.

60. Petersson, C.J. & Redlund-Johnell, I. (1983) Joint space in normal glenohumeral radiographs. *Acta Orthop. Scand.* **54:** 274.

61. Pollock, R.G., Higgs, J.B., Codd, T.P. et al. (1994) Total shoulder replacement for the treatment of primary glenohumeral osteoarthritis. Presented at the American Shoulder and Elbow Surgeons 10th Annual Open Meeting, New Orleans, LA. February 1994.

62. Kelly, I.G. (1994) Unconstrained shoulder arthroplasty in rheumatoid arthritis. *Clin. Orthop.* **307:** 94–102.

63. Clayton, M.L. & Ferlic, D.C. (1974) Surgery of the shoulder in rheumatoid arthritis. *Clin. Orthop.* **106:** 166.

64. Jonsson, E., Egund, N., Kelly, I. et al. (1986) Cup arthroplasty for the rheumatoid shoulder. *Acta Orthop. Scand.* **57:** 542–546.

65. Gschwend, N. & Bischof, A. (1991) Clinical experience in arthroplasty according to Neer. *J. Orthop. Rheum.* **4:** 135–143.

66. Dines, D.M., Warren, R.F., Altchek, D.W. & Moeckel, B. (1993) Posttraumatic changes of the proximal humerus: malunion, nonunion, and osteonecrosis. Treatment with modular hemiarthroplasty or total shoulder arthroplasty. *J. Shoulder Elbow Surg.* **2:** 11–21.

67. Pritchett, J.W. & Clark, J.M. (1987) Prosthetic replacement for chronic unreduced dislocations of the shoulder. *Clin. Orthop.* **216:** 89–93.

68. Tanner, M.W. & Cofield, R.H. (1983) Prosthetic arthroplasty for fractures and fracture-dislocations of the proximal humerus. *Clin. Orthop.* **179:** 116–128.

69. Flatow, E.L., Miller, S.R. & Neer, C.S. (1993) Chronic anterior dislocation of the shoulder. *J. Shoulder Elbow Surg.* **2:** 2–10.

70. Hawkins, R.J., Neer, C.S., Pianta, R.M. & Mendoza, F.X. (1987) Locked posterior dislocation of the shoulder. *J. Bone Joint Surg.* **69A:** 9–18.

71. Rowe, C.R. & Zarins, B. (1982) Chronic unreduced dislocations of the shoulder. *J. Bone Joint Surg.* **64A:** 494–505.

72. Bigliani, L.U., Weinstein, D.M., Glasgow, M.T., Pollock, R.G. & Flatow, E.L. (1995) Glenohumeral arthroplasty for arthritis after instability surgery. *J. Shoulder Elbow Surg.* **4:** 87–94.

73. Hawkins, R.J., Bell, R.H. & Jallay, B. (1989) Total shoulder arthroplasty. *Clin. Orthop.* **242:** 188–194.

74. L'Insalata, J.C., Pagnani, M.J., Dines, D.M. & Warren, R.F. (1994) Osteonecrosis of the proximal humerus: Natural history, long term follow-up and radiographic predictors of outcome. Presented at the American Shoulder and Elbow Surgeons Tenth Open Meeting, New Orleans, LA, February 27.

75. Samilson, R.L. & Prieto, V. (1983) Dislocation arthropathy of the shoulder. *J. Bone Joint Surg.* **65A:** 456–460.

76. Young, D.C. & Rockwood, C.A. (1991) Complications of failed Bristow procedure and their management. *J. Bone Joint Surg.* **73A:** 969–981.

77. Hawkins, R.J. & Angelo, R.L. (1990) Glenohumeral osteoarthritis: a late complication of Putti–Platt repair. *J. Bone Joint Surg.* **72A:** 1193–1197.

78. Fenlin, J.M., Ramsey, M.L., Allardyce, T.J. & Frieman, B.G. (1994) Modular total shoulder replacement. Design rationale, indications, and results. *Clin. Orthop.* **307:** 37–46.

79. Brems, J.J. (1994) Rehabilitation following total shoulder arthroplasty. *Clin. Orthop.* **307:** 70–85.

80. Bonutti, P.M., Hawkins, R.J. & Saddemi, S. (1993) Arthroscopic assessment of glenoid component loosening after total shoulder arthroplasty. *Arthroscopy* **9:** 272–276.

81. Bonntti, P.M. & Hawkins, R.J. (1992) Fractures of the humeral shaft associated with total replacement arthroplasty of the shoulder. A case report. *J. Bone Joint Surg.* **74A:** 617–618.

82. Boyd, A.D., Thornhill, T.S. & Barnes (1992) Fractures adjacent to humeral prosthesis. *J. Bone Joint Surg.* **74A:** 1498–1504.

83. Brems, J.J., Wilde, A.H., Borden, L.S. & Boumphrey, F.R.S. (1986) Glenoid lucent lines. *Orthop. Trans.* **10:** 231.

84. Moeckel, B.H., Altchek, D.W., Warren, R.F., Wickiewicz, T.L. & Dines, D.M. (1993) Instability of the shoulder after arthroplasty. *J. Bone Joint Surg.* **75A:** 492–497.

85. Kjaersgaard-Anderson, P., Frich, L.P. & Sojbjerg, J.O. (1989) Bone formation following total shoulder arthroplasty. *J. Arthroplasty* **4:** 99–104.

26

Surface Replacement Arthroplasty of the Shoulder

SA Copeland

The most common type of shoulder arthroplasty used today is the cemented stemmed humeral component in conjunction with a cemented glenoid of the Neer type (see Chapter 25). These have been generally successful, and longer-term studies are now becoming available. However, there are certain disadvantages to this type of design. The most common component to fail is the glenoid component with a high incidence of glenoid lucent lines on X-ray and a significant late glenoid loosening rate.[1] The humeral component has been more successful, and the long-term results for the cemented stemmed component are better than for the non-cemented stem.[2] Unfortunately if the humeral component becomes infected or loose, then the same problems arise in the proximal humerus that occur in the proximal femur when a femoral component loosens in total hip replacement. There may be gross loss of bone stock making revision an extremely difficult procedure. As with the hip joint, the shoulder prosthesis is most commonly indicated in the elderly patient whose bones may be osteoporotic and the patient liable to fall or stumble, sustaining fractures of the proximal humerus.[3] There is a stress riser at the tip of the prosthesis and cement such that the fracture may occur at this site which may be a difficult clinical problem to deal with. In the stemmed humeral component the prosthetic head is situated centrally to the longitudinal axis of the humerus. This is in fact not anatomical as the humeral head is offset by an average of 4 mm,[4] hence any shoulder replacement not specifically designed for left or right shoulder cannot accurately mimic the centre of rotation of the natural joint. Also, rarely because of malunion of the proximal end of the humerus or congenital abnormality a stemmed component may not be surgically possible. Because of the very success of joint replacements, patients are now presenting earlier with minimal arthritic destruction of the humeral head and glenoid, but gross loss of movement and severe pain. In these cases it seems illogical to remove the head completely and violate the humeral shaft purely for fixation of the prosthesis. It was for these reasons that a surface replacement was designed which has been used since the mid-1980s.[5] The purpose of this design was to have minimal bone removal, cementless fixation and as near as possible surface replacement only. Both components are fixed by a single peg of taper-fit fluted design (Figure 26.1A and B). The humeral head is made of cobalt–chrome and the glenoid component is metal backed with an ultra high molecular weight polyethylene (UHMWP). Three sizes of both components are available, standard, small and large. The radius of curvature of the humeral head and glenoid are conforming.

(A)
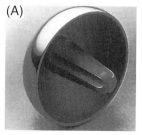

(B)
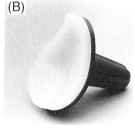

Fig. 26.1 (A) Humeral head prosthesis; (B) glenoid prosthesis.

INDICATIONS

The indications are the same for any shoulder replacement. The ideal shoulder for surface replacement would be one with minimal bone destruction, but severe loss of movement, pain and hence function. Approximately half of this series are rheumatoid arthritis and half primary and secondary osteoarthritis. Initially, almost universally, both humeral and glenoid components were implanted. However, during the period of this series, concern was raised in other unconstrained shoulder replacement series that glenoid loosening may be a late problem in the grossly rotator-cuff-deficient shoulder.[6] Hence, if there was upward subluxation of the humeral head in relation to the glenoid and the rotator cuff cannot be reconstructed at the time of surgery, then the humeral hemiarthroplasty alone is used. Sometimes glenoid erosion is so severe that any glenoid implant is impossible. If the erosion has medialized beyond the base of the coracoid, there is not enough bone left in the scapula for fixation of any component and a hemiarthroplasty again is used. Both components are now available with hydroxyapatite bone ingrowth coating and this is now universally used (since December 1994).

SURGICAL TECHNIQUE

The patient is prepared and draped in a beach chair position, with the arm draped free and supported on an arm board. The standard anterior deltopectoral approach may be used, but my present preference is for the anterosuperior approach.[7] Whatever approach is used, the subscapularis almost invariably needs to be lengthened, as the centre of rotation will be lateralized by the joint replacement causing a relative shortening of this muscle. At the end of the procedure external rotation must be passively possible as this will not be gained after the operation. The joint is exposed and the humeral head exposed superoanteriorly. All humeral head osteophytes are excised peripherally to visualize the alignment of the surgical neck of the humerus. Using a jig, a

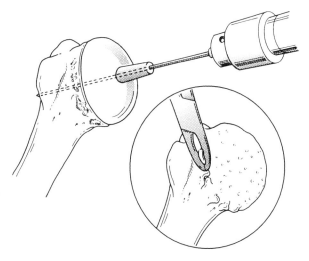

Fig. 26.2 Humeral head osteophytes are removed. A jig is used to centre the guide wire in the humeral head.

guide wire is drilled through the centre of the anatomical head (Figure 26.2). This automatically builds in the normal head retroversion approximately 30° in relation to the shaft. A cannulated humeral stem hole cutter is passed over the guide wire and the central drill hole made (Figure 26.3). This pilot hole is used for the humeral surface cutter to shape the humeral head to the exact shape of the undersurface of the prosthesis (Figure 26.4). The trial humeral head is inserted and then the glenoid exposed using a humeral head retractor on the trial prosthesis to prevent deformation of the bony humeral head. The glenoid is then

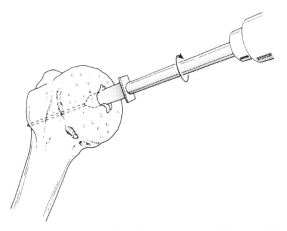

Fig. 26.3 Central drill hold made over guide wire. The bone is kept for later grafting.

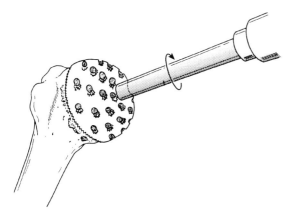

Fig. 26.4 Humeral head shaping reamer.

assessed for replacement. If the glenoid component is to be used, further capsulotomy may be
necessary to gain adequate visualization of the
glenoid *en face*. The centre of the glenoid is
located using the drill guide and a guide wire
drilled into the centre of the glenoid. This may
bridge the anterior cortex of the vault of the
scapula. The cannulated taper drill is passed over
the guide wire and a central taper hole made
(Figure 26.6). The glenoid surface cutter is passed
into the central pilot hole and the surface prepared
to leave bleeding subchondral bone (Figure 26.7).
The trial glenoid and humeral components are
inserted and the joint tested for stability and range
of motion (Figure 26.8). The glenoid prosthesis is
then impacted into the bone with a mallet and
impactor, such that there is a good metal-to-bone
contact. An excellent fix is usually achieved by
three taps of the mallet. The humeral component
is inserted in a similar way (Figure 26.5). Any

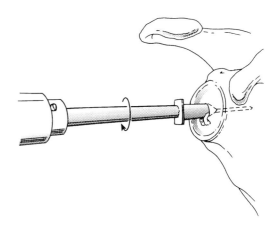

Fig. 26.6 Central glenoid tapered hole made over guide
wire. The bone is kept for possible later grafting.

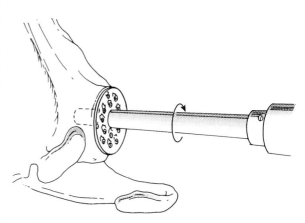

Fig. 26.7 Glenoid shaping reamer in central pilot hole.

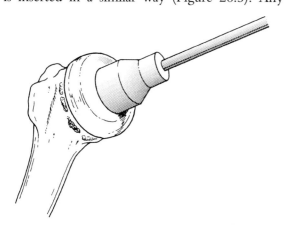

Fig. 26.5 Humeral component is compacted in place.

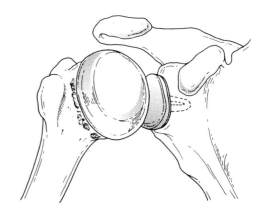

Fig. 26.8 Humeral and glenoid components *in situ*.

bone reamings from the central drill hole are used as auto-graft between the humeral component and the head. This may also be used to fill any defects in the head where there is not direct bone–prosthesis contact. Again, both components are tested for stability. If a rotator cuff tear is present, this is repaired with interrupted sutures at this stage and the scapularis muscle repaired. The wound is closed without drainage.

POSTOPERATIVE REHABILITATION

The postoperative programme is tailored to the individual patient. Patients with an intact rotator cuff begin early passive and assisted active mobilization exercises. After 3 weeks the patient is placed on a programme of range of movement

exercises, followed by a gradually strengthening cuff exercise programme (see Chapter 25).

RESULTS

From 1987 to 1995, 165 surface replacement arthroplasties have been implanted. In cases where the humeral head was too badly destroyed to accept the surface replacement, the stem design was used, but of all the cases presenting for total shoulder replacement, 85% were treated by the surface replacement technique alone. Figure 26.9 shows the results for pain relief function and the mean range of movements in osteoarthritis and rheumatoid arthritis. As with most total shoulder series, patient satisfaction was high and comparable with other series. Six patients have had to have revision surgery for loosening. Two of these

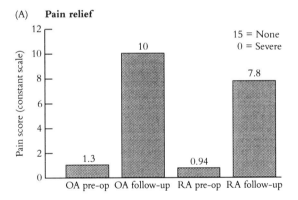
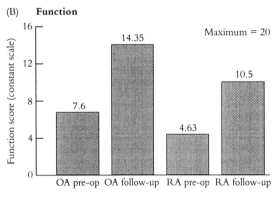
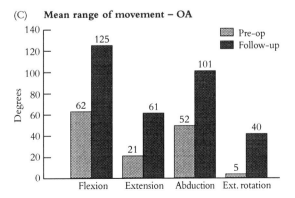
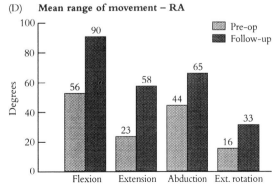

Fig. 26.9 Average 4-year clinical results of 69 patients following treatment with the Copeland shoulder. OA, osteoarthritis; RA, rheumatoid arthritis.

were related to severe trauma, one fracturing at the anatomical neck. All these patients were satisfactorily revised to a stemmed cemented prosthesis. The revision surgery presented little problem as bone loss was minimal. Two further patients have been revised to arthrodesis for persistent posterior dislocation and in retrospect the surgery was unwise. The initial indication in these patients was for long-standing persistent posterior dislocation with arthritic change in the dislocated posterior position. At the time of shoulder replacement an attempt was made to normalize the rotation of the glenoid and the humeral head. Both patients went on to immediate dislocation after surgery and in future this clinical situation will be considered a contraindication to this form of shoulder replacement.

Non-progressive lucent lines have been seen around 60% of prostheses. The patients requiring surgery for loosening presented within 2.5 years of surgery. One loosening was suspected to be due to infection, but was not proven at the time of revision surgery.

DISCUSSION

In glenohumeral arthritis, especially rheumatoid arthritis, the most solid bone is often in the subchondral area of the head.[8] This bone is not removed during surface replacement arthroplasty. It is believed that this produces better fixation for an uncemented component with reduced tendency towards sinkage and loosening.

The design of the humeral component in this study maximizes the contact between it and the glenoid component articulating surface. There are no bevels or collars and therefore there is a maximum spherical surface for contact with the glenoid in the functional range of movements. This may avoid unwanted translations and optimize the mechanics of the arthroplasty.[9] The ability to put the humeral head in its anatomical position allowing for the posterior offset may improve the mechanics of the rotator cuff action of the new joint. The newer modular off-set stem designs can achieve the same. However, modularity may present new complications, including component disassociation and metal-on-metal wear.

An intact working rotator cuff is important for a good functional result and good movement after shoulder arthroplasty. However, pain relief can be excellent in the cuff-deficient shoulder. This permits improved overall movement by allowing pain-free scapulothoracic motion and increased glenohumeral motion.

There is an increasing trend to use humeral head hemiarthroplasty alone and this is strongly advised if there is any doubt about the adequacy of glenoid fixation because of loss of bone stock. Also, in the presence of a good articulating surface on the glenoid side, glenoid replacement is unnecessary.

Medium-term outcome of shoulder arthroplasty is not yet comparable with that of hip or knee and therefore the possibility of revision within 10 years must be a consideration. Uncemented surface replacement of the humeral head may facilitate eventual revision of surgery. This is because the proximal humeral canal is virgin, making insertion of the stemmed prosthesis straightforward. However, if because of failure due to infection an arthrodesis is considered, the bone stock on the humeral head is preserved and arthrodesis is facilitated.

The 7-year results have been very encouraging and the use of the present design with hydroxyapatite coating appears to have been highly successful in the short term. The long-term results must be awaited.

REFERENCES

1. Brems, J. (1993) The glenoid component in total shoulder arthroplasty. *J. Shoulder Elbow Surg.* **2:** 47–54.
2. Cofield, R.H. (1994) Uncemented total shoulder arthroplasty. *Clin. Orthop.* **307:** 86–93.
3. Wright, T.W. & Cofield, R.H. (1995) *J. Bone Joint Surg.* **77A:** 1340–1346.
4. Roberts, S.N.J., Foley, A.P.J., Swallow, H.M., Wallace, W.A. & Coughlan, G.P. (1991) The geometry of the humeral head and the design of prostheses. *J. Bone Joint Surg.* **73B:** 647–650.
5. Copeland, S.A. (1990) Cementless total shoulder repla-

cement. In M. Post, B.F. Morrey & R.J. Hawkins (eds), *Surgery of the Shoulder*, pp. 289–297. St. Louis: Mosby Year Book.

6. Arntz, C.T., Jackins, S. & Matsen, F. (1993) Prosthetic replacement of the shoulder for the treatment of defects in the rotator cuff and the surface of the glenohumeral joint. *J. Bone Joint Surg.* **75A:** 485–491.

7. MacKenzie, D.B. (1993) The anterosuperior exposure of the total shoulder replacement. *Orthop. Traumatol.* **2:** 71–77.

8. Saitoh, S., Nakatsuchi, Y., Latta, L. & Milne, E. (1994) Distribution of bone mineral density and bone strength of the proximal humerus. *J. Shoulder Elbow Surg.* **3:** 234–242.

9. Ballmer, F.T., Lippitt, S.B., Romeo, A.A. & Matsen, F.A. (1994) Total shoulder arthroplasty; some considerations related to glenoid surface contact. *J. Shoulder Elbow Surg.* **3:** 299–306.

27

Nerve Injuries of the Shoulder

R. Birch

SOME LESIONS OF NERVES TO THE THORACOSCAPULAR AND GLENOHUMERAL JOINTS

The complex of joints within the shoulder girdle permits an extraordinary range of movement for the upper limb, and the function of the whole upper limb, particularly the hand, rests on this. The sixth cervical nerve is perhaps the most important in cutaneous innervation in the hand and it is a spinal nerve which contributes much to the shoulder. The shoulder–hand syndrome is one instance of the interdependence of these two segments of the upper limb; the severe impairment of hand function from paralysis of the shoulder is another. One spinal and three peripheral nerves are of particular interest to those engaged in shoulder work: the spinal component (accessory) of the eleventh cranial nerve, the nerve to the serratus anterior (long thoracic), and the suprascapular and circumflex nerves. Ruptures of the suprascapular and circumflex nerves form about 5% of larger series of peripheral nerve injuries. Partial injury to these nerves with incomplete recovery is a common complication of injuries to the shoulder.

The spinal accessory and long thoracic nerves are particularly at risk from surgeons, and the tally of injuries to these from operations in the neck or axilla is too high. It may even be increasing. Furthermore the number of gunshot and knife wounds in this country is increasing. Our understanding of the significance of these lesions has been increased by studies of shoulder function notably by Comtet et al,[1] Narakas[2] and Coene

and Narakas,[3] by renewed attempts to re-innervate the paralysed shoulder after lesions of the brachial plexus and by renewed interest in the birth lesion of the brachial plexus. I shall describe some experiences in the treatment of the four main nerves, particularly the cause of injury and consequences, difficulties in diagnosis and methods of treatment with their attendant difficulties. Palliative operations involving muscle transfer produce results that are inferior to the normal state and to the results of successful repair of the nerve. Damage to the subclavian and axillary vessels is common in open wounds of the shoulder. Adequate methods of exposure were developed in the First World War, and successful and reliable techniques of repair were developed in the Second World War and later conflicts. It is as well for shoulder surgeons to remember these facts and to consider that vascular lesions are not infrequent in high-energy lesions of the forequarter and also in the more severe fracture dislocations of the shoulder itself.

ANATOMY

It is said that 25% of the nerves of the brachial plexus pass to the shoulder girdle. The fifth cervical nerve is entirely destined for this structure, and the sixth and seventh cervical nerves substantially so. The cervical plexus contributes to cutaneous innervation and possibly to the trapezius muscle. Now is the time to dispel a common misconception that the spinal accessory, suprascapular and long thoracic nerves are 'motor'

Table 27.1. Classification of nerve injuries

Injury	Consequence	Presence of distal conduction
Neurapraxia	Conduction block: short term or prolonged	Present
Axonotmesis	Rupture of nerve fibres: Wallerian degeneration	Lost
Neurotmesis	Rupture of nerve trunk: Wallerian degeneration	Lost

nerves implying that their fibres pass solely to skeletal muscle. This is quite wrong. It is inconsistent with the severe pain that follows injuries to these nerves; it does not admit proprioceptive function. Biopsies from all three show large numbers of non-myelinated C-fibres and A delta fibres, responsible for pain and other afferent modalities. Biopsies from the suprascapular nerve weeks after proven preganglionic injury show that at least 30% of the myelinated fibres survive: these fibres must have cell bodies within the dorsal root ganglion and are presumably responsible for proprioception for intrafusal fibre function and for pain and temperature sense.

This chapter follows Seddon's (1975) classification[4] of nerve injuries and also his modification of his MRC system in discussion of results. His classification is based on the recognition of the physiological consequences of nerve injury (Table 27.1).

Neurapraxia or conduction block is often a diagnosis of wistful 'hoping for the best' and it is often further muddled by the meaningless term 'neuropraxia'. It is a very precise diagnosis and it falls into two parts. Conduction block may be short term or it may be prolonged. Most surgeons will have noted that nerve conduction is lost when a suprasystolic cuff is placed around the limb. The response of muscles to stimulation of the nerve trunks exposed disappears at about 40 min and then rapidly returns on the release of the tourniquet. In contrast is the deeper compression lesion of the unconscious patient. There is no Wallerian degeneration but recovery takes months or even years. The distinction between the two types of conduction block is an important one for shoulder surgeons, for the transient loss of conduction after dislocation is usually speedily recovered after reduction. If reduction is delayed, then the lesion to the nerve is deeper. Examples of early recovery after prompt reduction of a fracture or dislocation or evacuation of a haematoma show that timely intervention leads to full and early recovery of the nerve. Delaying such intervention leads to progression of the nerve lesion to a degenerative one.

The critical distinction lies between non-degenerative and degenerative lesion and this is an easy matter in such nerves as the median, ulnar and sciatic which have a large cutaneous component and a major element of sympathetic fibres responsible for vaso- and sudo-motor functions. It is admittedly less easy in the nerves to the shoulder, and neurophysiological investigations, accurately performed and accurately interpreted, are extremely useful.

SPINAL ACCESSORY NERVE

This, the external ramus of the eleventh cranial nerve, arises from the second to sixth cervical segments and it enters the neck through the jugular foramen in company with the tenth nerve. It traverses the retrospinal space between the mastoid and mandible and usually deep to the internal jugular vein to enter the sternomastoid muscle in its upper one-third. It passes into the posterior triangle of the neck at the junction of the upper and middle one-third of the posterior margin of the sternomastoid where it is in close and constant contact with sensory branches of the cervical plexus. The transverse cervical and greater auricular nerves wind around the sternomastoid muscle 1 cm caudad. The accessory nerve is about 2 mm in diameter and contains about 2000 myelinated nerve fibres. The proportion of

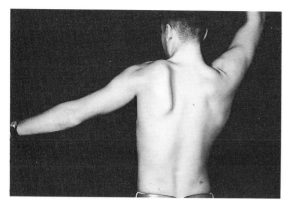

Fig. 27.1 Iatropathic section of spinal accessory nerve at the apex of the posterior triangle. Note the loss of active abduction.

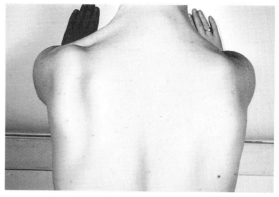

Fig. 27.2 Iatropathic section of spinal accessory nerve at the apex of the posterior triangle. Note the apparent winging of the shoulder blade.

non-myelinated and A delta fibres is about 50%.[5] The nerve crosses the levator scapulae undulating in fatty tissue before passing obliquely towards the anterior margin of the trapezius. There are between three and six rami to the upper fibres of this muscle. The nerve leaves the posterior triangle to pass medially and caudally innervating the middle and lower fibres. Just above the clavicle, slender branches from C3 and C4 join it. Observations from stimulation of the nerve here suggests that there are few motor fibres within these contributions.

Damage to the nerve causes paralysis of the trapezius, resulting in profound disturbance of the function of the shoulder girdle and glenohumeral joint (Figures 27.1 and 27.2). The shoulder droops, abduction is usually limited to between 70 and 90° and the scapula wings, sometimes causing an erroneous diagnosis of paralysis of the serratus anterior. Williams et al[6] studied 40 cases. In 23 the nerve was damaged by the surgeon working in the posterior triangle, and in two others irradiation was the cause. Delay in diagnosis was usual, ranging from immediate to 32 months. Twenty-six of these 40 patients had severe pain at rest which disturbed sleep; in eight more there was significant pain brought on by movement of the shoulder. In 24 cases the nerve was repaired by grafting, and useful recovery was seen in 19 of these, with relief of pain and improvement in the range and strength of

shoulder movement. What are the causes for the severity of pain so characteristic of injury to this nerve? Traction upon the brachial plexus from the unsupported shoulder is not a wholly adequate explanation. The onset of pain is too early and those patients who suffered damage to the nerve during operation with local anaesthetic described a severe shooting pain coursing into the neck and shoulder. Some patients note relief of pain within days of repair of the nerve, long before any return of function to the trapezius.

There is a large volume of literature about the spinal accessory nerve and it is astonishing and shaming that iatropathic injuries are so frequent (Table 27.2), and the consequences of these injuries so often unrecognized. It is likely that the trend towards day-care surgery performed by unskilled surgeons with inadequate follow-up of the patient will see a continuing rise in these severe injuries.

LONG THORACIC NERVE

This is formed from constant branches which arise from the most proximal segment of the anterior primary rami of the fifth and sixth cervical nerves. A branch from the fourth cervical nerve occurs in 30% of patients and from the seventh cervical nerve in over one-half. These pass deep to the

Table 27.2. Nerve injuries at the shoulder (1979–1995)

Nerve	Cause or type of injury	No.
Spinal accessory	Iatropathic	42
	Wounds	6
	Irradiation	2
	Neuralgic amyotrophy	11
Long thoracic	Iatropathic	14
	Wounds	8
	Neuralgic amyotrophy	45
	Traction lesion of the brachial plexus	700+
Suprascapular	Iatropathic	11
	Wounds	13
	Neuralgic amyotrophy	31
	Fracture or dislocation	38
	Brachial plexus lesion	700+
Circumflex	Iatropathic	8
	Wounds	14
	Neuralgic amyotrophy	22
	Fracture or dislocation	79
	Brachial plexus lesion	700+

From the Peripheral Nerve Injury Unit, St Mary's and the Royal National Orthopaedic Hospitals, London.

scalenus medius. The nerve, which is between 1.5 and 2 mm in diameter, courses laterally to the scalenus medius to enter the axilla. It is particularly vulnerable to accidental damage where it crosses the first and second ribs.

The serratus anterior muscle holds the scapula against the chest and protracts it. When the muscle is paralysed the inferior pole of the scapula does not move forward but slides medially and cranially (Figure 27.3). Deep aching pain is common and it is sometimes severe. The nerve was repaired in four cases of stab wounds and in three iatropathic injuries. Re-innervation of the muscle is an essential element in the treatment of patients with preganglionic injury of the fifth, sixth and seventh nerves by means of nerve transfer, using a branch of the dorsal scapular nerve or deep division of the third or fourth intercostal nerves. Useful function, at least MRC 3+, followed all grafts and in 10 of 12 repairs by nerve transfer.

SUPRASCAPULAR NERVE

The suprascapular nerve springs from the upper trunk at the junction of the fifth and sixth cervical nerves about 3 cm above the clavicle. It passes laterally and posteriorly deep to the omohyoid to the scapular notch, entering the supraspinatus fossa deep to the superior transverse ligament. It traverses the fossa deep to the supraspinatus muscle winding around the lateral border of the spine of the scapula to enter the infraspinous fossa. The nerve contains between 3000 and 4000

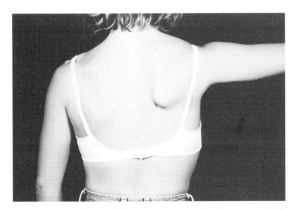

Fig. 27.3 Paralysis of the serratus anterior from neuralgic amyotrophy.

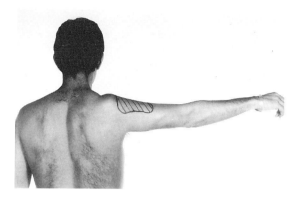

Fig. 27.4 Patient with rupture of circumflex nerve. Full abduction was maintained.

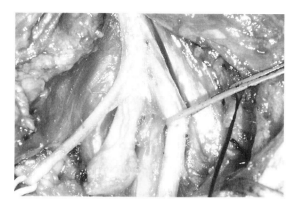

Fig. 27.5 Stab wound in the posterior triangle of the neck: section of the posterior division of the upper trunk and long thoracic nerve. Slings displace the anterior division and the suprascapular nerve.

myelinated nerve fibres; at least 30% of these do not degenerate in preganglionic injury. Their cell bodies must be in the dorsal root ganglion and are afferent. The suprascapular nerve is essential for abduction and lateral rotation of the glenohumeral joint. Patients with isolated paralysis of the deltoid in whom the suprascapular and rotator cuff are normal are usually able to abduct fully and retain lateral rotation (Figure 27.4).

CIRCUMFLEX NERVE

This is the terminal branch of the posterior cord, springing from it just distal to the thoracodorsal nerve. It contains between 6000 and 7000 myelinated nerve fibres which pass through the fifth and sixth cervical nerves. The nerve divides into two branches within the quadrilateral tunnel, the anterior division continuing around the neck of the humerus to innervate the anterior deltoid, and the larger posterior branch innervating the teres minor and posterior deltoid muscles. One cutaneous branch, the upper lateral cutaneous nerve of the arm, is a useful landmark where it pierces the deep fascia over the posterior border of the deltoid. Spilsbury and Birch[7] have reviewed 129 nerve injuries in 98 patients. There were 62 ruptures of the circumflex and 22 of the suprascapular nerves. Lesions in continuity were dis-

played in 26 circumflex and 19 suprascapular nerves. In 31 patients there was a combined lesion of the two nerves, and in at least eight more there was an associated rupture of the rotator cuff.

Most lesions occurred in closed injuries and were associated with fractures or fracture dislocations of the shoulder. Stabbing, gunshot or iatropathic injuries accounted for 25 nerves in 16 patients (Figure 27.5).

Results were measured by the systems of Seddon[4] and by the scoring system introduced by Narakas[2] and used by some surgeons engaged in repair of the brachial plexus. Myometric measures of strength and stamina were made in 28 cases.

Of the 56 circumflex nerve grafts, results were considered good in 27 and fair in 23. They were good or fair in 18 of 20 grafts of the suprascapular nerve. A good result was seen in only six of the 23 lesions in continuity of the circumflex nerve, but in eight of 16 lesions in continuity of the suprascapular nerve. Some causes of the poor results are set out in Table 27.2. MRI scanning is particularly useful for analysing this complex group of injuries, not only in demonstrating damage to the rotator cuff but also indicating the extent of denervation of the deltoid and supraspinatus muscles. Both suprascapular and circumflex nerves may be seen, respectively at the notch and in the quadrilateral space.

Myometric measurements of strength and stamina reveal a rather more unfavourable picture. The stamina of the shoulder with paralysis of the deltoid was no more than 30% of the normal side, and ranged between 40 and 45% in those where there had been some recovery in the lesions in continuity. Shoulder stamina after successful repair of the suprascapular nerve with an intact circumflex nerve reached 70% of normal. Where the circumflex nerve had been grafted, the shoulder achieved only 50% of normal stamina. On the whole, paralysis of the deltoid muscle affects extension most markedly and in many patients extension behind the plane of the body was impossible with the shoulder abducted. With the arm adducted, the latissimus dorsi muscle can compensate.

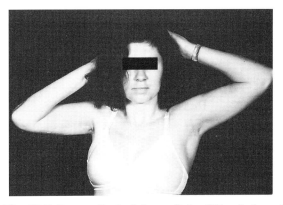

Fig. 27.7 Preganglionic injury of the fifth, sixth and seventh cervical nerves. Nerve transfers included: a part of the dorsal scapular to the long thoracic; spinal accessory to suprascapular; intercostal to circumflex; one bundle from the ulnar nerve to the biceps. Function was regained at 20 months.

THE SHOULDER IN INJURIES OF THE BRACHIAL PLEXUS

In 40% of 1200 cases of injury to the brachial plexus the upper roots were involved, i.e. the fifth, sixth and seventh cervical nerves (Figures 27.6 and 27.7). Until about 10 years ago the treatment of patients with an intact lower trunk but with avulsion of the upper three roots was by reconstruction surgery and included muscle transfer for elbow flexion and arthrodesis of the shoulder; the results were rather poor.[8] The re-

introduction of nerve transfers has proven promising. The current method in my unit for re-innervating the shoulder in cases of preganglionic injury includes transfer of intercostal or dorsal scapular nerve to long thoracic nerve, spinal accessory to suprascapular nerve, and intercostal nerves to circumflex nerves. Results are encouraging and the spinal accessory to suprascapular nerve transfer has proved to be the most consistently reliable of all nerve transfers in reconstruction of the brachial plexus.

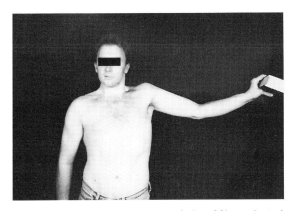

Fig. 27.6 Preganglionic injury of the fifth and sixth cervical nerves. Repair was by spinal accessory to suprascapular nerve transfer and intercostal to circumflex nerve transfer. Function was regained at 18 months.

REFERENCES

1. Comtet, J.J., Herzberg, G. & Alnaasan, I. (1993) (English translation) Biomechanics of the shoulder and the scapulothoracic girdle. In R. Tubiana (ed.), *The Hand*, vol. 4, pp. 99–111. Philadelphia: W.B. Saunders.
2. Narakas, A.O. (1991) Compression and traction neuropathies about the shoulder and arm. In R.H. Gelberman (ed.), *Operative Nerve Repair and Reconstruction*, pp. 1147–1176. Philadelphia: J.B. Lippincott.
3. Coene, L.N.J.E.M. & Narakas, A.O. (1992) Operative management of lesions of the axillary nerve isolated or combined with other nerve lesions. *Clin. Neurol. Neurosurg.* **94** (Suppl.): S64–S66.
4. Seddon, H.T. (1975) *Surgical Disorder of the Peripheral Nerves*, 2nd edn. London: Churchill Livingstone.
5. Williams, W., Unwin, A. & Smith, D. (1995) Fibre

content of the accessory nerve. Presented at the Reading Shoulder Course.

6. Williams, W., Twyman, R., Donnel, S. & Birch, R. (1996) The spinal accessory nerve (abstract). *J. Bone Joint Surg*. In Press.

7. Spilsbury, J. & Birch, R. (1996) Injuries of the supra-scapular and circumflex nerves. *J. Bone Joint Surg*. **73B:** 1–59.

8. Ross, A. & Birch, R. (1993) (English translation) Reconstruction of the paralysed shoulder after brachial plexus injuries. In R. Tubiana (ed.), *The Hand*, vol. 4, pp. 126–133. Philadelphia: W.B. Saunders.

28

The Shoulder in Obstetric Brachial Plexus Palsy (OBPP)

R Birch

INTRODUCTION

Seddon in 1975[1] reported the following: 'the decline in the incidence of these injuries during the last 40 years, which is not confined to what we are pleased to call advanced countries, is one indication of widespread improvement of the standard of obstetrics. Whereas Sever, an American, writing in 1925 could report 1100 cases my own experience is limited to under 50 cases over a period of almost 40 years.' It is no longer true to say that OBPP is a rare condition. We have seen a dramatic increase in referrals over the last 5 years so that new cases now exceed those in adults. Rational discussion of the British experience is marred by the inadequacy of our central statistical service. In the Office of Population Censuses and Surveys (OPCS) birth lesions of the plexus are lumped together with congenital deformities. The deterioration of our statistical service is further exposed by Power[2] who commented 'it is regrettable that figures for birth weights were no longer kept in England and Wales from 1986.' We start from two weak points in the British experience: the incidence is unknown and one of the most important risk factors cannot be measured.

Serious study of this disorder began over 150 years go, significantly earlier than equivalent work in the adult lesion. The history of this study is marked by controversy about causation, the natural history and treatment, and the cause of secondary deformity. These controversies persist. Duchenne[3] confirmed that the lesion of the brachial plexus caused during birth is not a con-

genital injury. In the following decade other writers described the main patterns of injury, risk factors and mechanisms of injury, and early in this century there was already significant experience of operative repair; however, postoperative deaths and the difficulty of demonstrating any benefit led to disenchantment with this pioneering work. In the late 1970s Morelli and Narakas[4] encouraged by their experience with adults made a disciplined start in describing the indications for and techniques of operative repair. Gilbert, who now has the largest experience of any, carefully described the natural history of an untreated population and, with his colleague Tassin, proposed a system of classification which is now widely used.[5]

There are two significant risk factors. The birth lesion breech delivery is severe and often bilateral. Giddins et al[6] in their study of risk factors in 230 consecutive babies confirmed that the birth weight was significant: the mean birth weight in their series was 4.5 kg, substantially higher than the mean for North West Thames region of 3.88 kg. These writers found that the more severe neural injuries were associated with even higher birth weights, and that shoulder dystocia had been recorded as a complication of delivery in over 60%.

The detailed prospective study from Gilbert and Tassin[5] of 44 children reported complete recovery in 14 (32%). Eleven children (25%) showed useful recovery but not of active lateral rotation, and 19 babies (43%) made a far from full recovery. These authors proposed a new and relatively simple classification of OBPP replacing earlier eponymous or regional systems and we follow it. It is as follows.

Group 1: the fifth and sixth cervical nerves are damaged. There is paralysis of the deltoid and biceps muscles. About 90% of babies proceed to full spontaneous recovery, with clinical evidence of early recovery no later than 2 months.

Group 2: the fifth, sixth and seventh cervical nerves are damaged. The long flexor muscles of the hand are working from the time of birth but there is paralysis of extension of the elbow, wrist and digits. Perhaps 65% of these children make full spontaneous recovery, but the remainder persist with serious defects in control of the shoulder.

Group 3: paralysis is virtually complete although there is some flexion of the fingers at or shortly after birth. Full spontaneous recovery occurs in less than one-half of these children, and most are left with substantial impairment of function at the shoulder and elbow with deficient rotation of the forearm. Wrist and finger extension does not recover in about one-quarter.

Group 4: the whole plexus is damaged, Paralysis is complete. The limb is atonic and there is a Bernard–Horner syndrome. No child makes a full recovery, for the spinal nerves have been either ruptured or avulsed from the spinal cord. There is permanent and serious defect within the limb.

The disparity in limb length ranges from up to 2% in Group 1 to 20% in Group 4. Damage to the spinal cord, which occurs in 2% of Group 4 babies presents as delayed and unsteady walking and smallness of the ipsilateral foot.

This chapter now describes experience in my unit in the treatment of the single most important secondary deformity in OBPP, the medial rotation contracture of the shoulder, which if unrecognized and untreated progresses to posterior dislocation.

MEDIAL ROTATION CONTRACTURE AND POSTERIOR DISLOCATION OF THE SHOULDER

This problem required treatment by operation in about one-quarter of children referred with OBPP between 1990 and 1995. In 120 of these, hand function was good or normal. These were children who originally fell into Group 1 and 2 with some in Group 3. All had made full recovery through the eighth cervical and first thoracic nerves and at least useful recovery through lesions in continuity or grafts of the fifth, sixth and seventh cervical nerves.[7] In about 10% of these it seems likely that the dislocation occurred at birth or shortly after; in five cases the subscapularis muscle was densely fibrosed and the appearance consistent with ischaemia from acute compartment syndrome. We believe that this group are examples of the osteoarticular lesion described by Zancolli and Zancolli.[8] However, in no case did we find radiological evidence of separation of the epiphysis nor a fracture of the most proximal part of the metaphysis. In the great majority of these children, the deformity was provoked by muscular imbalance caused by the neurological injury. The medial rotators of the shoulder, notably the powerful subscapularis muscle, innervated by the seventh and eighth cervical nerves, recover early if indeed they were ever paralysed and overwhelm the weaker abductors and lateral rotators innervated by the fifth and sixth cervical nerves. The progression from simple medial rotation contracture to dislocation was seen in 12 children awaiting treatment. What was originally no more than a loss of 30–40° of passive lateral rotation had progressed to subluxation or dislocation. We agree with the analysis of Gilbert:[9] 'Contrary to traditional thinking, the surgeon should not wait to treat an internal rotation contracture. In the absence of surgical treatment, recovery is limited, abduction is impossible, the extremity is less functional, and, most importantly, osseous and articular deformities occur. Posterior subluxation and deformity of the humeral head permanently worsen the prognosis. These anomalies, which have long been considered a result of obstetrical palsy, are in fact simply a consequence of untreated contractures.' The reader is referred also to Goddard's analysis.[10]

Clinical presentation

Medial rotation contracture

The contour of the shoulder is normal. Passive lateral rotation is limited to 30–40°. There is a mild flexion pronation posture of the forearm but this deformity is not fixed. Radiographs are normal.

Posterior subluxation

The head of the humerus is prominent to palpation, and passive lateral rotation is possible only to 10°. There is a marked flexion pronation posture of the forearm which is not fixed. Radiographs may show a curved appearance of the proximal humerus (Figure 28.1).

Posterior dislocation

The contour of the shoulder is plainly abnormal. The head of the humerus can be seen as a prominence behind the glenoid. The arm cannot be laterally rotated at all and there may now be a fixed flexion pronation posture. Radiographs confirm the displacement with a characteristic wind-swept curved appearance of the proximal humerus.

Complex dislocation (Figures 28.2 and 28.3)

There are now secondary bone changes which are apparent on clinical and radiological examination. Foremost is an elongation of the coracoid which is

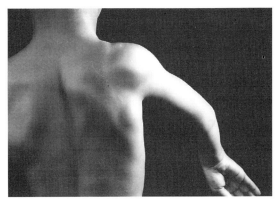

Fig. 28.2 The appearance in posterior dislocation of the head of humerus.

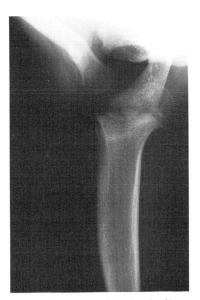

Fig. 28.1 Subluxation of the head of humerus.

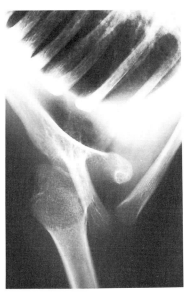

Fig. 28.3 Posterior dislocation.

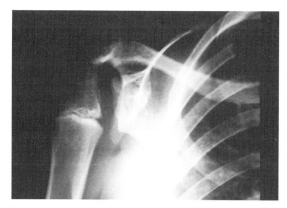

Fig. 28.4 Complex dislocation. Note the overgrowth of the acromion and coracoid.

easily noted by palpation. The acromion may be elongated and hooked downwards. Examination with an image intensifier shows a bifacet appearance of the glenoid; in abduction the acromion forces the humerus downward and the lesser tuberosity lies in the inferior facet to be allowed back into the superior facet in adduction. This leads to an apparent abduction contracture; if the head is held in the plane of the superior facet, the arm can only be brought to the side by forcing the spine of the scapula upward (Figures 28.4 and 28.5).

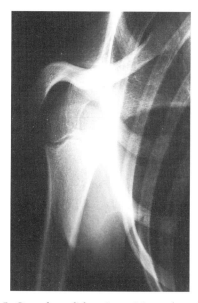

Fig. 28.5 Complex dislocation. Note the elongated coracoid and the bifacet appearance of the glenoid.

Progression of the defect: long-term outcome

We do not know why the coracoid becomes elongated nor can we offer an explanation for the hooking of the acromion and biconcave development of the glenoid in the late complex dislocation. A few young adults have been seen with complex dislocation (Figure 28.6). Function at the shoulder was extremely poor, indeed it was substantially impaired throughout the upper limb. There was pain from the disorganized glenohumeral joint. The compensatory thoracoscapular movement seen in many young children had diminished and the position and function of the shoulder was inferior to that following arthrodesis. Flexion at elbow and pronation of forearm had become fixed. In four of six of these older cases the head of the radius was dislocated. These patients presented very late and we were unable to offer any useful treatment. Relocation of the shoulder is out of the question, arthrodesis is technically impossible, and palliative lateral rotation osteotomy of the humerus is contraindicated because of the very small arc of rotation remaining at the shoulder. It seems logical to recognize and treat the deformity before secondary bone changes occur. We do not know at what age attempts at relocation should be abandoned; the oldest child in which it was performed was aged 13, and the result was useful.

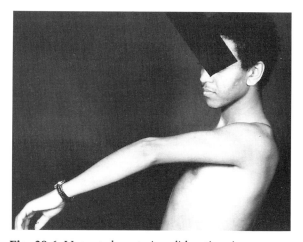

Fig. 28.6 Untreated posterior dislocation in a young adult.

Treatment

Prevention

Parents are taught a set of exercises which start soon after birth and progress must be regularly supervised. Many of the stretching regimes taught are valueless. *Both arms should be worked simultaneously in adduction.* The range of movement is recorded with particular attention to the arc of lateral rotation in abduction and adduction. The systems proposed by Mallet[11] and Gilbert[9] for shoulder assessment are both simple and useful. Active treatment is indicated when lateral rotation is diminshed by about 40°.

Subscapularis slide

In this operation the subscapularis muscle is dis-inserted from the scapula which is approached by an incision in the mid-axillary line. The pedicles are respected and the capsule not opened. Full lateral rotation is achieved. The shoulder is immobilized for 6 weeks in the corrected position. The operation is indicated when there is a significant loss of lateral rotation. It is contra-indicated if the head of humerus is not fully reduced or if the coracoid is overgrown.

Posterior subluxation

Simple dislocation. The extent of bone abnormality can be determined by examination of the shoulder by plain radiographs before operation and by screening the shoulder with an image intensifier after induction of anaesthesia. In some of my early cases, I was able to relocate the shoulder by subscapularis recession. There were some failures, and I now recommend the anterior approach.

The shoulder is approached through the delto-pectoral groove, without interfering with the origin of deltoid and the insertion of the pectoralis major. The subscapularis tendon is exposed and lengthened. Detachment of the coracobrachialis tendon from the tip of the coracoid makes this a lot easier. In most cases the capsule of the shoulder is so adherent to the tendon that it is opened. With the shoulder fully located and moved into full lateral rotation, the relation of the head of humerus to the coracoid and acromion is checked. The subscapularis is the most powerful medial rotator of the shoulder and it must be repaired. The limb is immobilized for 6 weeks or a little longer in older children.

Complex dislocation. The object of the operation is to secure reduction of the head of the humerus into the glenoid by removing the obstructing deformities. There are two of these. The coracoid is always shortened by between 1.0 and 2.5 cm. Sometimes osteotomy of the outer lip of the acromion was necessary. The subscapularis tendon is formally lengthened, and the pectoralis minor and coracobrachialis are reattached to the stump of the coracoid.

Difficulties and complications

First amongst these is failure to reduce or secure reduction of the head of the humerus. A second operation proved necessary in cases of subscapularis recession. The arm should not be splinted with the shoulder in abduction. Repair of the subscapularis muscle is essential; loss of active medial rotation can occur when tenotomy alone is performed, and a later operation of transfer of pectoralis major to the lesser tuberosity is necessary to overcome this defect. Four older children with established bone deformity lost medial rotation after successful relocation. A medial rotation osteotomy of the humeral shaft performed no earlier than 6 months after relocation restored functional medial rotation so that the hand could come to the face and behind the back whilst permitting a useful range of lateral rotation. It is best not to perform osteotomy of the humerus at the same time as the relocation as it is difficult to predict which children will need it.

Results

It seems that there is significant and lasting improvement in function at the shoulder after operation. The long-term outcome is not known but I have seen remarkable remodelling of the head of humerus and of the glenoid at 5 years after

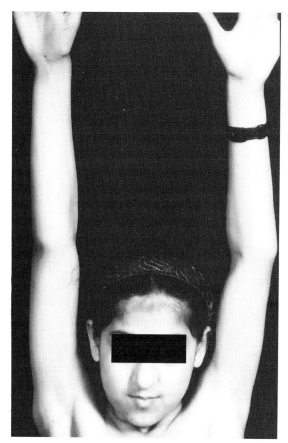

Fig. 28.7 A 13-year-old girl 6 years after relocation of the head of the humerus which required shortening of the coracoid and osteotomy of the acromion.

relocation. An unexpected finding was the improvement in the function of forearm and hand observed in 50% of cases (Figure 28.7).

We suspect that this deformity of the shoulder is more common than is appreciated. It seems that dislocation of the shoulder is a preventable condition. Regular and careful stretching exercises of the shoulders reduce the risk of dislocation. A timely subscapularis slide is indicated when the last 30–40° of lateral rotation are lost. The elongated

coracoid forces the humerus posteriorly, and the overgrown acromion forces it inferiorly; it seems that both of these deformities can be corrected. The spontaneous correction of flexion deformity of the elbow and active supination of the forearm after successful treatment considerably improves overall function of the limb.

REFERENCES

1. Seddon, H.J. (1975) *Surgical Disorders of the Peripheral Nerves*, 2nd edn, p. 130. Edinburgh, London and New York: Churchill-Livingstone.
2. Power, C. (1994) National trends in birth weight. *Br. Med. J.* **308**: 1270–1271.
3. Duchenne, G.B.A. (1872) *De l'électrisation localisée et de son application à la pathologie et à la thérapeutique*, 2nd edn, p. 353. Paris: J.B. Ballière.
4. Narakas, A. (1987) Obstetrical brachial plexus injuries. In D.W. Lamb (ed.), *The Paralysed Upper Limb*, pp. 116–135. Edinburgh, London and New York: Churchill-Livingstone.
5. Gilbert, A. & Tassin, J.L. (1984) Réparation chirurgicale du plexus brachial dans la paralysie obstétricale. *Chirurgie* **110**: 70.
6. Giddins, G.E.B., Taggart, M., Singh, D. & Birch, R. (1994) Risk factors in obstetric brachial plexus palsy (abstract). *J. Bone Joint Surg.* **76B** (Suppl. II and III): 156.
7. Chen, L. & Birch, R. (1996) The medial rotation contracture in OBPP (abstract). *J. Bone Joint Surg.* In Press.
8. Zancolli, E.A. & Zancolli, E.R. (1993) (English translation) Palliative surgical procedures in sequelae of obstetrical palsy. In R. Tubiana (ed.), *The Hand*, vol. 4, pp. 602–623. Philadelphia: W.B. Saunders.
9. Gilbert, A. (1993) (English translation) Obstetrical brachial plexus palsy. In R. Tubiana (ed.), *The Hand*, vol. 4, pp. 575–601. Philadelphia: W.B. Saunders.
10. Goddard, N. (1993) (English translation) The development of the proximal humerus in the neonate. In R. Tubiana (ed.), *The Hand*, vol. 4, pp. 624–631. Philadelphia: W.B. Saunders.
11. Mallet, J. (1972) Paralysie obstétricale. *Rev. Chir. Orthop.* **58** (Suppl. 1): 115.

29

Fractures of the Clavicle and Scapula

PT Calvert

CLAVICLE

Introduction

Fractures of the clavicle are common, easy to recognize and, in the majority of cases, heal rapidly with a good funtional outcome. As a result the management of clavicular fractures tends to be given little consideration. Most of the time this approach produces acceptable results but on occasions healing is not so straightforward and complications can occur. An awareness of the possible difficulties will ensure that those fractures which are more likely to cause problems are recognized and given appropriate attention.

History

In Grecian times Hippocrates noted that clavicular fractures heal rapidly with good callus. He further observed that initially the patient attaches a great deal of importance to the fracture believing that the outcome will be worse than is the reality, but that quite quickly finds there is little restriction of function. At this stage the patient stops worrying about the fracture and the physician, unable to improve the appearance, disappears. At the other end of the spectrum there have been famous persons who have died as a result of clavicular fractures, William III in 1702 and Sir Robert Peel in 1850 being the most celebrated. Over the centuries a number of elaborate devices have been used to treat these fractures but Dupuytren observed that most were unnecessary. Malgaigne stated that the absence of residual deformity was so unusual that he had never seen a case!

Incidence

Recent studies by Nordqvist and Petersson[1] in a well-defined urban population in Malmo have helped to define the incidence of clavicular fractures. The overall annual incidence of shoulder injuries was 219/100 000 with the most frequent being fracture of the proximal humerus (53%). Most of the proximal humeral fractures occurred in elderly women. In children (0–14 years) and adults (15–64 years) the most common injury was fracture of the clavicle with an incidence of 87 and 37% respectively. Clavicular fractures made up 4% of all fractures seen in Malmo. The overall incidence of these fractures was 64/100 000 population in 1987 and this had increased from 45/100 000 in 1952. Rowe[2] found that fracture of the clavicle was the most frequent shoulder girdle injury constituting 43% of the injuries. However, his population is not well defined and it may well have included a lower proportion of elderly female patients.

Classification (Figure 29.1)

The most useful classification is division into the three Allman groups.[3] Group I is a midshaft fracture, Group II a fracture of the lateral third and Group III a fracture of the medial third. In Nordqvist and Petersson's study[4] Group I accounted for 76% with a median age of 13 years, Group II for 20% with a median age of 47 years and Group III for 3% with a median age of 59 years. Each fracture type can be further divided into undisplaced (A), displaced (B) and, for midshaft fractures, comminuted (C). The most

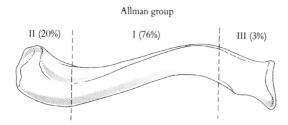

Allman group

II (20%)   I (76%)   III (3%)

Fig. 29.1 Classification of clavicle fractures into Allman groups.

common fracture in children is the undisplaced midshaft clavicle fracture.

Fractures of the outer end of the clavicle have been classified by Neer[5,6] into three types (Figure 29.2). Type I is undisplaced, Type II has ruptured coracoclavicular ligaments and is displaced and Type III is an intra-articular fracture into the acromioclavicular joint but with intact ligaments. The clinical significance of this classification is that Type I has a good prognosis with conservative treatment whereas Type II has a high incidence of non-union and may require operative fixation. Type III may lead to later degenerative change. Fractures of the medial third have been similarly divided into three types, undisplaced, displaced with ruptured ligaments and intra-articular.

In children there is a further type of fracture which can occur at either end of the clavicle. At the outer end the periosteal sleeve may remain

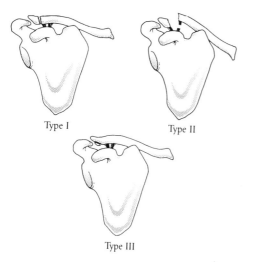

Type I   Type II

Type III

Fig. 29.2 Fractures of the lateral clavicle – Neer classification.

attached to the coracoclavicular ligaments while the bone displaces superiorly out of the periosteal sleeve. This has been called a pseudodislocation of the acromioclavicular joint. At the medial end the epiphysis is the last to ossify, appearing during the teenage years, and fuses at about 22 years. In children and young adults injuries to the medial end of the clavicle tend to be epiphyseal fracture separations and these can look exactly like a sternoclavicular dislocation in the adult. Prior to ossification it can be extremely difficult to diagnose.

Mechanism

It used to be thought that most fractures of the clavicle were caused by a fall on the outstretched hand. At least one study, however, has demonstrated that the majority result from a fall directly on to the shoulder.[7] In adults the majority are related to road traffic accidents or are sports-related injuries whereas in the elderly they are caused by a fall.[1] In children both aetiologies are common. In addition, there are a number of midshaft clavicular fractures which occur as a result of birth trauma.

Anatomy

The clavicle is **S**-shaped and entirely subcutaneous. It is crossed only by the suprascapular nerves which supply sensation to the infraclavicular region. Operations on the clavicle may result in loss of sensation in this area; it does not cause any functional loss but it is worth warning patients about the possibility. More important are the neurovascular structures passing underneath the clavicle. These are the subclavian vessels and divisions of the brachial plexus which may be damaged acutely with midshaft fractures. In addition malunion or exuberant callus may occasionally cause narrowing of the thoracic outlet and subsequent late compression.

The ligaments (Figure 29.2) linking the clavicle to the scapula are particularly important when considering fractures of the lateral third. The coracoclavicular ligaments consist of two strong bands, the conoid and trapezoid ligaments. The acromioclavicular ligaments are really condensations of the joint capsule. Although the coracoacromial ligament contributes nothing towards the stability of the clavicle it may be useful for late reconstruction and should be respected.

Presentation and assessment

Birth fractures

Other than the history of a traumatic birth or a crack heard during delivery a clavicular fracture may go undiagnosed until a swelling caused by the callus appears about 1 week later. Sometimes the fracture is only noticed during a routine examination of the infant. A more common presentation is the infant who moves the affected limb less than the contralateral uninjured side (pseudoparalysis). When a search is made for the cause of the apparent lack of movement, the fracture of the clavicle is found. It is important to remember that a brachial plexus palsy may be associated with a clavicular fracture caused by birth trauma and the limb should be carefully examined to confirm or refute this.

Children

These are often caused by relatively minor injury and are frequently greenstick in type. Consequently this fracture may be missed. After a few days the parents may notice that the child has been protecting the injured limb or that handling induces crying. Clearly if the fracture is complete or displaced the diagnosis is obvious; it is usually in the midshaft.

Adults

In adults there is usually no difficulty in making the diagnosis. The fracture is caused by more significant trauma. If it is in the midshaft it is frequently displaced; the medial fragment is pulled upwards so that its lateral end can tent the skin (Figure 29.3). Occasionally this medial spike compromises the viability of the overlying skin and may even be compound. The clinical appearance of fractures at the lateral end mimics acro-

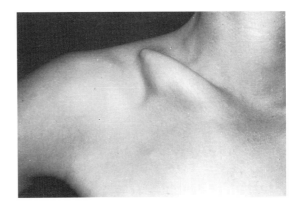

Fig. 29.3 Fractured clavicle tenting the skin.

mioclavicular joint dislocations so that an X-ray is required to distinguish between them.

Most clavicular fractures are isolated injuries and not associated with major complications. As a result additional injuries, when they do occur, are often missed. It is essential to always examine the whole upper limb for evidence of neurovascular compromise. Brachial plexus damage, although rare, is well described. It may be associated with injury to the subclavian vessels. Other injuries, particularly in the victim of high-speed trauma, include those to the head and neck, fractures of the first rib and pneumothorax.

Radiographs

As with any other fracture radiographic assessment of the clavicle should include two views in different planes. The usual combination for a midshaft fracture is an AP view and a 45° cephalic tilt view. When there is doubt, at a later stage, as to whether a clavicular fracture has united it may be necessary to take several views with different tilt angles in order to visualize the non-union.

For a fracture of the lateral third an AP view and an axillary view are essential. The axillary view reveals the degree of posterior displacement of the medial fragment, which will not be seen on the AP view.

Fractures of the medial end are difficult to visualize and may require computed tomography (CT) for adequate definition. The fracture separation of the medial clavicular epiphysis is particularly difficult to image even with CT because the physis remains entirely cartilaginous until somewhere between 12 and 19 years of age. Careful clinical examination is most important with this rare injury.

Complications

Neurovascular compromise, malunion and non-union may be associated with midshaft fractures. The latter two and post-traumatic arthritis can occur with fractures of the outer end of the clavicle.

Acute injury to the brachial plexus or subclavian vessels is rare in association with clavicular fractures but can occur particularly in the victim of high-speed trauma with multiple injuries. A major vascular injury is clearly an indication for urgent exploration. Whether a brachial plexus injury on its own merits exploration is a debatable issue. To a certain extent it will depend on the total clinical picture, the severity of the plexus injury and the available expertise. If it is deemed necessary to expose the damaged plexus, then the clavicular fracture should be stabilized.

Malunion with overlap and shortening is the usual outcome in adults following displaced midshaft clavicular fractures treated conservatively. Fortunately shoulder function is rarely compromised despite the malunion. Occasionally the clavicle is sufficiently shortened that the whole shoulder girdle is protracted forwards. This can be cosmetically unattractive and in a few patients causes symptoms. These symptoms tend to be ill-defined, and it is difficult to be certain whether they arise from the malunion. I have corrected the malunion in four such instances and the symptoms have been relieved. Malunion and shortening can cause a thoracic outlet syndrome either by narrowing the outlet or because of protruberant callus on the inferior surface. In the former instance correction of the malunion is indicated whereas in the latter trimming of the callus is all that is required. It must be emphasized that the indications for correction of clavicular malunion are few and it is rarely required.

Non-union is unusual. The reported incidence for midshaft fractures treated conservatively is

Table 29.1. Factors predisposing to non-union

Inadequate immobilization
Severe injury
Large amount of displacement
Site of fracture (lateral one-third)
Primary open reduction
Refracture

between 1 and 4%. Factors said to predispose to non-union are listed in Table 29.1.

Although most non-unions occur in the midshaft because fractures in that area are the most common, fractures of the lateral third are associated with a higher incidence (30%). Not all non-unions require operative treatment. A number are asymptomatic and can be left alone. If symptoms are a problem, then open reduction, plating and bone grafting is the treatment of choice. The differential diagnosis for a non-union is a congenital pseudarthrosis; attempts to get this to join are unnecessary and doomed to failure.

Treatment[5–17]

Birth fractures heal extremely rapidly and require no specific treatment. Explanation to the parents about the healing process and the good prognosis is extremely important. Advice should be given about careful handling of the affected limb. It is also wise to warn them about the lump of callus which will appear and then disappear as remodelling progresses.

In children the treatment is symptomatic. Resting the arm in a broad arm sling is usually all that is required. Sometimes the child is more comfortable in a figure-of-eight type bandage, which is best constructed out of the material used for 'collar and cuff' supports. If a figure-of-eight bandage is used, then the parents need to be instructed on how to tighten it every 2 or 3 days. The child can start using the arm as comfort permits. Usually within 2 or 3 weeks the full range of movement has been regained and the sling or figure-of-eight bandage has been discarded. The speed with which this occurs depends on the age of the child and the degree of initial displacement. The younger the child and the less the displacement, the quicker the fracture heals and the faster that normal function returns.

In adults the majority of midshaft clavicular fractures can be treated conservatively. Over the years a wide range of devices have been used in an attempt to achieve and maintain a closed reduction. In some countries plaster spica immobilization is popular. However, there is no evidence that any of these methods achieve union in a better position than simple immobilization in a broad arm sling. Two studies comparing the efficacy of a figure-of-eight bandage with a simple sling demonstrated no difference in outcome between the two methods.[8,9] The overall conclusion throughout the literature is that the majority of midshaft clavicular fractures unite with some degree of cosmetic deformity and shortening but that the functional result is excellent. It is, therefore, difficult to justify more invasive methods of treatment except for specific indications. The indications for open reduction and internal fixation are listed in Table 29.2.

Table 29.2. Indications for operative treatment

Neurovascular compromise
Compound fracture
Multiple injuries
Type II distal third fracture
Symptomatic non-union
Symptomatic malunion

If operative treatment is selected then it is essential to use an adequate method of fixation. In my opinion the best method for midshaft fractures is plate fixation using a 3.5 mm reconstruction plate on the superior surface of the clavicle (Figure 29.4). This plate can be contoured in two planes allowing an accurate fit. There must be three screws gripping both cortices on either side of the fracture. Semitubular or one-third tubular plates are of inadequate strength and will break; the mini-plates illustrated in Figure 29.5 are totally inadequate. Dynamic compression plate (DCP) plates (3.5 mm) can be used[14] but are less easy to contour. A recent study[10] has demonstrated the efficacy of low-contact DCP plates. If

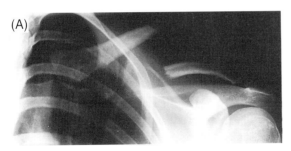 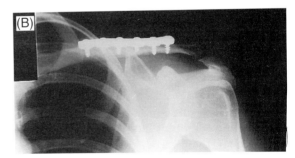

Fig. 29.4 Midshaft clavicular fracture with wide displacement. (A) Preoperative view. (B) Postoperative view showing fixation with 3.5 mm reconstruction plate.

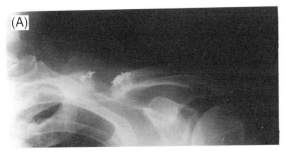 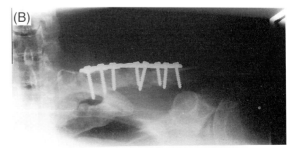

Fig. 29.5 (A) Inadequate plate fixation. (B) Plate fixation after revision.

one is going to plate the clavicle it is important to place the incision inferior to the bone and not along its surface; this reduces the chance of an unsightly keloid scar. It is also important to warn the patient that an area of loss of cutaneous sensation in the infraclavicular region is quite probable because the supraclavicular nerves pass directly across the operation site and cannot always be preserved; fortunately this seems to cause no functional deficit. It should be remembered that the subcutaneous position of the clavicle makes it quite likely that the patient will want the plate removed. This requires a second operation but should not be done until the bone is soundly united and probably not for at least 1 year to 18 months. If the operation is for symptomatic non-union, then autogenous bone graft is mandatory.

Although intramedullary devices have been described the shape of the clavicle does not lend itself to such methods and rotational control is difficult. At present a suitably tried and tested locking intramedullary device for the clavicle, which obviously has some cosmetic attractions in terms of the scar size, is not available. There are a few reports of the use of small external fixators for acute clavicle fractures which in terms of scar size may have some advantage but they have not been widely used.

Type II fractures of the lateral third have been shown, in several studies,[5,6,11–13] to have a high incidence of non-union if treated conservatively. Neer[5,6] found 30% non-union. In the series by Edwards et al[11] there was a 30% incidence of non-union and a 45% incidence of delayed union with only five of 20 in the non-operative group progressing to uncomplicated satisfactory healing. In their operative group all 23 patients had their fracture united by 6–10 weeks after the operation. Most authors advocate fixation of these Type II fractures. Recently one study has presented a contrary view;[13] in a study of 110 patients with fractures of the lateral clavicle treated without operation 95 shoulders were asymptomatic at follow-up; although there were ten non-unions eight were asymptomatic. It is difficult to reconcile this study with others in the literature, but it should be noted that 73 of their patients had Type I undisplaced fractures and there was a 22% non-union rate for Type II fractures; the difference lies in the observation that eight of the ten non-unions were asymptomatic.

A variety of methods have been used to stabilize this fracture. The precise method will depend on the fracture configuration. Open reduction and indirect stabilization with a coracoclavicular screw is one satisfactory method.[11,15] It is important to achieve a good repair of the deltotrapezius flap on the superior aspect; it is not necessary to repair the torn ligaments. Other methods have included K-wire fixation across the acromioclavicular joint, plates, cerclage wiring and suture techniques encircling the coracoid. K-wire fixation with or without tension band wiring has the potentially disastrous complication of wire migration; if this method is used, then the wires must be threaded and steps such as bending over the ends of the wires must be taken to avoid this problem; it is probably best avoided. Plates transgress the acromioclavicular joint and require a wide exposure both to implant and to remove. Cerclage wiring (Figure 29.6) is a

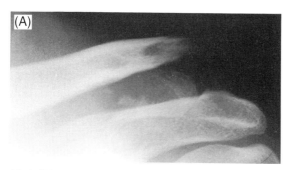

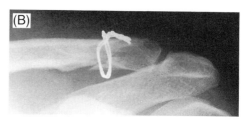

Fig. 29.6 (A) Type II fracture lateral third before surgery. (B) Type II fracture lateral third treated with cerclage wire.

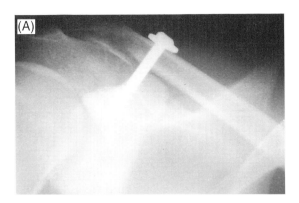

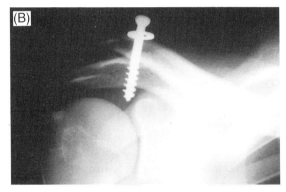

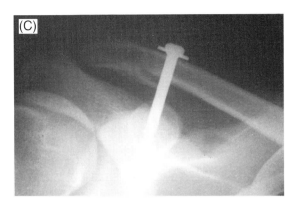

Fig. 29.7 (A) Lateral third clavicle fracture treated by poorly placed coracoclavicular screw. (B) Screw cut out. (C) Screw replaced correctly.

good technique but is only applicable if the fracture has an oblique configuration, which is infrequent. Suture techniques encircling the coracoid are similar to the coracoclavicular screw technique but are not removable and may result in erosion of either coracoid or clavicle. It is possible that the new absorbable cords and bands may solve this problem. If a coracoclavicular screw is used it is essential to place it centrally in the base of the coracoid; if this is not done there is a high rate of cut out (Figure 29.7). It is more difficult to place the screw than might appear because the superior surface of the base of the coracoid is not flat but somewhat angular and the drill tends to slide down the side of the coracoid between bone and the rather thick periosteum. Patient positioning is also important because the drill has to be angled slightly outwards and the patient's head can get in the way if this has not been considered.

SCAPULA

Introduction

The scapula is a flat triangular bone and is the link between the axial skeleton and the upper extremity. It is covered by muscle which affords considerable protection from injury. In addition its mobility on the chest wall allows energy from injury to be dissipated. Scapula fractures are, therefore, uncommon, often associated with other injuries, which dictate overall patient management, and usually treated conservatively. Fractures of the glenoid are even less common but need to be considered separately because of their intra-articular nature.

Incidence[18,19,20,21]

Scapula fractures represent 0.5–1% of all fractures and between 3 and 5% of shoulder fractures.

Table 29.3. Injuries associated with scapula fractures

Injury	Approximate incidence (%)
Rib fractures	25–50
Clavicular fractures	15–40
Pulmonary injuries	10–55
Skull fractures	25
Cerebral contusions	10–40
Humeral fractures	12
Brachial plexus	5–10
Tibial fractures	11
Major vascular injuries	11
Splenic rupture	8

Fractures of the glenoid cavity are about 10% of scapular fractures and about 10% of glenoid fractures are displaced. Therefore displaced fractures of the glenoid, if one excludes rim fractures associated with instability, are extremely rare and have a frequency of about one in ten thousand fractures. Any one individual cannot expect to have a large experience of these fractures.

Scapula fractures are more common in men than women and tend to occur most frequently under the age of 40 years. This is not surprising in view of the fact that they are usually caused by major trauma and have a high incidence (80–95%) of associated soft tissue injuries. On average there are 3.9 additional injuries and the mortality is around 2%.

The most frequent associated injuries are listed in Table 29.3.

The majority of scapula fractures are caused by direct trauma. There are a few fractures caused by indirect force. Most of these are avulsion fractures which result from sudden muscle contraction. Such fractures have been described for the coracoid (coracobrachialis), superomedial corner (levator scapulae), inferior angle (serratus anterior) and the spine of the scapula (deltoid). Stress fractures have also been reported.

Classification

Scapula fractures are usually classified according to their anatomical location but, in addition, intra-articular glenoid fractures have been separately classified by Ideberg.[22,23] The most common

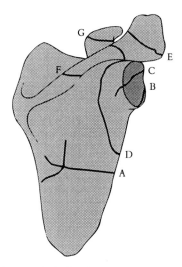

Fig. 29.8 Anatomical classification of scapula fractures. A, Body; B, glenoid rim; C, glenoid; D, neck; E, acromion; F, spine; G, coracoid.

scapula fracture is that involving the body; next is one involving the glenoid followed, in decreasing order of frequency, by the acromion or spine, the neck and finally the coracoid. The anatomical classification is illustrated in Figure 29.8. Ideberg's classification of intra-articular glenoid fractures was based on an analysis of 225 scapula fractures with 92 glenoid fractures. It is the most comprehensive classification. It is relevant for planning treatment, particularly the surgical approach, if open reduction and internal fixation is required. His classification has been slightly modified by Goss in an excellent review article[19] and is illustrated in Figure 29.9.

Presentation and assessment

Clinical assessment is directed initially at the potentially life-threatening associated injuries, which must be recognized and managed expeditiously. The scapula fracture is easily missed during the initial evaluation of the multiply injured patient because it is covered with soft tissue. It may be seen as an incidental finding on the trauma series chest X-ray. The fact that it is not identified immediately does not matter because there is no urgency to treat a scapula fracture. It is essential that any patient with multi-

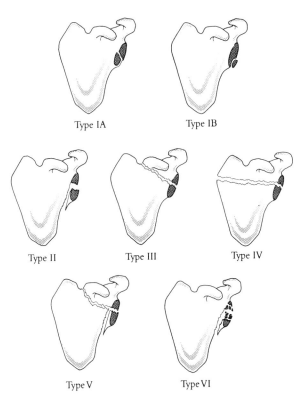

Type IA   Type IB

Type II   Type III   Type IV

Type V   Type VI

Fig. 29.9 Classification of displaced glenoid fractures (Goss's modification of Ideberg's classification).

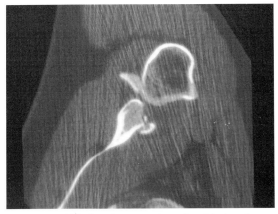

Fig. 29.10 CT showing anterior glenoid rim fracture lying posteriorly.

ple injuries is repeatedly examined so that all injuries, including any scapula fractures, are recognized in due course. The conscious patient may complain of pain around the shoulder girdle. There may be relatively little in the way of physical signs: bruising around the chest wall or over the scapula may not appear until later; there will be local tenderness. It is essential to do a full neurovascular assessment of the shoulder girdle and upper limb because of the close proximity of the neurovascular structures, particularly the brachial plexus. In addition the nerve to the serratus anterior, which courses over the chest wall, may be damaged more distally. The suprascapular nerve passes through the suprascapular notch under the supraglenoid ligament and can be damaged with fractures of the spine of the scapula or neck of the glenoid.

Proper assessment of scapula fractures requires good quality radiographs. These should be done once the patient is stable and other injuries have been treated. There is no place for spending time obtaining multiple views of the scapula when the patient needs resuscitation and stabilization. The definitive scapula X-rays can be obtained later. These should include an AP and tangential scapula lateral as a basic minimum. An axillary view is necessary to visualize fractures of the acromion. For the inexperienced it is easy to mistake a bipartite acromion, present in 3–8% of the population, for a fracture. Clinical examination will reveal no local tenderness in relation to the bipartite acromion; radiographically the edges tend to be well defined and may be sclerotic; the position varies but its direction is usually coronal. CT (Figure 29.10) is the best way of defining more precisely the configuration and displacement of scapula and glenoid fractures. Clearly this is only necessary if operative intervention is being considered; it is particularly useful for displaced glenoid fractures (Figures 29.10 and 29.11). If high-definition three-dimensional reconstruction is available, this can be extremely helpful. Magnetic resonance imaging is only required if it is thought that there might be an associated rotator cuff tear; this may occur with acromial fractures.

Treatment

The vast majority of scapula fractures can be managed conservatively.[18,20,21,24] Adequate analgesia, a sling and mobilization as comfort

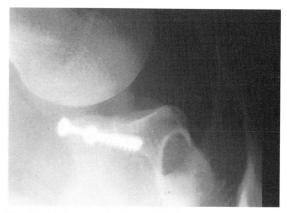

Fig. 29.11 Fracture in Figure 29.10 after open reduction and screw fixation.

permits are the mainstays of treatment. This should be used for all undisplaced fractures (Figure 29.12) and body fractures without involvement of the glenoid, coracoid or acromion. Reported results in the literature are universally good. Malunion of body fractures occurs but rarely results in any functional deficit.

Reported results of the conservative treatment of fractures of the neck, acromion and coracoid are variable. Non-operative treatment of displaced glenoid fractures produces about 50% poor results.

Hence the indications for operative treatment[19–21,25–27] are displaced glenoid fractures associated with instability or in which more than one-quarter of the articular surface is involved. Neck fractures in which there is more than 40°

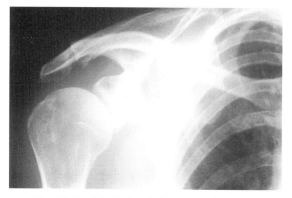

Fig. 29.12 Undisplaced glenoid neck fracture.

angulation or greater than 1 cm of medial translation may justify operation. If a neck fracture is associated with a fractured clavicle there is, in effect, a floating segment and stabilization is indicated;[27] provided that the coracoid and coracoacromial ligament are intact it is sufficient to plate the clavicle alone; if these latter structures are damaged then both the clavicle and scapula neck may require internal fixation. Acromial fractures which are displaced inferiorly will cause impingement on the rotator cuff and should be anatomically reduced and fixed. If the fracture is associated with an acute rotator cuff tear then both the tear and the fracture should be repaired. Occasionally acromial fractures fail to unite and require fixation with bone grafting (Figure 29.13). If the coracoid is widely displaced it should probably be treated by open reduction and internal fixation but most coracoid fractures, a rarity in any event, are minimally displaced and require no intervention.

Operative management

Accurate evaluation and classification of these fractures is important for determining the appropriate operative approach. An anterior deltopectoral approach is used for Type Ia (anterior lip glenoid) fractures, coracoid fractures and sometimes for Type III. A posterior approach is best for Types Ib (posterior lip glenoid), II, III, IV and usually for Type V. A superior approach is ideal for acromial fractures and may be used as a supplementary approach for Types III, IV and Va and Vc fractures. For posterior glenoid lip fractures a standard posterior approach splitting the deltoid and then exposing the shoulder joint between the infraspinatus and teres minor muscles is sufficient. It is important to remember that the axillary nerve emerges from the quadrilateral space under the teres minor and must be protected. The suprascapular nerve passes out of the suprascapular notch and around the base of the spine of the scapula to supply the infraspinatus; great care must be exercised with retractors in this region; if the infraspinatus is divided and retracted medially the nerve is at risk unless particular attention is paid to it. If a wide exposure of the body of the scapula is required it is probably best to detach the deltoid

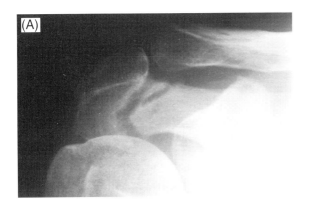

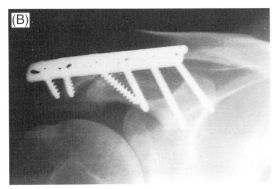

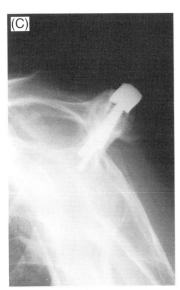

Fig. 29.13 (A), (B), (C) Non-union of acromial fracture treated by plating and grafting.

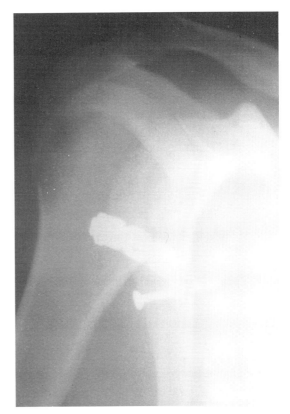

Fig. 29.14 Scapula fractures with glenoid displacement treated by open reduction and internal fixation.

tures. The precise method of fixation will depend on the fracture configuration but is likely to require a combination of interfragmentary screws and 3.5 mm reconstruction plates (Figure 29.14).

REFERENCES

Clavicle

1. Nordqvist, A. & Petersson, C.J. (1995) Incidence and cause of shoulder girdle injuries in an urban population. *J. Shoulder Elbow Surg.* **4:** 107–112.
2. Rowe, C.R. (1968) An atlas of anatomy and treatment of midclavicular fractures. *Clin. Orthop.* **58:** 29–42.
3. Allman, F.L., Jr. (1967) Fractures and ligamentous injuries of the clavicle and its articulation. *J. Bone Joint Surg.* **49A:** 774.
4. Nordqvist, A. & Petersson, C.J. (1994) The incidence of fractures of the clavicle. *Clin. Orthop.* **300:** 127–132.
5. Neer, C.S., II (1963) Fractures of the distal clavicle with

from the spine of the scapula and then raise the infraspinatus and teres minor muscles off the body of the scapula and retract them laterally paying attention once more to the neurovascular struc-

detachment of the coracoclavicular ligaments in adults. *J. Trauma* **3**: 99–110.

6. Neer, C.S., II (1968) Fractures of the distal third of the clavicle. *Clin. Orthop.* **58**: 43–50.

7. Stanley, D., Trowbridge, E.A. & Norris, S.H. (1988) The mechanism of clavicular fracture. A clinical and biomechanical analysis. *J. Bone Joint Surg.* **70B**: 461–464.

8. Anderson, K., Jensen, P. & Lauritzen, J. (1987) Treatment of clavicular fractures. Figure-of-eight bandage vs a simple sling. *Acta Orthop. Scand.* **57**: 71–74.

9. McCandless, D.N. & Mowbray, M. (1979) Treatment of displaced fractures of the clavicle. Sling vs figure-of-eight bandage. *Practitioner* **223**: 266–267.

10. Mullaji, A.B. & Jupiter, J.B. (1994) Low-contact dynamic compression plating of the clavicle. *Injury* **25**: 41–45.

11. Edwards, D.J., Kavanagh, T.G. & Flannery, M.C. (1992) Fractures of the distal clavicle: a case for fixation. *Injury* **23**: 44–46.

12. Jupiter, J.B. & Leffert, R.D. (1987) Non-union of the clavicle. Associated complications and surgical management. *J. Bone Joint Surg.* **69A**: 753–760.

13. Nordqvist, A., Petersson, C. & Redlund-Johnell, I. (1993) The natural course of lateral clavicle fracture. *Acta. Orthop. Scand.* **64**: 87–91.

14. Poigenfurst, J., Rappold, G. & Fischer, W. (1992) Plating of fresh clavicular fractures; results of 122 operations. *Injury* **23**: 237–241.

15. Ballmer, F.T. & Gerber, C. (1991) Coracoclavicular screw fixation for unstable fractures of the distal clavicle. A report of five cases. *J. Bone Joint Surg.* **73B**: 291–294.

16. Stanley, D. & Norris, S.H. (1988) Recovery following fractures of the clavicle treated conservatively. *Injury* **19**: 162–164.

17. Post, M. (1989) Current concepts in the treatment of fractures of the clavicle. *Clin. Orthop.* **245**: 89–101.

Scapula

18. Ada, J.R. & Miller, M.E. (1991) Scapular fractures. Analysis of 113 cases. *Clin. Orthop.* **269**: 174–180.

19. Goss, T.P. (1992) Fractures of the glenoid cavity. Current concepts review. *J. Bone Joint Surg.* **74A**: 299–305.

20. Wilber, M.C. & Evans, E.B. (1977) Fractures of the scapula. An analysis of forty cases and a review of the literature. *J. Bone Joint Surg.* **59A**: 358–362.

21. Zuckerman, J.D., Koval, J.K. & Coumo, F. (1993) Fractures of the scapula *Instr. Course Lect.* **42**: 271–281.

22. Ideberg, R. (1987) Unusual glenoid fractures: a report on 92 cases. *Acta Orthop. Scand.* **58**: 191–192.

23. Ideberg, R. & Myrhage, R. (1991) Fractures of the scapula. In M. Watson (ed.), *Surgical Disorders of the Shoulder.*

24. Nordqvist, A. & Petersson, C. (1992) Fracture of the body, neck or spine of the scapula. A long term follow-up study. *Clin. Orthop.* **283**: 139–144.

25. Hardegger, F.H., Simpson, L.A. & Weber, B.G. (1984) The operative treatment of scapula fractures. *J. Bone Joint Surg.* **66B**: 725–731.

26. Leung, K.S., Lam, T.P. & Poon, K.M. (1993) Operative treatment of displaced intra-articular glenoid fractures. *Injury* **24**: 324–328.

27. Leung, K.S. & Lam, T.P. (1993) Open reduction and internal fixation of ipsilateral fractures of the scapula neck and clavicle. *J. Bone Joint Surg.* **75A**: 1015–1018.

30

Four-Segment Classification of Proximal Humeral Fractures

CS Neer

INTRODUCTION

Most proximal humeral fractures respond satisfactorily to simple conservative treatment. It is only the displaced fractures and fracture dislocations that demand special treatment and judgement. However, earlier classifications were inadequate to identify these lesions. Failure to portray the specific fracture under consideration has led to confusion in the literature and difficulty in establishing guidelines for treatment. As will be emphasized, the four-segment classification is not an oversimplified arbitrary numerical system designed for easy roentgen classification, which fails to show the true anatomical problem. It was devised to correlate the roentgen appearance with the pathology for decisions on treatment of fresh fractures as well as to provide a meaningful terminology for use world wide for sorting lesions for analysis of results.

BACKGROUND

In 1944,[1] a study was made of fracture dislocations treated by removal of the humeral head. At that time there was marked confusion in the literature about proximal humeral fractures caused by the deficiencies of existing classifications.

Classification according to the level of the fracture[2,3] ('anatomical neck', 'pertuberous' or 'surgical neck') was of little assistance in depict-

ing the type of displacement because more than one level is usually involved. The fracture lines tended to occur, as Codman[4] had said, between one or all of four major fragments: the head, the greater tuberosity, the lesser tuberosity and the shaft. Fractures of both tuberosities can occur producing a lesion that is both an 'anatomical neck fracture' and a 'surgical neck fracture' (Figure 30.1). Furthermore a classification based merely on the level of the fracture permits a non-displaced lesion to be grouped with a serious displacement.

Classification based on the mechanisms of injury[5,6] was confusing. The terms 'abduction fracture' and 'adduction fracture' are misleading because the apex of angulation is usually directed anteriorly, occasionally in some other plane, but rarely in the coronal or scapular planes. Anterior angulation can produce the roentgen appearance of either an abduction fracture or an adduction fracture depending on the position of rotation of the upper humerus.

It was confusing to find opinions in the literature differ as to what constituted a fracture dislocation. Because the glenohumeral joint space is normally large enough to hold two heads, with muscle atony or detachment of one of the tuberosities, the articular surface might subluxate out of the glenoid cavity leading to such terms as 'fracture subluxation',[7,8] 'rotary dislocation'[9] and 'impacted fracture dislocation'.[5] However, these terms fail to specify specific lesions.

A classification of displaced proximal humeral fractures was needed because:

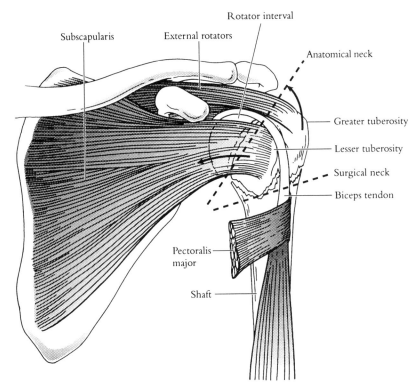

Fig. 30.1 The muscle forces acting on the four major segments of proximal humeral fractures: 1, the head; 2, the lesser tuberosity; 3, the greater tuberosity; 4, the shaft. The rotator cuff muscles tend to cause the tuberosities to separate at the rotator interval. Displacement of both tuberosities produces a lesion that is both an anatomical neck and surgical neck displacement. The pectoralis major is the major displacing force on the shaft segment.

1. These lesions are not rare. In 1970, when the first description of this classification was published, the incidence of proximal humeral fractures was 4.5%. A number of studies have shown a definite increasing incidence now estimated to be 70% as frequent as proximal femur fractures.
2. They occur in patients of all ages. The average age is about the prime of life (55 years) and not only in the elderly.
3. They are disabling.
4. Earlier classifications did not adequately identify the types of displaced fractures.

A classification was needed that would show the true pathology for proper groupings of these more complex lesions for results analysis in order to establish guidelines for optimum treatment.

Codman,[4] who actually never made a classification of proximal humeral fractures, made the important observation that in the upper humerus the fracture lines tend to occur between four fragments. My new classification was to use this fact and build upon it the effect of the muscles attaching in areas, the blood supply to the head, and the effect on the articular surface of the head (Figure 30.1). In addition optimum projections for roentgen evaluation and the results of treatment were studied. The term 'segment' was introduced to indicate zones of fracture fragments rather than a single fragment and the classification was termed the four-segment classification. As distinct anatomical patterns became evident, the classification was evolved (Figure 30.2). Knowledge about each category was based on the lesions seen on a large fracture service during a period of more than 20 years, as well as on a detailed study of 300 displaced fractures and fracture dislocations treated by closed reduction under anaesthesia or by surgery. The roentgeno-

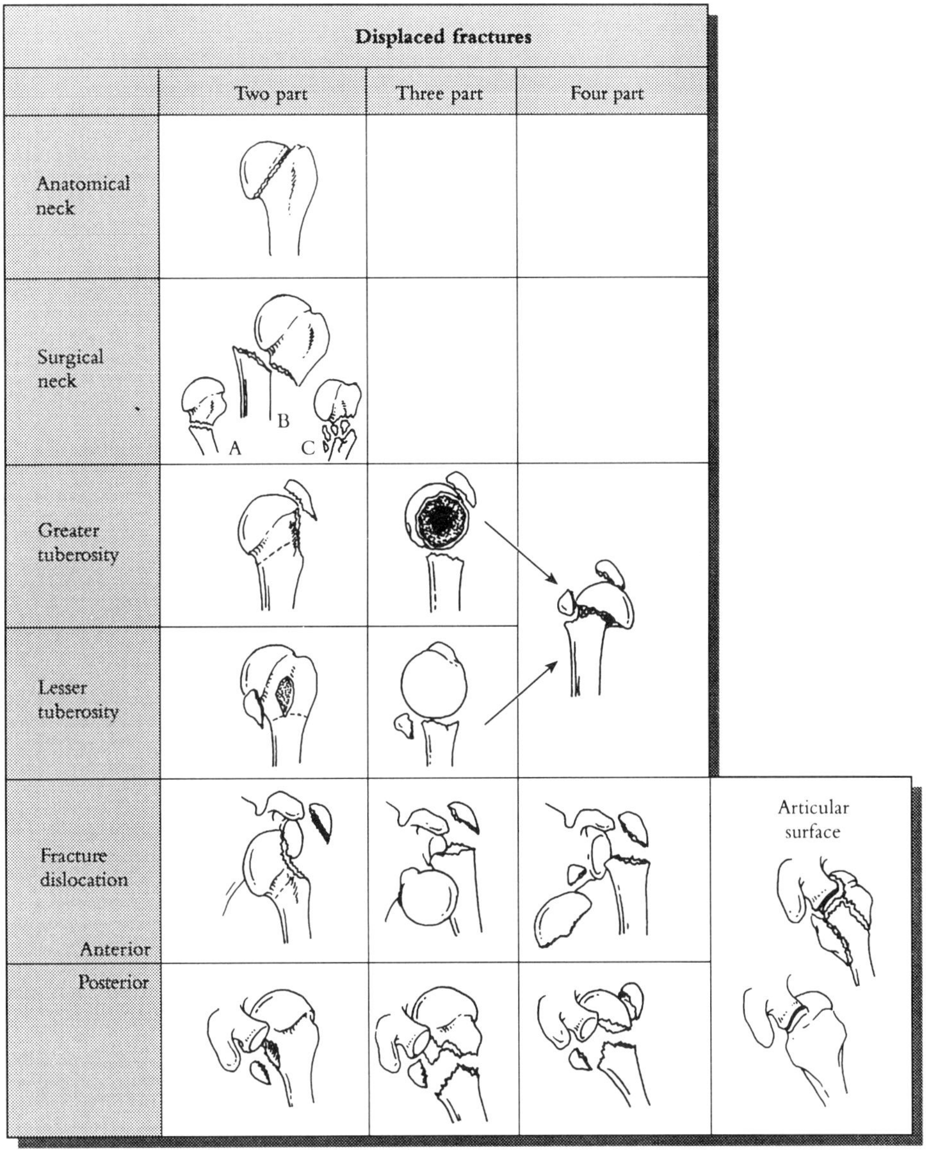

Fig. 30.2 Modification (1975)[8] of the original four-segment classification of displaced proximal humeral fractures. There is nothing to memorize but there are two requirements: (1) knowledge of the pathology and anatomy of proximal humeral fractures and (2) good roentgen evaluation (trauma series (Figure 30.3) for routine survey of displaced fractures supplemented with special views and imaging when in doubt). Non-displaced fractures (one-part) were defined for general purposes as less than 1.0 cm and angulated less than 45° (see the text). In two-part displacements, one segment is displaced. In a three-part displacement, there is always a displaced unimpacted surgical neck component that allows the articular segment to be rotated by one of the tuberosities that remains attached to it. In a four-part displacement, the head is displaced out of contact with the glenoid (i.e. dislocated) and detached from both tuberosities (Figure 30.4). Articular surface defects, crushing (impression fracture) and fragmentation (head-splitting fracture) receive special recognition.

grams, operative findings and treatment were analysed. Closed reduction had been performed in 162, open reduction in 75 (with removal of the head in five) and prosthetic replacement in 63 patients. The classification was not published for general use until 1970,[10] 26 years after the initial study began.

The original four-segment classification described in 1970[10] was simplified in 1975[11] by deleting the six subgroups designated with roman numerals. At that time it was stated that this is a concept of pathology with a continuum of displacement rather than merely a numerical, radiological classification.

It has been reiterated in the literature[11–13] and in numerous lectures that nothing need be memorized but there are two requirements: (1) a knowledge of the pathological anatomy of proximal humeral fractures and (2) good roentgen evaluation.

During the 25 years since the introduction of this classification, there have been improvements in roentgen technology. The Velpeau axillary view[14] became a part of the routine survey (trauma series; Figure 30.3). With the introduction of imaging, computed tomography (CT) has been used as a valuable supplementary study for evaluating doubtful lesions since the early 1980s. Magnetic resonance imaging (MRI) may have some practical application. Now with quality films and imaging, a knowledgeable reader can make the correct classification in the vast majority of cases. Occasionally, even the most experienced surgeon is in doubt and the final classification has to be made at surgery. In either case, the correct classification is eventually made for decisions on treatment and for meaningful results analysis.

REQUIREMENTS OF THE FOUR-SEGMENT CLASSIFICATION SYSTEM

Knowledge of the pathology

The objective is to find the four segments and determine the precise location of each. One of the patterns illustrated in Figure 30.2 is then usually obvious.

The inexperienced reader is helped by knowing that in all two-part displacements, only one segment is displaced, in all three-part displacements there is a displaced surgical neck component that allowed the head to be rotated, and in all four-part displacements, the head is dislocated out of contact with the glenoid.

The best way to develop a skill in correlating the roentgen appearance with the pathology is to re-review the films before, during and after surgery and then present the findings during fracture rounds. This should be routine for every shoulder service. There are a few radiologists who have a special interest in shoulder problems and can do well but they have the handicap of inadequate experience in the operating room.

Good roentgen evaulatuion

Oblique views of any fracture, for example the distal radius or distal femur, cause confusion. An oblique view of a proximal humeral fracture can cause confusion. The glenohumeral joint is in the scapular plane (not in the coronal or sagittal plane) and anteroposterior and lateral views of the upper humerus are made in the scapular plane (Figure 30.3). The Velpeau axillary view (Figure 30.3) is also a routine survey film. If doubt remains,

Fig. 30.3 Trauma series is made routinely when there has been an injury and the possibility of a fracture.[13] It includes (A) anteroposterior in the scapular plane, (B) lateral in the scapular plane and (C) Velpeau axillary view. The arm remains in a sling (without being moved). The anteroposterior and lateral views may be made with the patient standing or sitting, or, when multiple injuries are present, lying down. If after these studies the interpreter is in doubt, supplemental views and/or imaging are obtained (see the text). Reproduced with permission, from Neer, C.S., II (1990) *Shoulder Reconstruction*, 1st edn, p. 17, Philadelphia: W.B. Saunders.

(A)

(B)

(C)

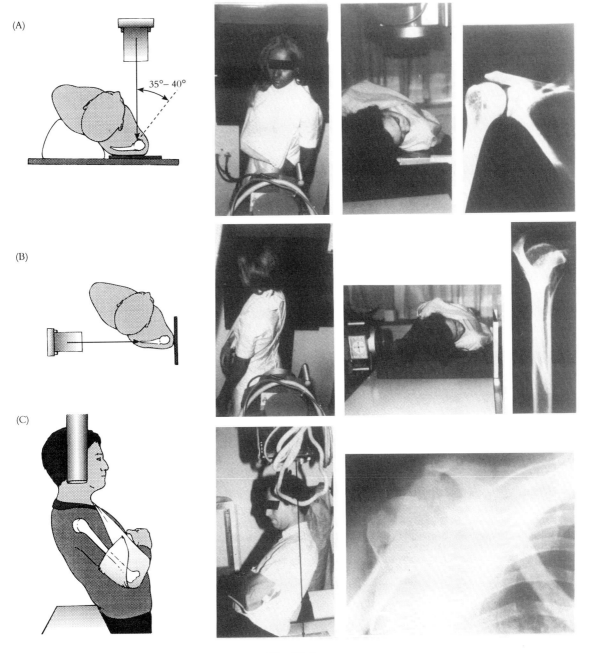

Fig. 30.3.

supplemental views (transthoracic or rotational), laminograms, or CT scans can be obtained. MRI has not been helpful enough to date to be used very often.

As with other fractures, one cannot accept films that cut off part of the pathology. The emergency room or fracture surgeon must strive to obtain regular X-ray technicians that are experienced with these views in injured patients.

APPRAISAL AND TREATMENT

Consider now some special points for each category regarding incidence, anatomical defect, details of roentgen classification and my preferred treatment when the patient is healthy and well-motivated.

One-part (minimal displacement)

Approximately 80% of upper humeral fractures are of this type. Thornton Brown, the editor of the first article on the four-segment classification,[10] thought it was important to specify the exact limits of displacement. I agreed and this group was arbitrarily defined as 'all fractures, regardless of the level or number of fracture lines, in which no segment is displaced more than 1.0 cm or angulated more than 45°'.

These lesions present similar problems in management. The fragments are usually held together by soft tissue or impacted, permitting early functional exercises. Occasionally, the fracture is disimpacted so false motion occurs. It is important to test for false motion as a guide to when exercises can be begun and, if present, the shoulder immobilized in a sling and swathe until the head and shaft rotate as one before exercises are begun.

In 1983 the authors of the AO Classification[15] objected to this category because, although they thought that it was reasonable to allow this amount of displacement, they thought that it was not well enough documented for it to be the standard for allowable deformity, since 'we have no information that ensures that less than 1.0 mm separation or 45 degrees angulation assures vascu-

lar continuity between fragments'. It was never intended that this definition of minimal displacement (1.0 cm and 45°) would guarantee a satisfactory result without avascular necrosis of the head. As has been shown in many lectures and in the literature,[10] avascular necrosis of the head and post-traumatic arthritis of the glenohumeral joint can occur in minimally displaced, one-part fractures.

There is a continuum of displacement and the specific limit of 1.0 cm and 45° was intended only as a practical guide for classification but not as a guarantee that the result of all of the lesions in this category would be good. Actually, it was deemed important to stress that unless these fractures are carefully treated with a well-directed exercise programme for a surprisingly long period of time, the result will be suboptimal and often very disappointing. Even then, late avascular necrosis occasionally occurs.

Two-part head (anatomical neck) displacement

Displacement of the head with intact tuberosities is a rare lesion. A good anteroposterior film is essential because this lesion can be missed with oblique views. At times, supplemental views made with the humerus in several positions of rotation are needed to show the extent of the displacement.

There is no extensive experience with the results of treatment but there appears to be a high incidence of avascular necrosis of the head. Furthermore, if this lesion is allowed to remain unreduced, a painful malunion may occur. To date, open reduction and internal fixation has usually been advised rather than immediate prosthetic replacement.

Two-part shaft (surgical neck) displacement

Displacement of the shaft (surgical neck displacement) is common and occurs in patients of all ages. Epiphyseal fractures are of this category. The pectoralis major is the deforming muscle and acts to pull the shaft forward and medially (Figure

30.1). The rotator cuff is intact and the tuberosities are not displaced so the proximal segments tend to be held in neutral rotation. It is helpful to recognize three clinical types: impacted, unimpacted and comminuted.

Impacted

There is more than 45° angulation. The apex is usually anterior. The periosteum is intact on the opposite side from the apex of angulation, i.e. usually on the posterior side. If union occurs in this position, elevation of the shoulder will be permanently limited in proportion to the amount of angulation and the greater tuberosity may impinge on the acromion, Therefore, I prefer to treat active patients by closed reduction. The periosteal sleeve affords sufficient stability so that the fracture may be disimpacted with traction and the angulation corrected by full elevation in the plane of the angulation. Fluoroscopic control with the image intensifier may be helpful. After alignment is corrected, the arm is immobilized for about 3 or 4 weeks (until the head and shaft rotate together). This is usually accomplished with a stockinette sling and an elastic bandage swathe to hold the arm in the Velpeau position (across the chest). An abduction cast puts tension on the pectoralis major and may cause the fragments to displace; however, in a few instances it has seemed to be more effective. A hanging cast allows angulation to recur, may distract the fracture and is not used.

Persistent symptoms due to a malunion of this type of fracture can usually be relieved satisfactorily with an anterior acromioplasty avoiding an osteotomy of the upper humerus.

Unimpacted

The pectoralis major acts to displace the shaft anteromedially and the head tends to be held in neutral rotation because the tuberosities are intact. The sharp calcar may damage the axillary artery or brachial plexus. Treatment may follow one of three courses.

1. Closed reduction may be obtained and is stable. Immobilization is then as after closed reduction of an impacted fracture as discussed above. Care is taken to defer exercises until the head moves with the shaft because non-union can occur.
2. Closed reduction can be obtained but is unstable and reduction cannot be maintained. Percutaneous pin fixation is then used, directing a stiff threaded pin through the deltopectoral interval and anterior shaft into the head. The sling and swathe is then applied with the arm in the Velpeau position. The pin is removed in about 3 weeks, before starting exercises.
3. Closed reduction may be unsuccessful. Interposition of soft tissue must be suspected. There are two types of interposition: deltoid muscle or long head of biceps and the subscapularis. Open reduction is required. In this case the fracture can be internally fixed.

Comminuted

Fragmentation of the upper shaft is present. The pectoralis major may displace some fragments anteromedially. Twist displacement of the fragments is usually present because the arm has been placed in a sling with the distal fragments internally rotated while the head is held in neutral rotation by the intact rotator cuff. A spica cast that holds the arm in neutral rotation, forward flexion and near the side is usually preferred. It is unnecessary to attempt internal fixation.

Two-part greater tuberosity displacement

There are three distinct facets for insertion of the supraspinatus, infraspinatus, and teres minor. This segment is usually fragmented and any, one, or all of these sites of tendon attachment may be retracted. The displaced fragment is associated with a tear of the rotator cuff and covers a portion of the articular surface of the head. Open reduction through a deltoid-splitting approach is advised and internal fixation with non-absorbable sutures along with repair of the cuff defect.

Three-part displacements

It is evident from Figure 30.2 that a displaced surgical neck component is present in every type of three-part displacement. One tuberosity remains attached to the head to give it blood supply, so careful open reduction through a deltopectoral approach and internal fixation is generally advised. In three-part greater tuberosity displacements the blood supply to the head is more tenuous; and, in this type, when at surgery the attachments to the head are in doubt and in the elderly, immediate prosthetic replacement seems preferable. This agrees with the experience of Tanner & Cofield.[16] I have seen some three-part greater tuberosity displacements that seemed initially to have been treated satisfactorily with open reduction and internal fixation that went on after 8 or 10 years to develop painful post-traumatic arthritis requiring a prosthesis.

Four-part displacement

In the original article on the four-segment classification, all four-part lesions were placed in 'Group VI: fracture dislocations'. This was because the head is displaced out of contact with the glenoid in every type of four-part displacement (Figures 30.2 and 30.4). The head may be anterior, lateral, posterior or inferior but it must be detached from both tuberosities to qualify as a four-part displacement (Figures 30.2 and 30.4). Since the articular segment is detached, the incidence of avascular necrosis of the head is high. Prosthetic replacement of the head with reconstruction of the tuberosities and cuff is advised.

In the initial report (1970) on prosthetic replacement for these lesions,[17] the results in 43 of 67 could be evaluated. The typical result was 'satisfactory but imperfect and many months were required for maximum recovery'. There have been tremendous improvements in the technique of humeral head replacement for four-part lesions[13] (Figure 30.5). The typical result in the report in 1988[18] was 'excellent' (near normal). Of 61, 51 were rated excellent, nine satisfactory and only one unsatisfactory. The extended deltopectoral approach, anchoring the prosthesis securely,

usually with cement, to hold it at the proper height to retain the normal length of the humerus, anchoring the tuberosities securely under the head of the prosthesis with non-absorbable suture, retaining all fragments to ensure bone union of the tuberosities, (Figure 30.5), early passive motion to recover the passive motion quickly, and a directed self-assisted exercise programme have all been important factors in the excellent results that are now achieved with this procedure.[13]

Some surgeons in the AO organization advise open reduction and internal fixation for 'valgus, impacted four-part fractures' believing that the prognosis is better than for other four-part lesions. In my experience, if the lesion under discussion is truly a four-part displacement (articular segment out of contact with the glenoid and detached from both tuberosities), there is no apparent difference in the incidence of necrosis of the head and post-traumatic arthritis following open reduction regardless of whether the head had been displaced laterally, anteriorly or posteriorly (Figure 30.4). Of course, if in the lesion under discussion the amount of displacement of the impacted head is insufficient to require disimpaction, the prognosis for survival of the head would be better. However, I believe such a lesion, without significant displacement of the articular segment, should not have been classified as a four-part displacement.

In some four-part lesions the tuberosities remain together while the detached head is dislocated out from under them (Figure 30.4). These, in my opinion, should be classified as four-part displacements because they conform to the definition given above and in Figure 30.2 in that the articular segment is displaced out of contact with the glenoid and detached from both tuberosities.

Fracture dislocations

All four-part displacements are fracture dislocations because the articular segment is dislocated and out of contact with the glenoid. Since there is bone extruded outside the joint, there is a greater risk of heterotopic bone formation and greater risk of injury to nerves and vessels.

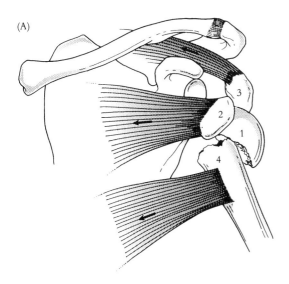

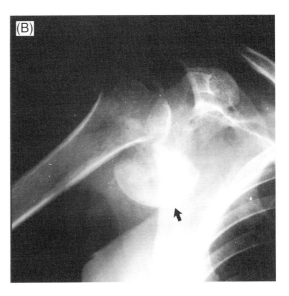

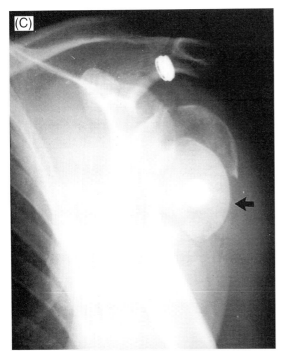

Fig. 30.4 Illustration of four-part displacements. In all of these lesions the articular segment (arrow) is dislocated out of contact with the glenoid and is separated from both tuberosities. The tuberosities may be retracted or may be held together by the soft tissue. The head may be anterior, lateral or posterior. (A) Drawing of a lateral four-part fracture dislocation showing the four segments. The tuberosity segments remain in contact in this illustration. (B) Anteroposterior view of an anterior four-part fracture dislocation in which the tuberosity segments remain in contact. (C) Anteroposterior view of a posterior four-part fracture dislocation in which the tuberosity segments are moderately retracted.

Articular surface defects

Crushing (impression fracture) and comminuted (head-splitting fracture) lesions of the head occur with at least some of the articular cartilage being displaced outside of the joint space.

Impression fractures pose a diagnostic pitfall that can be eliminated if the axillary view (Figure 30.3) is included as one of the routine initial survey films. Depending on the size of the head defect and the age of the lesion, treatment is by closed reduction, lesser tuberosity transfer to the head defect or a prosthesis.[13]

Head-splitting fractures are produced by a violent central impact that shatters the articular surface. For a healthy well-motivated patient a prosthesis is advised.

(A)

(B)

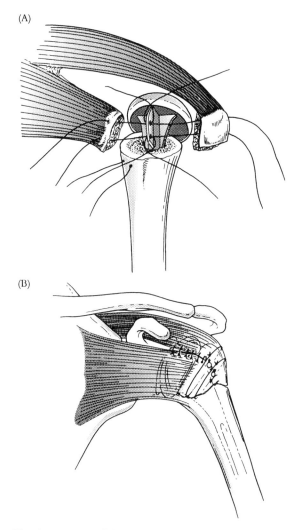

Fig. 30.5 Two of the many important steps accounting for why the great improvement in the results of prosthetic replacement of the humeral head with reconstruction of the tuberosities and repair of the rotator cuff for four-part displacements.[10,14] (A) After testing with a trial prosthesis to select the largest prosthetic head that will permit closure of the tuberosities and cuff and determining the proper version and height of the head, the prosthesis is securely anchored in the shaft (usually with acrylic cement) and the tuberosities are then anchored to the prosthesis and shaft. (B) Depicting final closure with the tuberosities secured beneath the head (to avoid detachment or impingement). The rotator cuff has been repaired. The long head of biceps is intact. Preservation of the origin of the deltoid muscle and earlier passive motion followed by a carefully directed rehabilitation programme are also of key importance for optimum results (see the text).

COMMENTARY

Now, after 25 years, this classification continues to be the method generally used all over the world. In 1987,[19] the original description of the four-segment classification[10] was designated a classic, and republished in its entirety by one of the leading orthopaedic journals in America.

In 1993, an editorial, written by a layman (not a physician)[20] and based on two confusing articles,[21,22] made a harsh surprise attack on the four-segment classification. Both studies used, for the most part, inexperienced interpreters and poor-quality films (not the present-day recommended roentgen routines and supplemental studies). The one experienced interpreter in each study classified the lesions with remarkably good reproducibility, especially considering the poor quality of the radiological material. A few issues later, the Board of Trustees of the journal that had published this editorial published a statement in a prominent place in the journal indicating that the deputy editor who wrote the editorial had expressed his personal views and not those of the journal.[23]

REFERENCES

1. Neer, C.S., II, Brown, T.H. & McLaughlin, H.L. (1953) Fracture of the neck of the humerus with dislocation of the head fragment. *Am. J. Surg.* **85**: 252–258.

2. Kocher, T. (1896) *Beitrage zur Kenntniss Einiger Praktisch Wichtiger Fracturen Formen.* Basel and Leipsig; Carl Sollman.

3. Böhler, L. (1929) Die Behandlung von Verren Kungsbruschen der Schulter. *Dtsch Z Chir.* **219**: 238–245.

4. Codman, E.A. (1934) *The Shoulder, Rupture of the Supraspinatus Tendon and Other Lesions in or about the Subacromial Bursa.* Boston, Privately Printed.

5. Watson-Jones, R. (1955) *Fractures and Joint Injuries*, 4th edn, vol. 2, pp. 473–476. Baltimore: Williams and Wilkins.

6. Dehne, E. (1945) Fractures of the upper end of the humerus. A classification based on the etiology of trauma. *Surg. Clin. North Am.* **25**: 28–47.

7. Fairbank, T.J. (1948) Fracture subluxations of the shoulder. *J. Bone Joint Surg.* **30B**: 454–460.

8. Thompson, F.R. & Winant, E.M. (1950) Unusual

fracture subluxations of the shoulder joint. *J. Bone Joint Surg.* **32A:** 575–582.

9. Silfverskiöld, N. On the treatment of fracture-dislocations of the shoulder joint with special reference to the capability of the head fragment, disconnected from capsule and periostium, to enter into bony union.

10. Neer, C.S., II (1970) Displaced proximal humeral fractures. Part I, classification and evaluation. *J. Bone Joint Surg.* **52A:** 1077–1089.

11. Neer, C.S., II (1975) Four-segment classification of displaced proximal humeral fractures. *Instr. Course Lect.* **24:** 160–168.

12. Neer, C.S., II (1984) Fractures about the shoulder. In C.A. Rockwood, Jr. and D.P. Green (eds), *Fractures in Adults*, 2nd edn, pp. 675–707. Philadelphia: J.B. Lippincott.

13. Neer, C.S., II (1990) *Shoulder Reconstruction*, 1st edn, pp. 363–403. Philadelphia: W.B. Saunders.

14. Bloom, M.H. & Obata, W. (1967) Diagnosis of posterior dislocation of the shoulder with use of Velpeau axillary and angle-up roentgenographic views. *J. Bone Joint Surg.* **49A:** 943–949.

15. Jakob, R.P., Kristiansen, T., Mayo, K., Ganz, R. & Müller, M.E. (1984) Classification and aspects of treatment of fractures of the proximal humerus. In J.E. Bateman & R.P. Welsh (eds), *Surgery of the Shoulder*, pp. 330–343. Philadelphia: B.C. Decker.

16. Tanner, M.W. & Cofield, R.H. (1983) Prosthetic arthroplasty for fractures and fracture-dislocations of the proximal humerus. *Clin. Orthop.* **179:** 116.

17. Neer, C.S., II (1970) Displaced proximal humeral fractures. Part II. Treatment of three-part and four-part displacement. *J. Bone Joint Surg.* **51A:** 1090–1103.

18. Neer, C.S., II & McIlveen, S.J. (1988) Replacement de la tete humerale avec reconstruction des tuberosities et de la coiffe dan les fractures deplacees. Resultats actuels et techniques. *Rev. Chir. Orthop. Suppl. II* **74:** 31.

19. Neer, C.S. II (1987) Displaced proximal humeral fractures: Part I. Classification and evaluation. (Reprinted with permission *J. Bone Joint Surg.* **52A:** 1077, 1970.) *Clin. Orthop.* **223:** 3–10.

20. Burstein, A.H. (1993) Editorial. Fracture classification systems: do they work and are they useful? *J. Bone Joint Surg.* **75A:** 1743–1744.

21. Sidor, M.L., Zuckerman, J.D., Lyon, T., Koval, K., Cuomo, F. & Schoenberg, N. (1993) The Neer classification system for proximal humeral fractures. *J. Bone Joint Surg.* **75A:** 1745–1750.

22. Siebenrock, K.A. and Gerber, C. (1993) The reproducibility of classification of fractures of the proximal end of the humerus. *J. Bone Joint Surg.* **75A:** 1751–1755.

23. Cooper, R.R. (1994) Statement by the Board of Trustees of the Journal of Bone and Joint Surgery. Reginald R. Cooper, Chairman, Board of Trustees. *J. Bone Joint Surg.* **76A:** 639.

31

Shoulder Rehabilitation

JA Bruguera and P Hourston

INTRODUCTION

The shoulder is the most mobile joint in the body. Motion is achieved from the combined movement of the glenohumeral joint and scapulothoracic region mainly, but with contributions from the acromioclavicular and sternoclavicular joints. Co-ordination of the muscular activity around the shoulder girdle is essential not only for movement but for stability of the joint. Capsule and ligaments act as passive restraints and contribute also to the stability and motion. Any disturbance in one or more of those anatomical structures will result in abnormal movements with pain, stiffness, instability, etc. The end result is inability of the shoulder to place the arm in different positions in space and to maintain them despite different forces acting on the arm at that precise moment.

Rehabilitation as a main treatment or in combination with any surgical technique aims to restore normality to the shoulder joint. This is achieved by addressing several aspects such as range of motion, strength, stability and pain control.

Good understanding and co-ordination between physiotherapist, patient and surgeon are essential in order to achieve maximum rehabilitation of the patient. A detailed assessment of the patient's condition is essential to determine the exact cause of the problem and to achieve the most desirable outcome. Every patient is different and the rehabilitation programme has to be tailored according to his or her needs. Different goals are established for different patients. A continued assessment is carried out throughout the whole

rehabilitation period and adjustments to the programme are made according to the findings.

DEFINITIONS

There are several terms used in daily practice in rehabilitation. It is important to understand the meaning of them in order to achieve smooth communication among surgeon, physiotherapist and patient. We will define them briefly.

Passive movements: the shoulder joint (glenohumeral or scapulothoracic joint) is moved by a physiotherapist or a continuous passive movement (CPM) machine, with no muscular activity from the patient. CPM machines are expensive and rely upon availability of the machine and patient co-operation before treatment is effective. However, in selected patients, the use of a CPM machine is beneficial and will release the therapist to perform other duties. Problems arising during manual passive movements performed by the therapist can be detected at the time of treatment and adjustments made accordingly during the delicate time of the immediate postoperative period.

Passive movements are designed to maintain, improve and/or regain motion. Passive movements are recommended in the postoperative period where maintaining the motion of the joint without disturbing the healing process is crucial. According to Neer,[1] motion must be re-established before the maturation of adhesions to prevent failure of the procedure. This rehabilitation period could start immediately after surgery, but depends on several factors such as the type of the operation, level of pain, staff or machines available, etc.

Active exercises: shoulder motion is achieved directly by the patient by contracting the muscles around the shoulder girdle. The aims are to increase/maintain range of movement, strength and/or stability.

Passive–active or **active-assisted exercises:** these are anatomical movements performed by the patient in conjunction with the therapist or assisted by other means, e.g. pulleys and sticks, using, in general, the opposite upper limb. During the period of rehabilitation this is a transitional phase between fully passive and active exercises.

Isotonic exercises: where muscle contracts against a constant resistance throughout the entire range of motion.[2]

Isometric exercises: where muscle contracts with no change in muscle length and no movement of the joint. They involve maximal force with no velocity.[2]

Isokinetic exercises: where muscle contracts at a constant velocity throughout the full range of motion.[2]

Another two terms frequently used in rehabilitation are **concentric** and **eccentric** contraction. In concentric muscle contraction there is movement in the direction of the contraction. In eccentric muscle contraction an external force causes movement opposite to the direction of muscle contraction. The muscle fibres are lengthened while the muscle develops tension.

STRETCHING EXERCISES

These exercises can be passive, active or passive-active. Stretching exercises are directed to improve the range of motion, concentrating the movement at its end of range. In the immediate postoperative period, they are aimed to avoid the adhesions of a normal healing process. During this period, exercises should be passive until the healing period is over, although the stretching programme can be progressed to passive-assisted or active.

Other indications for stretching exercises are in those cases where there is some residual stiffness of the shoulder with loss of few degrees of movement such as post-traumatic stiffness, chronic impingement syndrome, wrist fractures, etc.

Stretching exercises are also important before the operation in order to maintain the maximum range of movement while the patient is awaiting surgery.

The most common pieces of equipment used are pulley and sticks, but furniture, towels, etc. from around the house can be used as we will comment on below. The main advantage of these are that they are inexpensive, and patients can easily continue with a home exercise programme. Patients do need a reasonable range of movement and strength in the contralateral limb in order to be able to use active-assisted stretching techniques involving, for example, sticks or pulleys.

Hydrotherapy is also a very useful technique as the buoyancy and warmth of the water assists the patient to achieve optimum stretching.

There are several types of stretching exercises.

1. Forward flexion can be achieved with the patient lying supine with hands clasped, and lifting the arm up and over the head and holding it at the end of its range. Using this position, gravity assists the patient to stretch the joint a little bit further. Relaxation of the patient and adequate breathing control are very important. Forward flexion stretching can also be obtained with the patient standing with the arm elevated and leaning against a wall or with the patient sitting and the upper limb leaning against a table (Figure 31.1).
2. External rotation can be improved using a stick on the opposite side and pushing it against the hand on the affected side. If the patient is unable to use the 'normal' side, the affected side can be stretched against a door frame with the elbow in 90° of flexion (Figure 31.2).
3. Internal rotation can be improved by placing clasped hands behind the back and attempting to bring the affected limb further upwards using the unaffected hand. Another alternative is for the patient to grasp a towel behind his or her back with the affected limb and pull with the unaffected limb overhead (Figure 31.3).

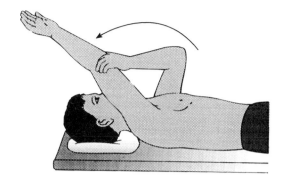

Fig. 31.1 Stretching in forward flexion.

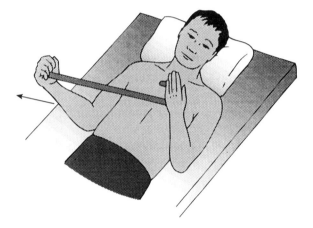

Fig. 31.2 Stretching in external rotation using a stick.

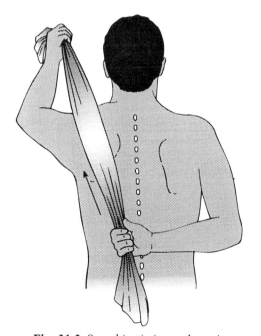

Fig. 31.3 Stretching in internal rotation.

4. Extension is an essential movement to recover particularly if internal rotation is reduced, and attention should be paid to this during the rehabilitation period. A simple exercise is to place both hands behind the body and with the help of a stick try to stretch the affected side.

STRENGTHENING EXERCISES

These are always active and are performed by patients at home or under physiotherapy supervision. Elastic bands with different strengths, springs and weights can be used. Proprioceptive neuromuscular facilitation (PNF) and hydrotherapy are two specialist techniques which can prove very effective. Special equipment for isotonic, isokinetic and isometric exercises as defined previously can be used during a strengthening rehabilitation therapy. The programme has to address the patient's needs, therefore constant assessment of the area of the weakness and rehabilitation tailored to this is essential.

Strengthening exercises can be incorporated into a rehabilitation programme at very different stages depending on the pathology involved, e.g. the last step in rotator cuff repair but one of the middle steps following a shoulder replacement.

STABILIZING EXERCISES

Muscle co-ordination and proprioception are important to prevent instability. There are groups of patients where muscle incoordination and reduced proprioception produce shoulder instability. Within this group of patients are the voluntary habitual dislocators, but there is another group where the muscle imbalance and diminished proprioception is not voluntary. In this group, quite often the alteration is triggered by a direct trauma to the shoulder or by psychological reactions. In all these patients, operative solutions will fail leaving the patient and the surgeon in a difficult situation. The only way to improve stability and proprioception within the shoulders of these patients is by an intensive rehabilitation programme involving muscle re-education, proprioceptive exercises, biofeedback and general cuff strengthening. These patients have lost the awareness of how their shoulder functions, therefore careful retraining and explanation throughout the rehabilitation are essential in order to obtain an understanding of the problem and the desired goal. Strapping and taping, brushing, icing and stroking can all aid proprioception, and are used frequently. The use of a mirror can also help to re-educate the patient. After a period of 3 months most of these patients regain normal muscle control, stability and proprioception. It is important that the patient continues with a general cuff-strengthening programme.

PAIN CONTROL

Pain can be due to a chronic or an acute process or arise from a postoperation period. Pain is a substantial factor in shoulder rehabilitation. It is important to record the level of pain and any changes in intensity, duration or cause relation during the programme. It cannot be measured objectively but there are several methods to establish its level, from a visual analogue scale, where the patient chooses the level according to his or her pain, to an evaluation of the analgesic level (Table 31.1).

Pain must be controlled in order to progress with the rehabilitation programme and achieve restoration of function. There are different methods that can be used to control pain in conjunction with rehabilitation.[3] The most commonly used are as follows.

1. **Transcutaneous electrical nerve stimulation (TENS).** There are two main groups: sensory stimulators and neuromuscular stimulators. The first ones are used in the treatment of pain and the second have the ability to contract muscle. Most of the TENS machines are portable, so patients can easily take them home. Different parameters, such as rate, intensity, pulse and frequency can be adjusted to control pain to suit patient needs.

2. **Cryotherapy.** Cold treatment is indicated when there is acute inflammation such as bursitis or tendinitis, in acute trauma haematoma formation or in the immediate post-operative period. Cold intolerance, peripheral vascular disease or Raynaud's syndrome are clear contraindications to this therapy. The basic principles upon which pain is controlled are vasoconstriction and decrease in neural conduction. There are several methods of giving cold treatments, but the most commonly used are ice packs, baths, sprays and cryocuffs.

3. **Heat packs.** They could be dry or wet. The main aim is to make the tissues more supple and relaxed before manipulation or stretching exercises. Because they increase vasodilatation and metabolic activity, they are contraindicated in acute trauma or the immediate post-operative period.

4. **Ultrasound.** This is a useful tool in rehabilitation. Its indications are pain relief, reduction of muscle spasm and inflammation and increased extensibility of connective tissue.[4] It is a technique that uses high-frequency acoustic energy and works by producing therapeutic effects of deep heat and vibration. If the heat effect is not required, pulsed ultrasound (PU) can be used. Two main effects of PU are dissipation of fluid and break up of scar tissue. Ultrasound should not be used to treat ischaemic or anaesthetized areas, in the first instance because of the lack of adequate blood flow, which helps disperse the heat effect, and in the

Table 31.1. Analgesic levels

Level	Analgesic requirement
1	Painkillers taken occasionally
2	Painkillers taken regularly
3	Association of regular painkiller with occasional NSAID
4	Regular NSAID in combination or not with a painkiller
5	Opioids

NSAID, non-steroid anti-inflammatory drug.

second because the patient has no perception of intensity or damage.

5. **Acupuncture/acupressure/auriculotherapy.** These techniques are based on stimulation of several points in the skin by means of needles, fingers or electrical stimulators in order to get adequate pain control.
6. **Interscalene block.** This is an invasive technique generally performed by anaesthetists. It can be carried out as a part of the operative anaesthetic procedure to control pain after the operation, e.g. shoulder replacement, and to help with the immediate rehabilitation programme. A catheter is left *in situ* and a continuous infusion pump is used for medium-term pain control in order to carry out shoulder rehabilitation in situations that otherwise would be painful and difficult for the patient.

PARAMETERS AND MEASUREMENT

Usually motion and strength are the most common parameters subjected to measurements around the shoulder. Their continuous reassessment by measurement devices is essential throughout the rehabilitation programme in order to quantify objectively a patient's achievements. Measurements should be done before, during and after the rehabilitation period. Normally, they are part of a scoring system giving an indication of the progress and outcomes. For instance, if the aim is to improve motion and after several sessions the range of movements has not improved, the patient will have to be reassessed to find out the cause.

Motion

Motion, both active and passive, can be measured by different techniques. From the clinical and practical point of view, a goniometer is used to determine the range of motion in the shoulder. Four parameters essential in assessing motion are: forward flexion or humeral elevation, abduction,

external rotation and internal rotation.[5] Forward flexion and abduction are measured as a continuum glenohumeral and scapulothoracic movement. It is important, however, to recognize any problem arising from those areas before or during the rehabilitation.

As well as the four ranges mentioned above, particular attention should also be paid to extension and adduction with certain patients. For example, during rehabilitation of a patient after shoulder replacement, extension and internal rotation are important. In the case of a patient with instability, the amount of external rotation in 90° of abduction after the surgery is important.

From the laboratory point of view, cinematic or optical techniques can be used.[6] However, they are expensive and time consuming. In addition, the markers on the skin could be misleading and bone markers are not accepted by patients. In the case of the shoulder, although it is possible to measure global displacement, it is very difficult to disclose the movements arising from the glenohumeral, scapulothoracic, acromioclavicular or sternoclavicular joints individually.

Strength

Co-ordination of muscles around the shoulder girdle is important, as muscle power provides strength and stability. Strength can be assessed subjectively or objectively.[7] Subjective clinical assessment is performed using a grading scale from 0 to 5 (Table 31.2).

This assessment has its limitations because of an ordinal base scale, interobserver errors and static testing conditions. During the rehabilitation programme it is useful to obtain objective data from

Table 31.2. Scale used for clinical assessment

Scale	Assessment
0	No muscular contraction
1	Muscular contraction but no limb movement
2	Active movements but not against gravity
3	Active movements against gravity but not resistance
4	Active movements against gravity and resistance
5	Normal

different muscle groups. Isokinetic testing provides the therapist with the possibility of objectively documenting muscular performance in a way that is both safe and reliable using either isolated or combined movement patterns. This objectivity ensures assessment, progression or regression of the patient.[8]

Isokinetic parameters include peak torque and torque acceleration energy. Peak torque is a measure of force or muscle strength and torque acceleration energy is a measure of work or muscle power.

Portable isometric dynamometers are used quite often during the rehabilitation assessment. According to Gerber[9] there is no proven superiority of isokinetic over isometric testing. In addition isometric dynamometers are smaller and cheaper.

SCORE SYSTEMS

There are several scoring systems designed to evaluate the shoulder. Most of them are designed to study the outcomes after conservative or surgical treatments. They incorporate some of the tools and parameters available, as already described in this chapter, to evaluate patients. So far none of the scoring systems are ideal. For instance, some of the scores are good for instability but not for the evaluation of a shoulder replacement. Ideally a scoring system should be easy to use and reproducible, with no interobserver errors. Complicated forms and expensive pieces of equipment should not be used. It should indicate, according to the score, the possibility of a certain pathology. Finally, the system should be flexible to be used before, during and after the treatment to provide not only the final result for a defined pathology and treatment but to evaluate the progress of the patient during the rehabilitation programme. We will describe briefly the most common scoring systems actually used.

1. **The simple shoulder test (SST).** This test was developed at the University of Washington by Matsen et al.[5] It is a questionnaire where the patient has to answer Yes or No to

12 practical questions about daily activities. It explores motion, strength, stability and pain. The authors claim 100% reproducibility in normal subjects. They conclude that the test is quick, practical and an inexpensive method for assessing patients.

2. **Rowe's score.** Rowe et al[10] published in 1978 the long-term results following Bankart operation using a rating sheet system. The score assesses stability, motion, function and pain but it does not test strength. This system evaluates only postoperative results in patients with instability but, obviously, it cannot be used to assess other shoulder pathologies.

3. **The Walch–Duplay Score**[11] is used to assess patients with shoulder instability. It scores motion, pain, stability and daily activities. Similarly to the Rowe score, it only can be used to evaluate patients with instability after a surgical procedure.

4. **The American Shoulder and Elbow Surgeons Shoulder Evaluation (ASES)**[12] evaluates pain, motion, strength, stability and function. Motion is assessed with the patient sitting and supine. Strength of the deltoid muscle and external and internal rotations are measured. This system is rather complicated and does not give a proper score of the patients subjected to this evaluation.[9]

5. **University of California at Los Angeles shoulder rating scale (UCLA).**[13] This scoring system considers pain, function, motion and patient satisfaction. Forward flexion is the only range in which motion and strength are evaluated. Strength is assessed by manual muscle testing, assigning degrees from 5 to 0. This score system is quite comprehensive but, like the Rowe and Walch–Duplay systems, it cannot be used to assess patients before surgery, in this case, because it is not possible to assess patient satisfaction at that stage.

6. **Constant–Murley score.**[14] This method was designed to evaluate shoulders from a subjective and objective point of view. The subjective assessment involves evaluation of pain and ability to perform the activities of daily living. The objective assessment evaluates strength and motion in different positions. Strength is

measured by a dynamometer with the arm in abduction up to a maximum of 90°. The method is, in theory, completely independent of the pathology of the shoulder. It was designed as a simple clinical method of shoulder evaluation. The equipment required is simple if a dynamometer is used, but could be more expensive if a microprocessor-controlled isometric muscular strength analyser is used. The method can be used to evaluate a patient's rehabilitation progress before and after surgery and it is reproducible. However, it may not be ideal to evaluate patients with shoulder instability. The Constant score is quite widely used in Europe.

HOW WE DO IT IN READING

In our unit, patients are assessed in the shoulder clinic by doctors and a physiotherapist. Once the diagnosis is made and if a patient needs a rehabilitation programme, this is discussed between doctors and physiotherapist and the plan explained to the patient. Although every case is different, we will give some guidelines of the protocols and rehabilitation programmes followed in Reading for the most common pathologies.

Frozen shoulder: manipulation under anaesthesia

After the manipulation, physiotherapy starts immediately in the recovery room. Active exercises, pendular exercises and passive stretches at least three times a day are encouraged. No sling is provided and the patient is warned about the pain he or she may experience through the first week.

Stability

We divide these patients into two major groups.

Those with multidirectional instability

Conservative treatment involves an intense programme of muscle re-education. On examination

these patients are often found to have one group of muscles that are hyperactive and another that are weak, leading to a gross muscle imbalance. Rehabilitation aims to restore normal balance of these muscle groups. A detailed and careful assessment is essential before the start of treatment in order to establish which muscles need retraining. Careful explanation, progressive active exercises, biofeedback training and proprioceptive exercises aid rehabilitation with this group. Treatment time varies from a few sessions as outpatients to several weeks of inpatient therapy.

Once patients have been re-educated, they are discharged with strengthening exercises to maintain their achievements. Some patients continue to have symptoms due to laxity despite the abolition of the voluntary component. On careful selection, some of these will undergo surgery, e.g. open capsular shift procedures or arthroscopic laser-assisted capsular shift (LACS). The rehabilitation programme for patients after capsular shift involves 6 weeks in a sling, 3 of those in a body belt. Pendular exercises begin at 3 weeks, progressing to active at 6 and strengthening thereafter. External rotation coupled with abduction are limited for the first 6 weeks. Patients who have undergone LACS also spend 3 weeks in a sling with no body belt. Pendular exercises start on day 1 and last for a period of 3 weeks. Active exercises and progressive strengthening exercises are carried out thereafter.

Those with unidirectional instability

The programme is the same as for patients undergoing open capsular shift with or without Bankart repair. Particular attention is required in strengthening of the internal rotators after 6 weeks.

Rotator cuff tears

Once the diagnosis is made, a preoperative rehabilitation programme starts while the patient is waiting for surgery. It is designed to maintain or improve the range of movement and to strengthen the remaining elements of the rotator cuff. Stretching and isometric exercises are done by the patient, normally at home, in order to obtain maximum benefit from the surgical procedure. The aim is to regain a full range of passive motion before the operation. This can be likened to flexor tendon surgery; it is pointless to repair a tendon to work on a stiff joint. In our experience a large number of patients improve their pain just with the preoperative exercises.

The postoperative regime for this operation varies according to the state of repair of the soft tissue found at surgery. At the end of the operation the surgeon should write some guidelines for the rehabilitation period. Aeroplane and abduction splints are not routinely used. A sling is used for a total of 6 weeks.

One to three weeks

Passive flexion and extension are started, as pain allows, the following morning after the operation. Attention is paid to the rest of the joints in the ipsilateral upper limb. The patient is encouraged to do regular active exercises with fingers, wrist and elbow. Patients are discharged from the ward with an appointment to attend the physiotherapy department in order to continue with the rehabilitation. Treatment is very intense initially as the patient is performing only passive movements.

Three to six weeks

Patients are reviewed in the clinic at 3 weeks after the operation. At that time they start with active-assisted exercises, keeping the sling during this period. They are taught a series of home exercises using techniques as previously described.

Six weeks

Active movements begin and patients are encouraged to use their limbs functionally. A strengthening programme is commenced starting with isometric work and progressing to resisted exercises as strength improves.

Patients with major cuff repairs are still encouraged to commence a passive movement programme, but active movement does not start for 8 weeks. The programme can be varied as to the security of repair.

Shoulder replacement (Copeland)[15]

The operated limb is placed in a master sling with a body belt. Pain control over the first 12–16 h is achieved by an interscalene block. The rehabilitation programme starts on day 1. Passive flexion and extension in the scapular plane and early pendular exercises are started if pain allows. The patient is encouraged to perform active exercises with fingers, wrist and elbow. Pendular exercises and passive flexion–extension are continued until the third week, when active-assisted and stretching exercises are begun. The sling is removed and gradually the patient progresses to active gentle resistance over next 3 weeks. At 6 weeks, the strengthening programme is started and the stretching programme is continued. Patients can start abduction with external rotation at 6 weeks. Patients are encouraged to continue with the exercises, especially stretching, for at least a year after surgery.

Arthroscopic acromioplasty. Arthroscopic acromioclavicular joint excision

The sling provided after the operation is for pain relief and the patient is advised to discard it after 3 or 4 days. Exercises are encouraged immediately after the operation and patients are advised to continue with these at home. They are seen in the clinic at approximately 3 weeks by which time they should be comfortably moving the joint below shoulder height and able to lift the arm above the head, although this may be uncomfortable. At this stage outpatient physiotherapy may be indicated in order to achieve maximum range of movement, strength and stability. By 3 months they should be at least 80% improved, but they are advised that improvement will continue for up to 1 year.

Open acromioplasty

Patients leave theatre with a sling for pain relief, but gentle passive and pendulum exercises are started the following day as pain allows. At 1 week, they are encouraged to increase the range of active exercises. Three weeks after the operation patients are seen in the clinic and strengthening exercises are started. There are two important points. First, the surgeon should indicate the timing of active exercises because he or she will know how extensively the deltoid muscle was detached and how strongly it was reattached. Detachment of the deltoid constitutes a serious complication. Secondly, active forward flexion should be carried out with the hand supinated to avoid maximum contact of the greater tuberosity with the operated area.

SUMMARY

The shoulder is a complex layered gliding mechanism and the results of surgery are dependent on a sound supervised rehabilitation regime if optimal results are to be achieved.

REFERENCES

1. Neer, C., II (1990) Shoulder rehabilitation. In *Shoulder Reconstruction*, pp 487–533. London: W.B. Saunders.
2. Anshel, M.H., Freedson, P., Hamill, J. et al (1991) *Dictionary of the Sports and Exercise Sciences*. Champaign, Illinois: Human Kinetics Books.
3. Souza, T.A. (1994) General treatment approaches for shoulder disorders. In T. Souza (ed.) *Sports Injuries of the Shoulder. Conservative management*, pp. 487–508. Edinburgh: Churchill-Livingstone.
4. Ziskin, M.C. & Michlovitz, S.L. (1986) Therapeutic ultrasound. In Michlovitz, S.L. (ed.) *Thermal Agents in Rehabilitation*, p. 141. Philadelphia: F.A. Davies.
5. Matsen, F.A., III, Lippitt, S.B., Sidles, J.A. & Harryman, D.T., II. (1994) Evaluating the shoulder. In *Practical Evaluation and Management of the Shoulder*, pp. 1–17. London: W.B. Saunders.
6. Sidles, J.A. & Pearl, M.L. (1992) Description and measurement of shoulder motion. In F.A. Matsen III, F. Fu & R.J. Hawkins (eds) *The Shoulder: A Balance of Mobility and Stability*, pp. 129–140.
7. Lephart, S.M. & Kocher, M.S. (1992) The role of exercise in the prevention of shoulder disorders. In F.A. Matsen III, F. Fu & R.J. Hawkins (eds) *The Shoulder: A Balance of Mobility and Stability*, pp. 597–619. Rosemont: American Academy of Orthopedic Surgeons.
8. Wilk, K.E. & Arrigo, C.A. (1994) Isokinetic testing and exercise. In T.A. Souza (ed.) *Sports Injuries of the Shoulder. Conservative Management*, pp. 237–255. Edinburgh: Churchill Livingstone.
9. Gerber, Ch. (1992) Integrated scoring systems for the functional assessment of the shoulder. In F.A. Matsen III, F. Fu & R.J. Hawkins (eds), *The Shoulder: A Balance of Mobility and Stability*, pp. 531–550. Rosemont: American Academy of Orthopaedic Surgeons.
10. Rowe, C.R., Patel, D. & Southmayd, W.W. (1978) The Bankart procedure. A long-term end-result study. *J. Bone Joint Surg.* **60A:** 1–16.
11. Walch, G. (1987) Directions for the use of the quotation of anterior instabilities of the shoulder. Abstracts of the First Open Congress of the European Society of Surgery of the Shoulder and Elbow, Paris, 1987, pp. 51–55.
12. Barrett, W.P., Franklin, J.L., Jackins, S.E., Wyss, C.R. & Matsen, F.A. (1987) Total shoulder arthroplasty. *J. Bone Joint Surg.* **69A:** 865–872.
13. Amstutz, H.C., Sew Hoy, A.L. & Clarke, I.C. (1981) UCLA anatomic total shoulder arthroplasty. *Clin. Orthop.* **155:** 7–20.
14. Constant, C.R. & Murley, A.H.G. (1987) A clinical method of functional assessment of the shoulder. *Clin. Orthop.* **214:** 160–164.
15. Copeland, S. (1995) *Operative Shoulder Surgery*. Edinburgh: Churchill Livingstone.

32

Outcomes in Shoulder Surgery

A Carr

INTRODUCTION

Outcome is defined by the *Oxford English Dictionary* as a visible or practical result. Assessment of outcome in orthopaedic surgery is becoming increasingly important. As the pioneering days of joint replacement and minimally invasive surgery come to an end orthopaedic surgeons are moving into a phase of increasing evaluation of the success and failure of the treatments they provide.

A pioneer of shoulder surgery E.A. Codman from the Massachusetts General Hospital described a method in 1910 of recalling all patients treated 1 year after surgery to see if their treatment had achieved the initial objective.[1] His classic paper the 'Product of a Hospital' concluded with the question 'What happens to the patient?' This question can still be asked today. Essential to all evaluation of outcome is the establishment of an end point or criterion by which success and failure can be assessed. The simplest of these is life or death. Thankfully in shoulder surgery this is rarely an issue. Assessment of outcomes must therefore be based on other criteria. These must evaluate outcome not only from the perspective of the doctor but also from the patient's point of view. They must determine not only what is efficacious, i.e. a procedure that has worked well in a particular patient, but also what is efficient, i.e. how well does that particular treatment work across a population of patients. In this chapter, I will outline methods of undertaking surgical trials and methods of assessing outcome using outcome instruments. I will also review the existing outcome measures used in shoulder surgery and describe some of their strengths and weaknesses.

TYPES OF SURGICAL TRIAL

As a general principle any surgical trial may be described as being either observational or experimental. An observational trial is the simplest form of trial and reports that which has occurred in surgical practice. In an experimental trial the environment of the trial has to be thought out ahead of time and usually involves comparing one type of treatment with another thus establishing the experimental nature of the trial. An alternative would be to apply one type of treatment to different groups of patients. The most straightforward patient population is a cohort. This need not necessarily include all the patients operated on, as some may be excluded using criteria set at the beginning of the trial. This cohort of patients may be followed prospectively and form part of a prospective study. Alternatively, as is common in orthopaedic surgery, the cohort of patients may be reviewed retrospectively. Prospective studies have the advantage that the data can be collected carefully as the trial is progressing. Often in retrospective studies various pieces of information are not adequately collected thus weakening the results of the trial. Nevertheless retrospective studies have an important part to play in orthopaedic surgery, particularly when rare syndromes or treatments are reviewed.

If the success of a particular treatment is to be studied in more detail then a case control study is required. In this type of study a particular treatment is compared with another treatment. The best method of case control study requires the use of a contemporary control treatment population where confounding variables are likely to be minimized. A historical case control study is of value but very often the historical controls have received treatment in a completely different environment and this makes an accurate comparison difficult. Scientifically the most effective method of comparing one treatment with another is to use a randomized control trial. Ideally both the experimenter and the patient should be blinded to which treatment is being used. The aim of this methodology is to avoid bias. Bias can be introduced by the patient, by the experimenter and also from the design of the study. The problem with a randomized surgical trial is that it is very difficult to blind the surgeon and the patient to the type of treatment being used. Because of this, very few blinded randomized control studies have been undertaken in surgery. Also surgeons tend to be happier with one form of operation than another and therefore comparing the success of two operations in a randomized study may be judging the skill of the surgeon rather than the effect of the operation itself. Another problem with surgical trials is that very often quite large numbers of patients need to be recruited in order to demonstrate differences between different types of treatment. This inevitably requires multicentre studies with significant cost and organizational implications. Despite all these difficulties with the establishment of surgical trials, much important information could be gained if they were adopted in a more widespread fashion in orthopaedic surgery and particularly in shoulder surgery.

METHODS OF ASSESSING OUTCOME

An outcome assessment instrument can involve a number of separate criteria including pain, range of movement, function, satisfaction and general health status.

Pain

A fundamental feature of orthopaedic disability is the presence of pain. Probably not enough attention has been directed by orthopaedic surgeons to how pain is best evaluated. Often simple binary scales are used. Such scales are fundamentally flawed and a much better method of assessing pain is to use a categorical verbal rating scale. These usually contain four or five possible words to describe the magnitude of the pain. Figure 32.1 shows categorical verbal rating scales describing pain intensity and pain relief. The main advantage of categorical scales are their simplicity and ease of scoring. An alternative is to use a visual analogue scale where a line is presented to the patient with the ends labelled with extreme descriptions of a dimension. Theoretical advantages of these scales are that they are simple and quick to score and do not involve imprecise descriptive terms. However, the disadvantages are that they require more concentration and more visual and multi-coordination by the patient. These criticisms are felt to outweigh the advantages over a categorical verbal rating scale.

Other methods of measuring pain include the use of questionnaires such as the McGill pain questionnaire.[2] The reliability and sensitivity of this questionnaire is now well established. Modifications have been developed such as the multidimensional assessment of pain suggested by Chapman et al.[3] In this, pain descriptors were reduced into three sets, sensory, intensity and unpleasantness and painfulness. It is also possible to measure pain indirectly using behavioural measures such as the effect of pain on sleep, the use of pain medication or engagement in recreational activities. It may also be possible to establish level of pain by enquiring how easy it was for a patient to walk a fixed distance or move an affected joint. This has some problems in orthopaedic surgery where there may be reasons other than pain why a patient is unable to achieve these objectives. The use of analgesic consumption and time to next analgesics (TNA) have also been assessed quite thoroughly in the literature (Figure 32.2).[4]

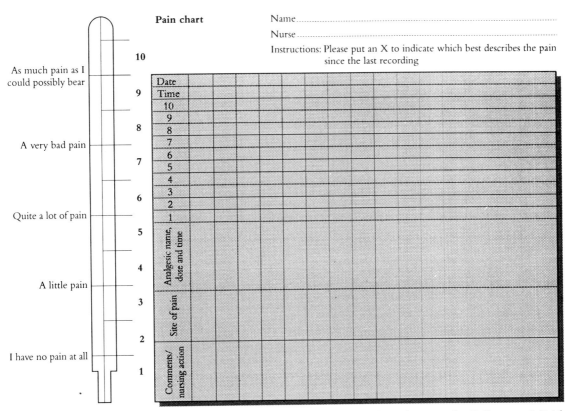

Fig. 32.1 Modified Burford pain chart. Reproduced from *Outcomes in Orthopaedic Surgery* by P. Pynsent, J. Fairbank and A. Carr, with permission from Butterworth–Heinemann.

Name.. **Oxford Pain Chart** Treatment week..........................

Please fill in this chart each evening before going to bed. Record your pain intensity and the amount of pain relief. If you have had any side-effects please note them in the side effects box.

	Date							
Pain intensity How bad has your pain been today?	Severe							
	Moderate							
	Mild							
	None							
Pain relief How much pain relief have the tablets given today	Complete							
	Good							
	Moderate							
	Slight							
	None							
Side effects Has the treatment upset you in any way?								

How effective was the treatment this week? *poor fair good very good excellent* Please circle your choice.

Fig. 32.2 Oxford pain chart. Reproduced from *Outcomes in Orthopaedic Surgery* by P. Pynsent, J. Fairbank and A. Carr, with permission from Butterworth–Heinemann.

Range of movement and function

Another important assessment of disability involving the shoulder is range of movement and function. Range of movement is a particularly difficult issue in the shoulder where a complex interaction between thorax, scapula and humerus occurs. The majority of evaluations therefore use an assessment not only of range of movement but also of the ability to perform activities of daily living. These activities of daily living might include the ability to brush hair or tuck-in a shirt. These assessments are also confounded by another significant problem which occurs in the field of surgery and that is co-morbidity. The ability of a patient to brush their hair not only depends on adequate function in the shoulder but also in the elbow, wrist and hand and to some extent the neck. I will discuss these in a little more detail later in the chapter.

Satisfaction and quality of life

Another important aspect of an outcome measure is an assessment of patient satisfaction and quality of life. Such issues have become very important in recent years and a number of new methods of assessing patient satisfaction have been developed. One important dimension of satisfaction is that patients may not necessarily be dissatisfied with the particular operation but may be dissatisfied with the process of the operation, i.e. delays in obtaining appointments or admissions and waiting for long periods in clinics and receiving inadequate information or impersonal or unfriendly care.[5] A number of different techniques have been developed to try to assess quality of life and how it may be changed by treatment. Rosser and Kind[6] used a magnitude estimation to assess quality of life. They produced a range of scores from (1) no distress and no disability to (0) severe distress and disability. In fact some states were rated as worse than the end of the scale, 'dead'. So-called quality-adjusted life years (QALYs) have become popular. Implicit in these scores is the acceptance of the fact that 1 year of healthy life for five people is equivalent to 50 years of life lived by one person with a quality of life of 0.1! It

is for this reason that these measures are unlikely to be embraced by people evaluating the relative success of different surgical procedures.

General health status

Another important set of measurement instruments are the so-called 'general health status measures'. These include the sickness impact profile,[7,8] the Nottingham Health Profile[9] and the SF36.[10] These measurements are used extensively by public health physicians and are being applied to studies on some surgical operations. A certain amount of care and circumspection needs to be employed in assessing the results of these studies. These instruments may not apply particularly well to surgical treatments.

So what then are the features of an ideal measurement instrument?

1. Repeatability: repeatability or reliability requires that measurement produces the same results on two separate administrations when no significant changes occurred in the object of measurement.
2. Validity: validity of an instrument requires that it accurately measures what it is claiming to measure. In the case of shoulder surgery it may be that a measurement that assesses movement and pain does not accurately and validly assess shoulder instability.
3. Practicality and feasibility: any measurement must be practical and feasible to use. If it is impossible to administer the measurement in clinical settings, then it is highly unlikely that it will provide any useful results.
4. Sensitivity to change: the measurement must be sensitive to change with treatment.

OUTCOMES MEASURES USED IN SHOULDER SURGERY

The shoulder is a complex joint with various afflicting disorders occurring within it which require different treatments. I have subdivided the assessment scores into the following sections: (1) the acromioclavicular joint; (2) the rotator cuff; (3) shoulder instability; (4) proximal humeral fractures; (5) generic shoulder instruments used in shoulder replacement surgery. Reviews of outcomes measures on shoulder surgery may also be found in Pynsent & Fairbank.[11,12]

The acromioclavicular joint

In 1946 Urist first reported the use of an acromioclavicular joint score by describing whether or not an individual was able to return to military duty within 2–3 months of injury. A slightly more sophisticated approach was adopted by Arneret et al[14] in Sweden in 1957 when they distinguished between subluxation and dislocation of the joint. In 1961, Lazcano et al[15] reported the use of a functional analysis. The first point scale for evaluation of the acromioclavicular joint was proposed by Imatani et al[16] (Table 32.1). This scale is based on pain, function and motion. In 1985 Walsh et al[17] devised another evaluation method which included the use of strength assessment.

Rotator cuff tears

A number of assessment schemes have been described for rotator cuff tears.[18–20] One of the more widely used methods was described by Wolfgang et al[21] which assesses the shoulder in terms of pain, movement strength and function and awards points to the various sections. As bedevils many assessments in shoulder surgery, no consistent scoring system has been used and Hawkins et al[22] in 1985 reviewed 100 patients who had had rotator cuff surgery and used a different rating scale.

Table 32.1. The Imatani scoring system, a clinical evaluation system for acromioclavicular separation

No. of points	Distribution
	Pain (40 points)
40	None
25	Slight, occasional
10	Moderate, tolerable, limits activities
0	Severe, constant, disabling
	Function (30 points)
20	Weakness (percentage of preinjury)
5	Use of shoulder
5	Vocational change
	Motion (30 points)
10	Abduction
10	Flexion
10	Adduction

Reproduced from *Outcomes in Orthopaedic Surgery* by P. Pynsent, J. Fairbank and A. Carr, with permission from Butterworth-Heinemann.

Shoulder instability

Assessment systems in shoulder instability have proved to be very difficult to establish. Rowe[23] in 1956 described probably the best used assessment methodology (Table 32.2). Other authors have devised their own evaluation systems including Hovelius et al,[24] Sillar et al,[25] Symeonides[26] and Varmarken & Jensen.[27]

Proximal humeral fractures

The classic description of fractures of the proximal humerus was given in 1970 by Neer.[28] This was based on Codman's earlier observation[1] that fractures of the proximal humerus tend to separate into four segments. Although Neer has described a specific outcome scoring system for fractures, a

Table 32.2. Evaluation of function following Bankart procedures

Poor	Fair	Good	Excellent
Marked limitation in all motions Limited in many activities and all sports Patients not satisfied	50% limitation in external rotation 30% limitation of elevation Limited in certain overhead work and sports Patients satisfied	25% limitation in shoulder motion Moderate limitation in sport Useful shoulder for work Patients satisfied	Essentially normal motion Very slight limitation in sports No limitation in work Patients very satisfied

Reproduced from Rowe.[23]

number of surgeons routinely employ the generic scoring systems used also in shoulder replacement surgery. These are described in the paragraph below.

Generic shoulder instruments

A variety of generic shoulder instruments have been devised for use in the shoulder and these are most usually applied to assessment of shoulder replacement surgery. The system devised for the Hospital of Special Surgery was reported by Warren.[29] This awards a total of 100 points, of which pain accounts for 30 and power and motion are each given 25 points with function being allocated 20 points. The most widely used scoring system in Europe is that described by Constant & Murley.[30] This also has a cumulative score and allocates a large proportion to assessments of movement and function. Other scoring systems described are those of Swanson,[31] the UCLA system,[32] the scoring system of Neer & Stanton[33] and that of Barrett.[34] Unfortunately, very few of these scoring systems have described any adequate repeatability and validity testing. The most widely accepted scoring system in Europe is the Constant–Murley score described in Chapter 31.

Patient-based assessments of shoulder function

A number of systems of assessing shoulder function using questionnaires which the patient completes are now being developed. Such patient-based questionnaires have the advantage that they can be administered to large numbers of patients without necessarily requiring the patients to attend clinic. This has obvious advantages in terms of allocation of resources. The other advantage is that such systems avoid bias introduced by surgeons or clinicians assessing the patients themselves. A recent development of this is described by Dawson[35] (Figure 32.3).

The use of survival analysis in shoulder replacement surgery

In any study where patients are recruited sequentially and where the final outcome cannot be judged for many years, then survival analysis techniques should be employed. These were first described by Kaplan and Meier.[36] They have since been adopted quite widely in orthopaedic surgery and descriptions can be found by Carr et al.[37] Any surgical paper describing results of outcome in shoulder joint replacement surgery should include an assessment of survival. The reader of such papers should be aware that pitfalls can arise if account is not taken of patients lost to follow-up and when the end point or failure point is not described adequately. Nevertheless, survival analysis does provide a very good analysis of how well a particular procedure performs over a 5–20-year period.

COMPLICATIONS IN SHOULDER SURGERY

Any assessment of outcome in surgery in general must include a description of complications. All complications must be documented in order to obtain an overall view or audit. Frostick[38] suggested categories of complications, including complications that are life-threatening due to either pre-existing disease or surgery, major morbidity again due to either pre-existing disease or surgery, and minor morbidity. An additional system of classification has been suggested by the American Society Anesthesiologists which describes physical status as being Class I (no systemic disturbance), Class II (mild to moderate systemic disturbance), Class III (severe systemic disturbance), Class IV (life-threatening systemic disturbance) and Class V (moribund with little chance of survival). Assessment of complications should also try to record their severity either in response to trauma using scales such as the APACHE score or for specific complications such as thromboembolic disease. In the case of shoulder surgery, specific complications could quite reasonably be divided into general complications or complications specific to the shoulder itself. An important group of complications are infections. The Surgical Infection Group[39] suggested that all surgical specialties use the scoring

PROBLEMS WITH YOUR SHOULDER
nb. not suitable for *post*-operative patients until 6 months

Study number ☐☐☐

✓ tick **one** box for each question

1. *During the last 3 months,* how would you describe the *worst* pain you have had **from your shoulder?**

| None | Mild ache | Moderate | Severe | Unbearable |
| ☐ | ☐ | ☐ | ☐ | ☐ |

2. *During the last 3 months,* have you had any trouble (or anxiety) with putting on a T-shirt or pullover **because of your shoulder?**

| No trouble/ no worries | Slight trouble or worry | Moderate trouble or worry | Extreme difficulty | Impossible to do |
| ☐ | ☐ | ☐ | ☐ | ☐ |

3. *During the last 3 months,* how many times has your shoulder felt as if it slipped out of joint (or dislocated)?

| Not at all in 3 months | 1 or 2 times **in 3 months** | 1 or 2 times **per month** | 1 or 2 times **per week** | More often than 1 or 2 times/week |
| ☐ | ☐ | ☐ | ☐ | ☐ |

4. *During the last 3 months,* how much has the **problem with your shoulder** interfered with your sporting activities?

| Not at all/ not applicable | A little/ occasionally | Some of the time | Most of the time | All of the time |
| ☐ | ☐ | ☐ | ☐ | ☐ |

5. *During the last 3 months,* has **the problem with your shoulder** prevented you doing the things that are important to you?

| No, not at all | Very occasionally | Some days | Most days or more than one activity | Every day or many activities |
| ☐ | ☐ | ☐ | ☐ | ☐ |

6. *During the last 3 months,* have you felt 'self-concious' about your shoulder – worried about other people staring or making comments?

| Not at all | Occasionally | Some days | Most days | Every day |
| ☐ | ☐ | ☐ | ☐ | ☐ |

Fig. 32.3 The Oxford shoulder assessment.

✓ tick **one** box for each question

7. *During the last 3 months,* how much has **the problem with your shoulder** interfered with your social life (including sexual activity)?

Not at all   Occasionally   Some days   Most days   Every day

8. *During the last 3 months,* how much has **the problem with your shoulder** interfered with your usual work (including housework, school or college work)?

Not at all   A little bit   Moderately   Greatly   Totally

9. *During the last **4 weeks**,* how often has your shoulder been 'on your mind' – how often have you thought about it?

Never or only if someone asks   Occasionally   Some days   Most days   Every day

10. *During the last **4 weeks**,* how much has **the problem with your shoulder** interfered with your ability – or willingness – to lift heavy objects?

Not at all   Occasionally   Some days   Most days   Every day

11. *During the last **4 weeks**,* how would you describe the pain you **usually** had from your shoulder?

None   Very mild   Mild   Moderate   Severe

12. *During the last **4 weeks**,* have you avoided lying in certain positions, in bed at night, due to **concern about your shoulder?**

No nights   Only 1 or 2 nights   Some nights   Most nights   Every night

Fig. 32.3 Continued.

system known as ASEPSIS for the assessment of wounds.[40] Deep infection can also be a problem in shoulder surgery particularly in the case of infections around implants such as plates, nails or shoulder replacements. However, specific systems have not yet been devised for the shoulder. Thromboembolism is also an important complication of orthopaedic surgery, although less so in shoulder surgery than in surgery of the lower limb.

CONCLUSIONS

This chapter has attempted to review some of the basic principles of assessment of outcome in shoulder surgery. I have also described some of the shoulder instruments that are currently being employed by shoulder surgeons with a commentary on their possible uses. There is no doubt that the issue of outcome assessment is not going to go away and shoulder surgeons need to understand some of the benefits that can be obtained from adequate assessments of outcomes as well as some of the pitfalls that occur if the studies are not carried out carefully.

REFERENCES

1. Codman, E.A. (1914) The product of a hospital. *Arch. Dis. Child.* **18:** 491–496.
2. Melzack, R. (1975) The McGill pain questionnaire: major properties and scoring methods. *Pain* **1:** 277–299.
3. Chapman, C., Casey, K., Dubner, K.M. et al (1985) Pain measurement: an overview. *Pain* **22:** 1–31.
4. McQuay, H., Carroll, D. & Moore, R.A. (1988) Postoperative orthopaedic pain: the effect of opiate premedication and local anaesthetic blocks. *Pain* **33:** 291–295.
5. Fitzpatrick, A. (1991) Surveys of patient satisfaction. *Br. Med. J.* **302:** 287–289.
6. Rosser, R. & Kind, P. (1978) A scale of valuations of states of illness: is there a social consensus? *Int. J. Epidemiol.* **7:** 347–358.
7. Gilson, B., Gilson, J. et al. (1975) The sickness impact profile: development of a health status measure. *Am. J. Public Health* **65:** 1304–1310.
8. Bergner, M., Bobitt, R., Carter, W. & Gilson, B. (1981) The sickness impact profile: development and final revision of a health status measure. *Med. Care* **19:** 787–805.
9. Hunt, S., McEwen, J. & McKenna, S. (1985) Measuring health status: a new tool for clinicians and epidemiologists. *J. R. Coll. Gen. Pract.* **35:** 185–188.
10. Stewart, A., Greenfield, S., Hays, R. et al. (1989) Functional status and well-being of patients with chronic conditions. *J. Am. Med. Assoc.* **262:** 907–913.
11. Pynsent, P. & Fairbank, J. (1993) *Outcome Measures in Trauma.* Oxford: Butterworth-Heinemann.
12. Pynsent, P. & Fairbank, J. (1994) Outcome measures in trauma. Oxford: Butterworth-Heinemann.
13. Urist, M.R. (1946) Complete dislocations of the acromioclavicular joint. *J. Bone Joint Surg.* **28A:** 813–837.
14. Arner, O., Sandahl, U. & Ohrling, H. (1957) Dislocation of the acromioclavicular joint. *Acta Chir. Scand.* **113:** 140–152.
15. Lazcano, M., Anzel, S. & Kelly, P.J. (1961) Complete dislocation and subluxation of the acromioclavicular joint. *J. Bone Joint Surg.* **43A:** 379–391.
16. Imatani, R., Hanlon, J. & Cady, J.J. (1975) Acute, complete acromioclavicular separation. *J. Bone Joint Surg.* **57A:** 328–332.
17. Walsh, W.M., Peterson, D.A. & Inglis, A.E. (1985) Shoulder strength following acromioclavicular injury. *Am. J. Sports Med.* **13:** 153–158.
18. McLaughlin, H. (1962) Rupture of the rotator cuff. *J. Bone Joint Surg.* **44A:** 979–983.
19. Heikel, H. (1968) Rupture of the rotator cuff of the shoulder. *Acta Orthop. Scand.* **39:** 477–492.
20. Godsil, R. & Linscheid, R. (1970) Intratendinous defects of the rotator cuff. *Clin. Orthop. Rel. Res.* **69:** 181–188.
21. Wolfgang, B.G., Simpson, L.A. & Hardegger, F. (1984) Rotational humeral osteotomy for recurrent anterior dislocation of the shoulder associated with a large Hill–Sachs lesion. *J. Bone Joint Surg.* **66A:** 1443–1450.
22. Hawkins, R., Misamore, G. et al. (1985) Surgery for full thickness rotator cuff tears. *J. Bone Joint Surg.* **67A:** 1349–1355.
23. Rowe, C. (1956) Prognosis in dislocations of the shoulder. *J. Bone Joint Surg.* **38A:** 957–977.
24. Hovelius, L., Thorling, J. et al. (1979) Recurrent anterior dislocation of the shoulder. *J. Bone Joint Surg.* **61A:** 566–569.
25. Sillar, P., Cser, I. & Kery, L. (1983) Results of the Putti–Platt operation for recurrent anterior dislocation of the shoulder. *Acta Chir. Hung.* **24:** 31–35.
26. Symeonides, P. (1989) Reconsideration of the Putti–Platt procedure and its mode of action in recurrent traumatic anterior dislocation of the shoulder. *Clin. Orthop. Rel. Res.* **246:** 8–15.
27. Varmarken, J.E. & Jensen, C.H. (1989) Recurrent anterior dislocation of the shoulder. *Orthopaedics* **12:** 453–455.
28. Neer, C. (1970) Displaced proximal humeral fractures. *J. Bone Joint Surg.* **52A:** 1077–1089.

29. Warren, R.F., Ranawat, C.S. & Inglis, A.E. (1982) Total shoulder replacement indications and results of the Neer nonconstrained prosthesis. In *The American Academy of Orthopaedic Surgeons: Symposium on Total Joint Replacement of the Upper Extremity*. Inglis A.E. (ed.). St Louis: C.V. Mosby.

30. Constant, C. & Murley, A. (1987) A clinical method of functional assessment of the shoulder. *Clin. Orthop. Rel. Res.* **214:** 160–164.

31. Swanson, A.B., de Groot Swanson, Sattel, G. et al. (1989) Bipolar implant shoulder arthroplasty. *Clin. Orthop. Rel. Res.* **249:** 227–247.

32. Amstutz, H.C., Sew Hoy, A.L. & Clarke, I.C. (1981) UCLA anatomic total shoulder arthroplasty. *Clin. Orthop.* **155:** 7–20.

33. Neer, C.I.W. & Stanton, F.J. (1982) Recent experience in total shoulder replacement. *J. Bone Joint Surg.* **64A:** 694–697.

34. Barrett, W.P., Franklin, J.L., Jackins, S.E., Wyss, C.R. & Matsen, F.A. (1987) Total shoulder arthroplasty. *J. Bone Joint Surg.* **69A:** 865–872.

35. Dawson, J.F. & Carr, A.J. (1995) A questionnaire on the perception of patients about shoulder surgery. *J. Bone Joint Surg.* **76B:** 593–600.

36. Kaplan, E. & Meier, P. (1958) No parametric estimation from incomplete observations. *J. Am. Stat. Assoc.* **53:** 457–481.

37. Carr, A., Morris, R., Murray, D.W. & Pynsent, P.B. (1993) Survival analysis in joint replacement surgery. *J. Bone Joint Surg.* **75B:** 178–182.

38. Frostick, S. (1993) Complications. In P. Pynsent, J. Fairbank & A. Carr (eds), *Outcomes in Orthopaedic Surgery*. Oxford: Butterworth-Heinemann.

39. Surgical Infection Group (1991) Proposed definitions for the audit of postoperative infection: a discussion paper. *Ann. R. Coll. Surg. Engl.* **73:** 385–388.

40. Wilson, A.T., Sturridge, M.F. & Gruneberg, R.N. (1986). A scoring method (ASEPSIS) for postoperative wound infections for use in clinical trials of antibiotic prophylaxis. *Lancet* **i:** 311–313.

Index